THE ENEMY WITHIN

THE HIGH COST OF LIVING NEAR NUCLEAR REACTORS

BREAST CANCER, AIDS, LOW BIRTHWEIGHTS,
AND OTHER RADIATION-INDUCED
IMMUNE DEFICIENCY EFFECTS

BY JAY M. GOULD

WITH MEMBERS OF
THE RADIATION AND PUBLIC HEALTH PROJECT

ERNEST J. STERNGLASS
JOSEPH J. MANGANO
WILLIAM MCDONNELL

FOUR WALLS EIGHT WINDOWS
NEW YORK/LONDON

Published in the United States by
Four Walls Eight Windows
39 West 14th Street, Suite 503
New York, NY 10011

U.K. offices:
Four Walls Eight Windows/Turnaround
27 Horsell Road London, N51 XL, England

Library of Congress Cataloging-in-Publication Data:
The enemy within: the high cost of living near nuclear reactors:
breast cancer, AIDS, low birthweights, and other radiation-induced
immune deficiency effects / by Jay M. Gould, with members of the
Radiation and Public Health Project, Ernest J. Sternglass, Joseph J.
Mangano, William McDonnell.

p. cm.
Includes bibliographical references and index.
ISBN 1-56858-066-5
1. Nuclear reactors—Health aspects. 2. Radioactive fallout—
Health aspects. 3. Immunosupression—Risk factors.
4. Immunodeficiency—Complications. I. Gould, Jay M.
II. Radiation and Public Health Project.
RA569.E55   1996
616.9'897—dc20   96–789
                         CIP

10 9 8 7 6 5 4 3 2 1

TABLE OF CONTENTS

FOREWORD

After a long and productive career as an economic and statistical consultant to many public and private agencies, in recent years I switched my professional focus to exploring the health effects of environmental abuses, including low-level radiation. Because of its politically sensitive nature, some may find this a puzzling change, but in reviewing my professional career over a span of 50 years, I can discern a logical progression of events that has finally led to this change of focus. Whatever success I have had resulted from several fortuitous incidents that beneficially changed the course of my life, and which may explain how I came to write this book.

Although I had majored in mathematics at college, when I came to do my graduate work at Columbia University in the late 1930s, I switched to economic statistics. I was inspired by a truly charismatic teacher—Professor Wesley Clair Mitchell. Probably the greatest of all American economists, Mitchell founded the National Bureau of Economic Research after World War I. At that time, he was head of the War Production Board, which made evident the United States' need to develop such modern statistical measures as the national income accounts and the time series required to trace the changing course of the American business cycle.

Each of Mitchell's famous lectures on the development of economic thought were attended by as many as 200 students from all parts of the world. The most popular "text" at that time was a mimeographed set of "Mitchell's Lecture Notes," a stenographic transcription of his 1933 lectures. After the war I edited the lecture notes with Mitchell's blessing, and they ultimately emerged as part of a series of economic classics published by my good friend and class-mate Augustus Kelley.[1]

Mitchell saw the work of each of the great economists as an outgrowth of the changing historical, economic, and social conditions of their times. He thought that only with the development of the necessary statistical tools could the relevance of any economic theory be really tested. As one who came to intellectual maturity in the depression years, I found this materialist emphasis so compelling that I succeeded in getting a job at the National Bureau in 1938. I spent eight wonderful years there while pursuing my graduate studies, and I developed a valuable statistical expertise that I was able to put to good use as a business consultant after completing my doctoral degree in 1946.

It was at the National Bureau that I first encountered the work of Dr. Wassily Leontief, who later won the Nobel prize in economics for developing the new econometric discipline of input/output analysis, which subsequently became the central focus of my own work. Leontief, as a young Russian mathematical economist, had been invited by Mitchell to come to the National Bureau in 1934 to develop a model of the American economy as a set of statistical equations that relate the input requirements of each industry to its output. As in construction of the national income accounts, input/output analysis required detailed statistical measures based on business census records plus a sophisticated knowledge of the mathematical techniques necessary to solve many simultaneous equations.

Leontief went to Harvard in 1937, where, with the help of a few graduate student assistants, he completed the construction of the first input/output model for the 1939 U.S. economy, which, despite its primitive nature, proved to be an important planning tool during World War II. For example, it showed that President Roosevelt's rash promise to deliver 50,000 planes to the Allied forces was unrealistic, and the model indicated the bottleneck obstacles that must be first overcome.

My own doctoral dissertation—a study of productivity trends in public utilities—was published by the National Bureau in 1946,[2] after which I began work as a business consultant specializing in the analysis of consumer and industrial markets. Here my knowledge of Leontief's input/output economics proved especially useful.

In an input/output chart of the U.S. economy, every industry is arrayed both horizontally and vertically so that any intersection can indicate the input requirements of the vertical (buying) industry from the selling industry, which is arrayed horizontally. Each intersecting cell represents a specific market, as for example the purchase of corrugated boxes by the glass industry. I was the first to demonstrate in articles in the business press that such data could be used to define and measure thousands of different industrial markets. For those markets that were dominated by a few major buyers and sellers, it would be possible to identify them in an economy in which the top Fortune 500 companies accounted for the bulk of economic output.

This insight not only proved to be extremely useful to me as a statistical expert in the postwar wave of antitrust litigation, but also eventually led to the establishment of a successful database company that gave me the financial independence necessary to investigate the environmental implications of the hazardous inputs and outputs of certain industries.

My antitrust activity began in 1955 with a visit from two young Department of Justice attorneys who sought my help in the measurement of the market for shoes in certain metropolitan areas. The Sherman antitrust laws were strengthened in 1950 to enable the Department of Justice to oppose mergers that would restrain trade in regional as well as national markets. The first case chosen to test the new law involved the merger of two shoe manufacturers with retailing affiliates, which in some metropolitan areas could be shown to account for perhaps 25 percent of the retail market.

The Department of Justice had no authority to retain an outside consultant, but in pretrial hearings with the opposing Sullivan and Cromwell attorneys, they felt the need for help to calculate the market shares that would not otherwise be available when the two companies merged.

Feeling some sympathy for their plight, I agreed to spend the two or three days (for which they could only pay a witness rate of $50 per day) necessary to provide the requested market share estimates, although I thought this to be a rather trivial application of the new antitrust legislation. I was therefore greatly surprised when several years later they called to ask me to defend my estimates in a hearing at a St. Louis Federal District Court—at the same *per diem* rate but with my travel expenses covered.

When I arrived, I was astonished to find I was to be cross-examined by Arthur Dean, senior partner of Sullivan and Cromwell. I was told he had interrupted discussions in Geneva with Gromyko on a moratorium on Soviet/American bomb tests in order to come to St. Louis to defend the Brown Shoe Company in what was to become the first postwar antitrust case in which the government position, based on a few days of work on my part, was ultimately upheld by the Supreme Court.

My estimates, based on the same common sense reasoning used in estimating the components of national income, were challenged as hearsay evidence because they were not based on surveys specifically undertaken for the purpose at hand. But both the Appellate and Supreme Courts ruled that prudent business decisions could be made on the basis of the best available statistical estimating procedures in the absence of the theoretically perfect information from expensive surveys.

And so as a result of what I consider to be a modest good deed, my career as an expert statistical witness blossomed. I have since been retained in over two dozen major private antitrust and several toxic tort cases. Over a period of more than 30 years, I have never lost a case. I developed the ability, which is demonstrated repeatedly in this book, to analyze quantitative data with the use of charts, which offered juries an immediate visual understanding of complex statistical relationships.

Most recently, for example, my associates and I have been retained in a class action by 2,500 plaintiffs suing the operator of the stricken Three Mile Island reactor. The anomalous increase in the mortality data available both before and after the 1979 near melt-down easily demonstrates the magnitude of the damage. Based on information taken from death certificates, such vital statistics are far more reliable than most economic statistics, particularly when the observed mortality increase can be shown to be too large to be due to chance. Unfortunately, perhaps because our case is so strong, the defendant has succeeded in postponing the trial, so that after 14 years the case remains unresolved.

After the successful use in World War II of Leontief's primitive 1939 input/output model, the government mounted the first full-scale input/output study of the U.S. economy in 1947, an effort requiring many millions of dollars and six years of labor for dozens of statisticians and economists. Unfortunately, when the results finally appeared in 1952, at the height of the McCarthy anticommunist hysteria, they were denounced as socialistic attempts at central planning, and the federal input/output team was disbanded. In 1960 President Kennedy revived it.

In 1965, I was retained by IBM to direct a joint research program to develop a computerized commercial application of input/output. With the help of the Dun and Bradstreet Company credit file, which carried information on the employment size and industrial classification of each of some 5 million establishments, I proposed to identify the major buyers and sellers in each of the industrial markets designated by the intersection of hundreds of vertical (buying) and horizontal (selling) industries. I had already demonstrated that Census Bureau data indicated that in most markets, plants belonging to a relatively small number of large companies accounted for the bulk of the output, and correspondingly, of the input requirements.

For example, 25 large chemical companies accounted for 80 percent of all chemical output, and therefore of all chemical inputs, as well as toxic chemical wastes. I proposed that there would be sufficient public information available to identify all plants belonging to these companies, but the Dun and Bradstreet file failed to provide adequate data, since such large plants were not subject to credit inquiries. After two years, IBM withdrew from the project when I reported that it would take several more years to develop, from various state directories, a file of about 300,000 establishments belonging to the top 3,000 industrial companies to meet the required quality standards.

I was able to carry on with the help of a $500,000 venture capital grant. By 1970, with the help of a fellow consultant, Bentley H. Paykin, we created the Economic Information Systems (EIS) Company, which, with a staff of no more than 28 persons, succeeded in achieving the necessary quality standards. We could now offer rough estimates of market shares for some 3,000 companies in thousands of specific industrial markets.

Both the Federal Trade Commission and the Department of Justice quickly found our market share estimates a good guide in their choice of possible antitrust investigations. Previously they had no access to the confidential Census Bureau reports. The Census Bureau published statistics on the degree of concentration in each industry, without plant or company identification. We found such census data useful as statistical controls for our plant estimates, a procedure that was perfectly legal for a private information company, since we could only achieve a rough approximation of the true figures.

We were also able to use our files to identify, by name and address, including the ZIP code, those plants engaged in the manufacture of petroleum, chemicals, plastic, and rubber, which accounted for the bulk of all hazardous chemical wastes. This proved to be helpful for geographic investigations of potential pollution problems by the Environmental Protection Agency and led to my appointment to the EPA's Science Advisory Board in 1977.

Large chemical companies such as DuPont and Monsanto, on the other hand, could use our files to find thousands of potential customers in various industries thanks to our rough estimates of the volume of potential sales, which was based on the employment size of the purchasing plant. As a small company, our own marketing problem was solved when our files were carried on the Lockheed DIALOG on-line information system. Thousands of on-line users could now get instantaneous answers to questions on who makes what, how much, and where.

The DIALOG service was a powerful computerized information retrieval system, but it was not equipped to handle input/output ratios used to calculate and instantaneously answer such questions as who *buys* what, how much and where.

By 1979, we decided that the Control Data Company offered an on-line service that could make full use of our unique ability to provide instantaneous answers to perhaps millions of marketing questions. As the result of a successful antitrust suit against IBM in 1970, Control Data had acquired the IBM Service Bureau based in Greenwich, Connecticut, which by the late 1970s was offering on-line access, via telephone-linked modems, to giant IBM mainframe computers. We made them an offer they could not refuse. We would mount our files on their system at our expense, write the necessary software to offer their users our full services, share the revenue equally, and at the end of one year, if they wanted, they could buy EIS for what we considered a sufficient figure.

They agreed, but said we could forget about the option—they could not imagine any success that would warrant so high a purchase price. At the end of the year, however, the joint venture did so well that in 1981 EIS was sold to Control Data for a figure close to our original option price. I believe this happy outcome was accelerated by the following incident.

Just as our joint venture was nearing its end, I received an urgent call from Leontief, who over the years had closely followed my efforts to promote the business use of input/output. After he was awarded the Nobel prize in 1973, he was invited to establish the well-endowed Institute for Economic Analysis at New York University. At the time of our conversation, he had just returned from abroad to find that in his absence his budget has been drastically reduced. Ironically, the Japanese who had just honored Leontief, were now spending hundreds of millions of dollars on their input/output tables, making it the centerpiece for their economic plans to achieve international dominance in certain key industries.

I decided to contact the Control Data headquarters in Minneapolis on Leontief's behalf. I knew that its chief executive officer, William Norris, had spoken publicly about the need for large corporations to exercise social responsibility. And indeed, within about a week Norris invited Leontief to Minneapolis. As one of the engineers working on the first ENIAC computer, Norris recalled that among the early accomplishments of the first computer was the simultaneous solution of the 200 equations underlying the 1947 input/output model of the U.S. economy. Aware of the potential national importance of input/output, he offered Leontief a large, generous grant.

In celebration, Gerard Piel, the publisher of *Scientific American*, decided to host a dinner in New York to honor both Norris and Leontief, which gave me my first opportunity to meet Norris. I had been retained by Piel in the mid-1960s to help develop a large input/output wall chart that promoted *Scientific American'* s ability to reach executives, who, like Norris, had the technological background to make strategic business decisions. For example, the amount of steel sold to the automobile industry in a given year was not the result of good salesmanship but rather rested on changing technological factors that were best captured in periodic input/output tables.

This insight enabled and inspired me to write a book entitled *The Technical Elite*,[3] which my friend Augustus Kelley published in 1966 to accompany the reprint of Thorstein Veblen's *The Engineer and the Price System*,[4] the first book to point to the strategic role of science and technology in modern capitalist enterprise. In my book I stressed that the revolutionary postwar impact of both the computer and nuclear technology on business showed that good scientific ideas had become more important than capital in accounting for economic growth. The new "captains of industry" were more likely to come from the ranks of scientists and engineers. (I did not then realize, as I do know now, how badly nuclear technology has been used.)

After meeting Norris I sent him a copy of *The Technical Elite*, and he soon wrote back that he found it a delightful surprise, a reaction that may have contributed to the sale of my company in 1981. By 1984, upon completion of a management contract with Control Data, I was in a position to utilize my experience on environmental problems, which I first encountered during my service on the EPA Science Advisory Board.

In 1981 I read a remarkable book when seeking answers to a puzzling problem concerning the nuclear industry—*Secret Fallout: Low-Level Radiation from Hiroshima to Three Mile Island*,[5] by the radiation physicist Dr. Ernest J. Sternglass, who was at that time head of the Radiology Department at the University of Pittsburgh Medical School. He had previously led the Westinghouse Lunar Station research program, where he devised much of the imaging equipment now used in space satellites. He left Westinghouse when he began to have doubts about the safety of nuclear reactors. I read his book seeking answers to a puzzling problem that had been given to me concerning the nuclear industry.

In 1979 I had been retained by the law firm Donovan and Leisure on behalf of Westinghouse, who on antitrust grounds was suing several uranium mining companies alleged to have formed a uranium cartel to control the price of uranium. My job was to examine the forces of supply and demand that would justify a six-fold increase in the price of uranium in the 1970s, which matched an equivalent rise in the price of oil during the oil embargo years. Westinghouse had contracted with utility companies to supply uranium at a fixed price, but because of the extraordinary price increase they were forced in 1977 to make a default payment of 1 billion dollars to their customers. But after some memoranda from an Australian uranium mining company surfaced, indicating possible collusion, Westinghouse instituted its antitrust suit.

I found the government data on the output and consumption of uranium inexplicably confusing but finally found the answer to the puzzle in the trade press. McGraw-Hill publishes *Nucleonics Week* and *Nuclear Fuel* (annual subscription price about $3,000), which furnish operating statistics for every civilian power reactor. From a study of the years 1970 to 1977 when most large reactors began to come on line, I discovered there were so many forced stoppages and unforeseen problems that by and large the industry was working at less than half its rated capacity for those years. I concluded that if the forces of supply and demand were operating freely, the price of uranium would have dropped rather than increased six-fold. Unfortunately, as soon as I reached this conclusion, the case was settled out of court, much to my disappointment. I was left with the notion that this was a strange industry indeed and that the doubts expressed by Sternglass might warrant further investigation.

While serving on the EPA Science Advisory Board, I discovered that state and federal epidemiologists were reluctant to explore the politically sensitive reasons for the widespread variation in county cancer mortality rates, which were dramatically revealed by county cancer mortality maps published by the EPA during the 1970s. For example, rates appeared to be extremely high in counties in New Jersey and Louisiana that had high concentrations of petrochemical employment and wastes.

With the time and resources on hand, I decided to investigate the reasons for variation. And so I began a new career in 1984, first working with a small New York nonprofit agency called the Council on Economic Priorities. With their help, I published a book in 1986 entitled *Quality of Life in Residential Neighborhoods: Levels of Affluence, Toxic Waste and Cancer Mortality in Residential Neighborhoods.*[6] In this book I established correlations between ZIP code areas with high cancer rates and high concentrations of chemical wastes. I also discovered that other cofactors had to be considered. For example, breast cancer mortality rates in Texas and Louisiana were extremely low despite exposure to the nation's highest levels of petrochemical pollution, while the suburban counties of Westchester and Long Island, with low exposures to chemicals, had among the nation's highest breast cancer rates, for reasons which are discussed in the present study.

The mystery began to be resolved when in 1986 I finally met Sternglass. He suggested that exposure to reactor emissions might be the missing cofactor. Indeed, in this book we show that the breast cancer rates in affluent New York suburban counties in the late 1980s reflect the nation's highest *per capita* exposures to radioactive emissions from civilian reactors, whereas Texas and Louisiana—with much more chemical pollution—have no such exposures. In other words, radiation makes chemicals doubly carcinogenic, as Rachel Carson first pointed out in her book *Silent Spring*.[7]

Sternglass encouraged me to use my professional skills in analyzing large computer databases to ascertain whether mortality rates were significantly higher in counties that were downwind of nuclear power reactors. Although initially somewhat skeptical, I was surprised to find significant mortality increases in 175 counties located northeast of about 50 such reactor sites, which I published in a December 1986 CEP newsletter entitled "Nuclear Emissions Take Their Toll."[8]

These findings were presented to Senator Edward Kennedy's Senate Public Health Committee in 1987 on behalf of plaintiffs suing the operator of the Three Mile Island reactor. (Their claims of injuries sustained in the 1979 accident have yet to come to trial.) In January of 1988 Senator Kennedy asked the National Institute of Health to examine cancer mortality rates near nuclear reactors. This formal request resulted in a three-volume report published by the National Cancer Institute in July of 1990, which concluded that "if . . . any excess cancer risk was present in U.S. counties with nuclear facilities, it was too small to be detected with the methods employed."[9]

This book will show that in reaching this erroneous conclusion, the NCI misrepresented their own data, chiefly by defining only 107 counties as "nuclear." Such small samples of the nation's 3,000-odd counties would not be large enough for any divergent mortality trend to prove statistically significant.

Our findings imply that women living near reactors are at greater risk of contracting breast cancer, which does not mean that women living further away from reactors are safe. It does suggest that some malevolent force of mortality is being emitted from reactors and that this force could interact with pesticides and other chemical pollutants, thus affecting residents of all counties to a varying degree.

In 1987 we discovered that fallout from the Chernobyl accident, which reached the United States in the second week of May 1986, had a significant immediate adverse impact on the mortality of Americans— young and old—with failing immune response. For example, the number of AIDS-related deaths in May 1986 was double that of May 1985. Our report, published by the American Chemical Society in January 1989[10] offered epidemiological support for the ominous predictions made by Linus Pauling and Andrei Sakharov in 1958. Only in 1995 have we come to know, thanks to the efforts of DOE Secretary Hazel O'Leary, that thousands of human guinea pigs were used by the Pentagon to test the health effects of the ingestion of man-made fission products.

We know from the Chernobyl accident that radiation clouds can travel thousands of miles to come down in the rain, contaminating local food and water—exactly as predicted by Rachel Carson. Over long periods of time the contamination might be reflected in the form of statistically significant increases in cancer mortality, but there are also other far more immediate indicators of the biological harm done by radiation.

In 1990 I established the nonprofit Radiation and Public Health Project and published *Deadly Deceit: Low-Level Radiation High Level Cover-Up*,[11] which details many of the epidemiological anomalies that can only be adequately explained in terms of the biological harm of ingested or inhaled fission products. In addition, this book, written as a companion volume to *Deadly Deceit*, offers a popular exposition of material presented in articles recently published in the peer-reviewed *International Journal of Health Services* (Johns Hopkins School of Public Health) by members of the Radiation and Public Health Project, as follows:

"Breast Cancer: Evidence for a Relation to Fission Products in the Diet," by E.J. Sternglass and J.M. Gould.[12]

"Nuclear Fallout, Low Birthweight, and Immune Deficiency," by J.M. Gould and E.J. Sternglass.[13]

"Cancer Mortality Near Oak Ridge, Tennessee," by J.J. Mangano.[14]

"A Response to Comments on 'Cancer Mortality Near Oak Ridge,'" by J.J. Mangano.[15]

"A Response to Comments on 'Breast Cancer: Evidence for a Relation to Fission Products in the Diet,'" by E.J. Sternglass and J.M. Gould.[16]

In addition, we can add the following:

"Breast Cancer Mortality Near Nuclear Reactors," by J.M. Gould and E.J. Sternglass, presented on April 30, 1995, to the Berlin meeting of the Berlin Radiological Protection Society.[17]

"Thyroid Cancer in America since Chernobyl," by J.J. Mangano and W. Reid, published in the *British Medical Journal* in August 1995.[18]

"A Post-Chernobyl Rise in Connecticut Thyroid Cancer," by J.J. Mangano, published in the *European Journal of Cancer Prevention* in January 1996.[19]

These articles and this book represent the collective output of all four members of the Radiation and Public Health Project, with the aid of generous grants from the CS Fund, the Deer Creek Foundation, and the Friedson Philanthropic Foundation. As senior members of the project, Sternglass and I are particularly proud to have attracted the support of a younger generation of environmental scientists, including Joseph Mangano and Dr. William Reid, whose work we will discuss in some detail.

The fourth member of the RPHP team is William McDonnell, whose mastery of the personal computer made this book possible. The information is based on a massive data-processing effort that would have been prohibitively expensive if we had to use large mainframe computers to produce the many maps and tables shown here. McDonnell is also the coauthor of *Deadly Defense: Military Radioactive Landfills*, published by the Radioactive Waste Campaign in 1988.

We have retained all the tables, figures, and references used in the original professional articles but try to explain in layperson's terms the concepts that are taken for granted by professional epidemiologists. Be forewarned, this book is not a primer and will not answer all possible questions about ionizing radiation that may occur to the lay reader. It cannot be regarded as easy or pleasant reading and is addressed to the large number of persons who would be reluctant to live near a reactor but don't really know why. By offering readers access (on floppy disks) to the giant database used here, along with instructions on how the data may be analyzed by those with personal computers, we hope to make our readers active participants in ensuring our fullest under- standing of why we are at risk.

We therefore dedicate this book to the 1 million questioning breast cancer victims who in the short space of 4 years have made the hun- dreds of chapters of the newly organized National Breast Cancer Coalition a potent political force. They and the 1 million victims of the AIDS epidemic may someday unite with all other young people who have borne the brunt of the damage from low-level radiation to put an end to the operation of all nuclear reactors.

OVERVIEW AND SUMMARY

> Who wants to live near a nuclear power plant? Probably, nobody, given a choice. Although nuclear installations pay a lot of property taxes, they often spark deep-seated worries over the effects of unseen radiation.

This is the opening sentence of an editorial entitled "Fact vs. Fear," which appeared in the *Minneapolis Star Tribune* on May 6, 1995—a sentiment which is widely shared by the American population. However, the editorial goes on to say, "Nevertheless living near a nuclear plant engenders no greater risk than living elsewhere in Minnesota," in an effort to refute the chief argument of this book—that women living close to reactors are at significantly greater risk of dying of breast cancer than those living further away. But this is a fact that was confirmed in a confidential memo circulated on January 5, 1995, by the National Cancer Institute (see appendix D, page 321). The memo was also intended to refute the argument of this book, but in it the author admitted that there was a significantly higher rate of breast cancer mortality in counties within 50 miles of a reactor site than in all other counties of the nation. We show that this same statement is true of women living within 100 miles of a reactor site.

This book uses National Cancer Institute county data collected since 1950 on white female breast cancer mortality to prove that the popular fear of living near a reactor is well grounded. The aforementioned editorial suggests we have a choice in the matter; we were in fact given no choice. Although Black women are experiencing a greater breast cancer mortality than white women today, the present study focuses on the latter group because in most counties, the number of Black or other minority women is too small to allow statistically significant effects to be observed at the county level. (We hope in the future to do a separate study of cancer rates among Blacks.) We also use official data from state health departments and from the Center for Disease Control to show that ionizing radiation from bomb tests and reactors play an important role not only in the current epidemic rise of breast cancer but also in that of AIDS and low-birthweight live births.

The NCI, which used our methodology in an attempt to disprove our findings, estimated the current age-adjusted mortality rate for "nuclear" counties within 50 miles of a reactor site at 26.9 deaths per 100,000 women, based on 69,554 deaths in the years 1985–89, compared with 23.3 deaths for all other counties. The probability that so great a difference could be due to chance is infinitesimal. This means that the cause of the current epidemic increase in breast cancer involves geographical factors that must be environmental and cannot be ascribed to differences due to genetic factors. We must therefore discard all the "blame the victim" and lifestyle factors invoked by the authorities to conceal the true man-made causes of this epidemic.

In the 50 years since 1945, when the Nuclear Age began with the first atomic bomb explosion, over 1.5 million American women have died of breast cancer. The incidence of breast cancer has risen almost three-fold in this period in some areas. We will show that the major overlooked cause is man-made ionizing radiation—either from low-level internal radiation due to nuclear fallout or from external sources of unnecessary overexposure to X rays, exacerbated by the interaction of nuclear fallout with chemical pollutants. Low-level nuclear radiation (unlike natural sources of ionizing radiation) harms our immune defenses against cancer that results from ingesting fission products like bone-seeking radioactive strontium—which did not exist in nature prior to 1943. As Rachel Carson foresaw in *Silent Spring*, strontium 90 is a "sinister partner" interacting with industrial chemicals and air pollution to accelerate the process of human carcinogenesis.

This book validates Carson's prediction by using official data compiled by the National Cancer Institute since 1950 to show that of the 3,000-odd counties in the United States, women living in about 1,300 "nuclear" counties (located within 100 miles of a reactor and most directly exposed to man-made ionizing radiation) are at the greatest risk of dying of breast cancer. The largest source of such radiation since 1945 has been fallout from U.S./U.S.S.R. above-ground nuclear weapons testing, which ceased in 1963—but which has been estimated to be equivalent to setting off some 40,000 Hiroshima bombs.

Most of this fallout came down in heavy rainfall counties, because radiation clouds can more easily bypass dry areas. It turns out that these heavy rainfall counties were also exposed to continuing emissions of man-made fission products from nuclear reactors. They are also generally the most affluent counties, whose residents have comprehensive health care, and therefore have most likely been previously exposed to high doses of X rays in fluoroscopy and mammography. These same counties also have the highest concentration of industrial chemical wastes. All nonnuclear counties tend to be located between the Rocky Mountains and the Mississippi River. Even though these counties are in the mountain states closest to the Nevada test site—and the west south central states with high concentrations of petrochemical pollution—because they have little rain and fallout from nuclear reactors, they have the lowest mortality rates from breast cancer and AIDS. The highest rates are found in the New York metropolitan counties subject to the nation's highest *per capita* exposures to emissions from the Indian Point, Millstone, and Brookhaven nuclear reactors.

This book demonstrates that, based on official breast cancer mortality data for every county in the nation, women living near nuclear reactors—because of past and present exposure to such ionizing radiation—are at the highest risk of dying of breast cancer, no matter how proximity to reactors is defined.

For example, the National Cancer Institute defines a "nuclear" county as one in which a nuclear facility is located, based on the simple-minded assumption that emissions from a reactor would stop at the county line. With so limited a definition, there would be so few deaths involved since 1950, that no overall change for such a county could prove to be statistically significant—which is to say, the change could not be the result of chance. One of our most revealing findings concerns the 14 counties in which the 7 oldest Department of Energy reactor sites are located. The combined age-adjusted white female breast cancer mortality rate for all 14 of these counties rose by 37 percent from 1950–54 to 1985–89, when the corresponding rate in the United States rose by only 1 percent. Over that period, the number of breast cancer deaths in those 14 counties quintupled, whereas the number in the United States doubled. The probability that so great a divergence in mortality trends could be the product of chance is infinitesimal.

Proximity to a reactor can also be defined as residence within 50 or 100 miles (although, as demonstrated by the Chernobyl disaster, large-scale fallout can extend for thousands of miles). For each of 60 reactor sites in operation from 1943 to 1981, we have calculated the combined breast cancer mortality trends for an average of 7 contiguous rural counties located mainly downwind and within about 50 miles of the reactor sites. In the aggregate, there are 346 such counties that in 1950–54 registered an age-adjusted mortality rate well below that of the United States; but by 1985–89, these counties experienced a 10 percent increase. Today the combined rate for these rural "nuclear" counties is well above that of the United States. Again, the probability that so great a divergent trend could be due to chance is infinitesimal.

This definition is mainly limited to rural counties—because almost all nuclear reactors were located in rural areas—and these rural counties accounted for only 15 percent of all breast cancer deaths in 1950–54 and 21 percent in 1985–89. We chose this definition of "proximity" to demonstrate that when it was substituted for the limited NCI definition—involving only 1 or 2 counties per site—the breast cancer mortality increase in counties closest to each of 55 of the 60 reactors proved to be statistically significant.

Finally, we dropped the downwind requirement and extended the definition of proximity to a radius of 50 and then 100 miles. It turns out that east of the Mississippi River, the concentration of civilian power reactors, along with all other adverse environmental factors, is so great that we could define a radius of 100 miles around each reactor, which had a combined mortality rate that would exceed national norms by a statistically significant degree.

On this basis, it turns out that 1,319 of the 3,053 counties in the nation are "nuclear." These counties account for far more than half of all breast cancer deaths—because most of the nation's metropolitan counties in the Northeast and the Great Lakes states are included in this extended definition of proximity, and they tend to have the highest breast cancer mortality rates in the nation.

Therefore for these 1,319 "nuclear" counties, the current combined white female breast cancer mortality rate, adjusted to reflect the

U.S. age composition in 1950, is close to 26 deaths per 100,000 women as compared to a corresponding rate of 22 deaths per 100,000 for the remaining mainly rural nonnuclear counties—a difference too great to be attributed to either chance, genetics, or other factors shared to a comparable degree by the entire population.

For the large urban and suburban counties with the largest concentration of population, reactor emissions can be shown to have an exacerbating effect on women who have already suffered heavily from exposure to other environmental causes of the breast cancer epidemic, including a 100-year build-up of industrial chemical pollutants, a 50-year exposure to fallout from the manufacturing and testing of nuclear bombs, and the often unnecessary overexposure to X rays.

Individuals living in the large metropolitan areas of the Northeast also suffered disproportionately from low-level internal radiation for other reasons. They were dependent on surface waters from reservoirs, lakes, and rivers rather than on water from underground wells, so that urban counties, such as those in New York City, were the first to be exposed to drinking water contaminated by the early bomb test fallout. These metropolitan counties also had a disproportionately heavy exposure to industrial chemicals earlier than nonnuclear rural counties did. When exposure to toxic chemicals is combined with exposure to ionizing radiation, cancer mortality is exacerbated.

This is best illustrated by the fact that breast cancer mortality rates are 40 percent higher in the New York metropolitan counties than in Louisiana, Texas, and Oklahoma. These southern states have the nation's highest concentrations of petrochemical wastes, but they have no operating reactors during the period we studied, while Westchester and Long Island have been exposed to the nation's highest *per capita* levels of reactor emissions.

Perhaps the most shocking single revelation in this book is the large number of class action suits now underway by victims of large radiation releases, which have been studiously ignored by the mainstream media. There are, for example, 2,500 plaintiffs suing the operator of the stricken Three Mile Island reactor, which after 14 years has yet to be reported by the *New York Times*, despite the fact that about 300 cases have been privately settled. The *Times* has barely noted that 27,000 plaintiffs are suing the operators of the Hanford Nuclear Weapons plant in Hanford, Washington, after the Department of

Energy admitted in 1991 that an unknown number of thyroid cancer cases were caused by large releases of radioactive iodine from Hanford in the late 1940s. Finally, as this book was being completed, the Brookhaven National Laboratory in Suffolk County has conceded our claim that the southern flow of contaminated ground water under the laboratory, representing a 45-year build-up of radioactive and chemical pollutants, compromised the quality of private water wells in areas just to the south of the laboratory, causing an instantaneous drop in local home values. As this book was going to press, hundreds of prospective plaintiffs and attorneys were preparing for class action suits against the laboratory, which may eventually exceed the magnitude of the Hanford action. I believe that such suits will eventually drive a stake into the heart of the nuclear industry.

Civilian and military reactor emissions—although relatively small when compared with bomb test fallout—are thus shown to play a key role in the present epidemic rise of breast cancer incidence and mortality in some regions of the nation. Since 1980, major accidental releases from civilian power reactors, such as Three Mile Island and Chernobyl, have accelerated immune system damage for women born after 1945, whose immune response had already been damaged in utero, during the years of bomb test fallout, and who are now reaching the ages of 35 to 50. This is why young women are increasingly vulnerable to contracting breast cancer.

Such vulnerability could be greatly reduced by accelerating the shutdown of all reactor operations. Already the most dangerous Department of Energy reactor buildings have become so radioactive that the knowledgeable supervisory personnel will no longer enter them, and thousands of DOE plant workers are now unemployed. Many are dying prematurely of cancer and are therefore not regarded by insurance companies as suitable risks for alternative employment. Civilian reactors will soon reach the end of their operational life cycles, as have five in the recent past, and as foreshadowed by the judgment of Wall Street, which has taken a very dim view of the stocks and bonds of nuclear utilities.

With the end of the Cold War, which we will see was greatly accelerated by the 1986 Chernobyl disaster—the worst industrial accident in human history—the only supporters of continued reactor operation are the well-entrenched members of the international nuclear establishment. They ignore the fact that the resulting worldwide build-up of radioactive materials has left humankind with a legacy that must be monitored for hundreds of thousands of years. Here is a major example of an enormous environmental problem that cannot be blamed on the ecologically blind free play of market forces. Without the support of huge subsidies from governments, who still see nuclear bombs as offering the promise of unlimited power, the fearfully expensive and dangerous civilian reactors would find no acceptance by prudent business people.

Thirty-five years ago mothers took the lead in forcing the nuclear powers to ban above-ground bomb tests, because they knew from the warnings of the world's greatest scientists that fallout was harming their babies. One of our major findings is that they were right—from 1945 to 1965 there was an anomalous 40 percent rise in the percentage of live births weighing less than 5.5 pounds—and an equally sharp improvement when above-ground testing ceased. In 1963, when those born in 1945 reached the age of 18, there began an equally anomalous 20-year decline in SAT scores—perfectly synchronized with peak bomb tests 18 years earlier. We shall show that the SAT decline reflected the bomb test damage to the thyroid of the infant in the mother's womb—the key gland that controls the development of the brain in early childhood. This can now be seen most dramatically in the enormous rise of thyroid cancer in the former Soviet republics of Belarus and Ukraine.

We shall also show that in 1970, male baby boomers—whose glandular and immune systems were damaged at birth—on reaching the age of 25 began a 20-year period in which they increasingly dropped out of the labor force. By 1980, when they reached the age of 35, another 2-decade period began in which those engaged in unsafe sex—which heightens the transmission of infectious diseases—increasingly died of AIDS. Thus the 75 million young men and women under the age of 50 today belong to a generation born in the worst of all possible times.

How fitting it would be if they emulated their mothers, whose agitation against the bomb helped end above-ground testing. We must press for an end to the production of nuclear weapons and operation of nuclear reactors, which destroy the health and economic future of our nation.

Chapter 1

INTRODUCTION: FALLOUT AND COUNTY BREAST CANCER RATES

About 45,000 American women die each year of breast cancer—twice the number that died in 1950. This book uses official data to trace the differential growth of white female breast cancer mortality in each of the counties that make up the nation in order to analyze the environmental factors that have contributed to the epidemic rise of this disease over the past four decades. We have found that there is a great geographic variation in the degree to which our nation is in the grip of the current breast cancer epidemic.

A new database of county-by-county, age-adjusted breast cancer mortality rates, secured from the National Cancer Institute, permits us to examine the environmental differences between those geographic clusters in which cancer mortality is both most and least concentrated. (Age-adjusted county cancer mortality rates are what the rates would be if every county had the same age composition that the United States had in 1950.)

Since cancer mortality is a function of age, the use of age-adjusted breast cancer mortality rates means that differences among areas cannot be attributed to variations in age composition, and that we therefore will be able to show that the statistically significant variations over time and space from national norms must be attributed to environmental rather than genetic causes. Some of our findings will be surprising, because the environmental causes of geographic variations in cancer mortality rates raise sensitive political questions that governmental epidemiologists are reluctant to deal with.

We believe that an analysis of the official data on breast cancer mortality rates since 1950 must include an examination of all the environmental factors at work in different geographic areas, including one neglected factor—exposure to man-made fission products—that began with the birth of the Nuclear Age in 1945.

PROXIMITY TO REACTORS

We shall show that there are clusters of rural, suburban, and urban counties close to nuclear reactor sites with a current combined age-adjusted breast cancer mortality rate of about 26 or 27 deaths per 100,000 women. In sharp contrast, the remaining mainly rural counties have a corresponding rate of only 22 or 23 deaths per 100,000 women. Again, because these differences involve groupings of many millions, they cannot be due to chance. Epidemiologists cannot avoid the responsibility of ascertaining the cause. These rural counties are mainly concentrated in the states between the Rocky Mountains and the Mississippi River. It is as if the nation is divided into a "nuclear" sector with high cancer rates, and all remaining rural counties that are far enough away from reactors to be considered at relatively far less risk. The map shown on page 187 tells this story at a glance. The "nuclear" counties are shown with two degrees of shading; a heavy shading for those counties mainly in the Northeast and Great Lakes states that have breast cancer rates significantly greater than the national average, and a lighter shading for the "nuclear" counties within 100 miles of reactors in rural southern states. The lighter shading indicates that the increase in mortality rates since 1950–54 is significantly greater than the national average..

(See appendix A and B for computerized maps and data displaying the breast cancer mortality trends for exposed counties within a 50-mile and 100-mile radius of each of 60 nuclear reactor sites. All such data are available to anyone with a personal computer who wants to either replicate, extend, or dispute our findings.)

This book seeks to explain how the disproportion in breast cancer mortality risk has developed since 1950, when county age-adjusted breast cancer mortality rates first became available. Although it would have been ideal to have data beginning in 1940, before the Nuclear Age began, we do have sufficient state data on breast cancer mortality starting prior to 1950, from which we can make inferences about the rapid rise in breast cancer that began immediately after 1945.

We have examined how exposure to man-made fission products interacting with chemical pesticides and other toxins are particularly troublesome in heavy rainfall areas. Chemical pollutants are regarded by governmental epidemiologists as confounding factors that make it impossible to distinguish their effects from those of low-level radiation. We believe that the proper adjective is *exacerbating,* in accordance with the insight first given us by Rachel Carson on the way in which nuclear fallout interacts with chemical pollutants.

The extraordinary elevation of breast cancer rates relative to the national rate in the nation's largest affluent urban counties adds weight to a recent hypothesis that suggests that the current increase in breast cancer incidence also reflects frequent exposure of women to breast X rays decades ago when doses per examination were as much as 100 times larger than today. This practice was far more common in the past in affluent urban rather than poorer rural counties. But the fact that those rural counties near reactors have registered far greater increases in breast cancer mortality than nearby urban counties suggests that ingestion and inhalation of nuclear fission products must play an additional and exacerbating role.

The nation's highest age-adjusted breast cancer mortality rates for counties with over 100,000 population are found in New York City and the affluent suburban counties of Westchester and Long Island. These counties account for 5.4 percent of all white female breast cancer deaths, compared with only 3.9 percent of all white females—the highest mortality concentration in the nation. Large urban centers like New York, dependent on surface water reservoirs for their drinking water, are shown here to be the first to experience the adverse consequences of exposure to above-ground nuclear bomb tests.

The nation's largest statistically significant percentage increase in breast cancer mortality was registered by women living in the 14 counties that housed the nation's oldest Department of Energy reactors, which began in the years 1943 to 1950. For these women the age-adjusted mortality rate rose by 37 percent from 1950–54 to 1985–89, compared with a corresponding U.S. increase of only 1 percent.

Because the number of deaths in these 14 counties quintupled—from 371 to 1,926 over a 35-year period—the probability that so huge a divergence could be due to chance is only 1 in several million cases.

SOURCE OF COUNTY CANCER MORTALITY RATES

Our examination of clusters of rural, suburban, and urban counties that represent the nation's worst breast cancer problem areas make use of a county database secured from the National Cancer Institute. It is a sad fact that the government agencies charged with the task of collecting and analyzing these mortality statistics have been extremely reluctant to recognize the contribution of geographic environmental degradation to the inexorable increase in cancer rates over the past half century. So reluctant that a private nongovernmental nonprofit agency had to assume the task of acquiring and processing this official updated data. One reason for publishing our findings in a book written for popular consumption is to force the state and federal authorities to confront our arguments and offer an explanation for the extraordinary geographic differences in breast cancer mortality rates.

The good news is that the data have been carefully collected in the United States since 1950, and, unlike in any other nation, it can be secured either on the basis of Freedom of Information or similar requests. However, it does require expert processing and analytical skills not normally available to laypersons. It is the chief goal of this book to demonstrate that the personal computer has made these skills universally available—which is particularly important for those living in areas where such problems have literally become questions of life or death. These skills will be seen to be matters of common sense, and we will explain how to evaluate any large divergence of breast cancer mortality in a given county or cluster of contiguous counties from a national norm. If such a divergence cannot be attributed to chance, then we must go on to explore the specific causes of such a divergence if it proves to be statistically significant.

FALLOUT EFFECTS

Our findings were first anticipated by Rachel Carson, who died of breast cancer a few years after writing *Silent Spring* in 1962. Carson predicted that the nuclear fission products released in atmospheric bomb tests would interact with pesticides like DDT and other industrial chemicals to make the latter all the more carcinogenic. As she wrote in the opening page of chapter 2 of *Silent Spring*:

> In this now universal contamination of the environment, chemicals are the sinister and little-recognized partners of radiation in changing the very nature of life. Strontium 90, released through nuclear explosions into the air, comes to earth in rain or drifts down as fallout, lodges in soil, enters into the grass or corn or wheat grown there, and in time takes up its abode in the bones of a human being, there to remain until his death.[7]

Rachel Carson's bracketing of man-made radiation and chemicals echoed the extraordinary prescience of similar warnings made by two of the world's greatest scientists—Linus Pauling and Andrei Sakharov. In 1958, they both warned of the adverse health effects of man-made fission products that were first introduced into a then pristine atmosphere in 1945; both were subsequently awarded Nobel peace prizes for the courage required to counter the Cold War passions of those years.[20] [21]

Sakharov predicted that ingested fission products would do both immediate and delayed harm to the human immune response on a worldwide basis—a prediction that my associates and I have been able to validate. During the 1945–65 period of bomb test atmospheric fallout, there were extraordinary anomalous increases in infant mortality, neonatal mortality, stillbirths, and low-birthweight live births. But Sakharov also predicted that the man-made bomb test radiation would accelerate the mutation of all microorganisms, leading to the inference that the most vulnerable—baby boomers born between 1945 and 1965—would, when they grew to maturity in the 1980s, succumb to newly mutated sexually transmitted infectious diseases such as AIDS. Even diseases such as tuberculosis, because of mutation, now increasingly resist traditional antibiotics.

We have found that these predictions are validated by international mortality data broken down by age submitted by each nation to the United Nations. For the first time since World War II, the mortality rates of baby boomers aged 25 to 44 deteriorated in the 1980s for all nuclear powers except Germany and Japan. Having lost World War II, they were precluded from exposing their progeny to emissions from the manufacture and testing of nuclear weapons. Since this age-group is the most productive component of the labor force, their current lead in international productivity suggests that perhaps they did not really lose World War II!

Postwar radiation-induced damage to baby boomer immune systems affected women as well as men and explains why so many more young women are contracting breast cancer today. In a subsequent companion book we hope to analyze the environmental factors behind the current rise in such immune deficiency diseases as AIDS, tuberculosis, pneumonia, septicemia, and prostate cancer. The latter kills as many men today as the number of women dying of breast cancer, but with a longer latency period.

The warnings of Sakharov and Pauling, however, were so unwelcome to the major powers, intent on making use of nuclear technology for national defense, that both were treated, along with Carson, as scientific pariahs by their respective governments. Thus the true health effects of ingesting man-made fission products have been withheld from the public for nearly half a century. Nevertheless, the fact that President Kennedy signed the Partial Test Ban just prior to his death in 1963, ending U.S./U.S.S.R. above-ground tests, suggests that the pernicious health effects of ionizing radiation were known to our highest-placed public officials.

Humans have been exposed to natural forms of ionizing radiation from terrestrial sources and from cosmic rays for countless millennia, and so our immune systems have developed the capacity to resist cancer for the normal span of life. This is what is meant by background radiation, which should not be confused with low-level radiation. The latter refers to the internal radiation from man-made fission products that when ingested concentrate in certain organs of the body. It would be impossible for our immune systems to develop the capacity to resist the carcinogenic effects of low-level radiation in a mere 50 years.

Ingested nuclear fission products, such as radioactive iodine and strontium, have immediate and delayed adverse effects on hormonal and immune systems. Protracted low-dose exposures do most of their damage via free radicals, which are so dangerous to the cells of the immune system that defend against mutant cells. This is why antioxidants, such as vitamins C and E are so desirable to boost the immune response in the treatment of AIDS and breast and prostate cancer.

UNCOVERING LOW-LEVEL RADIATION HEALTH EFFECTS

The 1991 publication *Deadly Deceit: Low-Level Radiation High Level Cover-Up*[11] discusses in detail many of the epidemiological anomalies that can only be adequately explained in terms of the biological harm of ingested or inhaled fission products. The book's subtitle refers to the fact that governmental experts have concealed or misrepresented such dangers out of national security concerns. It has therefore become a matter of life or death for all of us—breast cancer victims particularly—to learn all we can about how ingested fission products do their damage, and how we can protect ourselves. To do this we must first learn exactly how officials lie to us. They rely on our inability to know when a given change in breast cancer mortality is too great to be attributed to chance. This said, we include a discussion of some basic concepts of statistical probability in chapter 4.

In this chapter we take great pains to describe how the factor of chance variation affects counties, which are generally too small to offer a meaningful trend. We must create combinations of contiguous counties to achieve statistically significant divergences from national norms. A notable exception would be Suffolk County, a large suburban county in New York State with the nation's highest current rate of breast cancer mortality for counties of similarly large population. Since 1950, its age-adjusted breast cancer mortality rates have risen 40 times more than the corresponding U.S. increase, and its current rate of 32.4 deaths per 100,000 is significantly higher than the current U.S. rate of 24.6 deaths. Suffolk is so large a county and has so many more breast cancer deaths than would be expected, there is no question that the increase in mortality since 1950 is statistically significant, and that therefore some environmental factor must be at work.

We have attributed this enormous difference in part to its exposure to emissions from reactors at Millstone on the Long Island Sound, only 15 miles away. But Suffolk County is also the home of the Brookhaven National Laboratory, which we now believe may have been contaminating the county's water supply with radioactive discharges since 1950. BNL has recently even admitted that private water wells just to the south of the laboratory may be contaminated. We have found in chapter 8, that there are also significant concentrations of high breast cancer incidence rates within 15 miles of the Brookhaven reactor.[22]

Generally, the women who live closest to reactors are in small rural counties. In order for any long-term mortality trend for these counties to achieve statistical significance, it is necessary to consider that reactor emissions do not stop at the border of the county in which the reactor is located. Local wind and rain patterns may affect a cluster of contiguous rural counties large enough to achieve statistical significance. Women living near reactors, or any other point source of dangerous toxins, can determine for themselves how to use our data and maps to combine several neighboring counties into larger clusters of sufficient size to measure the degree to which they may be at added risk.

If for any group of contiguous counties near a reactor, incinerator, or Superfund waste site, there has been a long-term statistically significant increase in breast cancer mortality, we think that unless some plausible alternative explanation can be found, local discharges may be judged to play a contributing role. The presence of a hazardous waste dump or any local concentration of toxic chemicals only enhances the probability that an interaction between radiation and the chemicals may be at fault, as Carson predicted.

Adjusting County Cancer Mortality Rates for Age

Another important epidemiologic concept that must be understood for environmental analysis is the difference between so-called "crude" mortality rates and those adjusted for age, which are used throughout this book. For example, the crude cancer mortality rate of a county in Florida that attracts retirees in large numbers would be high merely because it will have a larger than normal proportion of old people, say over 65.

By dint of a very laborious computational procedure, it is possible to replace a crude cancer mortality rate, which is derived by dividing the total number of cancer deaths in a county by its population, with an age-adjusted rate, which represents what the rate would be if the county had the same age composition as the nation had in a "standard" year, such as 1950. In this way an age-adjusted county mortality rate that rose significantly over time would reflect an environmental change rather than an influx of old people. The computational procedure requires a far greater database than the crude cancer mortality database. For each of 3,053 counties in the database, we must know the number of deaths and population for each of 18 different age-groups during each time period. While the federal government collects this data each year, the millions of separate computations required to calculate county age-adjusted rates was, until only recently, a monopoly of the National Cancer Institute.

IMPORTANCE OF PERSONAL COMPUTERS IN UNCOVERING THE TRUTH

The current generation of personal computers has become so powerful that the federal monopoly has been broken. For each of the 3 time periods discussed, spanning 35 years, we have secured the raw data necessary to calculate age-adjusted mortality rates for every county in the nation and for any desired combination of counties. (A confidential National Cancer Institute memo written on January 5, 1995, discussed in appendix D, completely validates both our methodology and major findings.)

We processed the data in a form that can be made available to anyone who wants to check our calculations or find other clusters of high-risk counties. All that is necessary is a standard personal computer and a standard spreadsheet program. As discussed in appendix A, for a small fee to cover duplication costs, we can offer readers floppy disks containing the necessary county data for any state or region, along with instructions on how to proceed.

While we believe that exposure to man-made fission products represents the most neglected single environmental factor linked to the breast cancer epidemic, we invite skeptical readers to use these floppy disks to do their own research. The disks show the change over 35 years in the number of breast cancer deaths and the female population in each 5-year age-group in every county. This information was compiled at a cost of billions of the tax payers' dollars. Fortunately, we live in the only nation in the world that makes such politically sensitive data publicly available. We would be foolish not to make good use of it.

Chapter 2

FALLOUT AND IMMUNE DEFICIENCY

The key to understanding the relationship between breast cancer and the ingestion of man-made fission products is to trace the impact of the latter on the immune response, which controls one's ability to cope with mutant cells.

We begin with an examination of data from the Connecticut Tumor Registry, the oldest and best facility of its kind in the nation. In a Tumor Registry, every case of cancer, whether first diagnosed in the office of a physician, hospital, or clinic, is recorded and traced until the time of death. The Connecticut data represents the largest sample of data on cancer incidence, which permits the examination of temporal changes over a span of 60 years.

Changing Rates of Breast Cancer Incidence Rates Since 1935

Since 1935 the incidence of breast cancer among women aged 50 to 74 in Connecticut has nearly tripled, and Connecticut represents a large enough sample of the United States to permit us to assume that a comparable increase has affected the whole nation.[23] If one examines the annual movement of the Connecticut breast cancer incidence rate since 1935, as in figure 2–1, one discovers the degree with which the postwar rise in breast cancer can be associated with man-made fission products, which were first introduced into a pristine atmosphere when the Nuclear Age began in 1945. That the atmosphere prior to 1944 or 1945 was pristine with respect to man-made fission products is clear from the fact that it can be shown that worldwide emissions from bomb tests and reactors since 1945 have amounted to millions of curies.

One curie is equivalent to a trillion picocuries, to use the unit in which dangerous concentrations of radioactive iodine and strontium in milk and water are measured.

In figure 2–1 we note that the breast cancer incidence rate in Connecticut was declining in the prenuclear years from 1935 to 1944 but only began its postwar incline in 1945 with the onset of nuclear bomb tests. The rate rose again even more sharply after the start-up of the Millstone reactors on Long Island Sound near New London, Connecticut.

Thus, the upward trend began at a rate of 2 percent each year during the years when the superpowers exploded hundreds of nuclear bombs into the atmosphere. There was another upward surge after 1970, at an annual rate of 3 percent, with the start-up of 4 troublesome civilian nuclear power reactors.

Figures 2–1 and 2–2, taken from the Connecticut Tumor Registry, show how low-level radiation from the fallout of nuclear fission products acts both as a promoter and initiator of breast cancer for younger women. Women born in 1945–54 reached their late thirties in the 1980s when the incidence rates for this age-group reached all-time peak levels. This may reflect immune system damage at birth, which was caused by their mothers' ingestion of man-made fission products. (In these figures we include the birth years of each age-group.)

Some may question why if a diagnosis of breast cancer may occur as long as 25 or 30 years after the initial insult to the immune response, the incidence rate rose so quickly after 1945. The answer is that we all carry a latent capacity to contract cancer as we age, so that for many people the immune insult acts as a promoter of carcinogenesis.

In figure 2–3 we trace the annual movement since 1935 (again from the Connecticut Tumor Registry) of the age-adjusted thyroid cancer rate, which has a much shorter latency period than breast cancer—only about five years. Thyroid cancer is a relatively rare disease. As in the case of breast cancer, the trend in the years before the introduction of man-made fission products was clearly declining, and prior to 1945, the rate was under 1 per 100,000. But thereafter it increased fivefold, reaching an all-time peak of nearly 4.5 per 100,000 in 1991, 5 years after the arrival of radioactive iodine in the United States from Chernobyl. All other peaks in figure 2–3 can also be associated with sudden

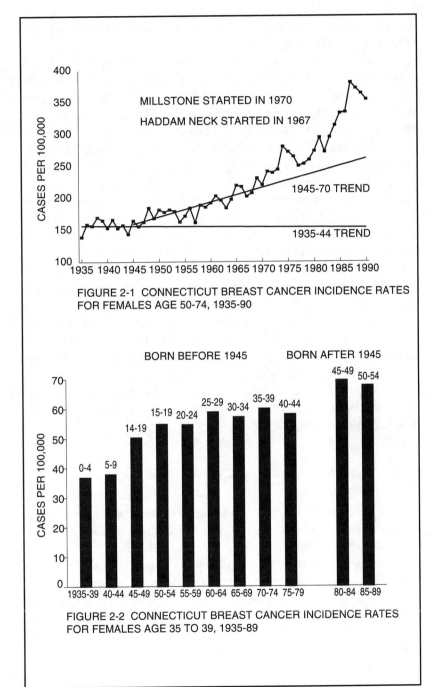

FIGURE 2-1 CONNECTICUT BREAST CANCER INCIDENCE RATES
FOR FEMALES AGE 50-74, 1935-90

FIGURE 2-2 CONNECTICUT BREAST CANCER INCIDENCE RATES
FOR FEMALES AGE 35 TO 39, 1935-89

upsurges of nuclear fallout five years earlier—from either bomb tests or from the Millstone and TMI reactors.

Figure 2–4 offers another dramatic view of the five-year lag of thyroid cancer after a large wave of ionizing radiation. The Connecticut age-adjusted rate doubled from 1945–49 to 1950–54 and again registered a 24 percent increase from 1985–89 to 1990–1992, when the rate for children under 15 doubled. The latter increases were attributed by the oncologist Dr. William Reid and epidemiologist Joseph Mangano to the arrival of Chernobyl radiation in Connecticut in April of 1986.[18]

Reid and Mangano noted that the concentration of radioactive iodine in Connecticut milk rose in April and May of 1986 from an average level of 2 picocuries per liter to a peak level of 53 on May 23, 1986. Thus the radiation-induced rise in thyroid cancer in Connecticut after Chernobyl could be compared to similar significant increases in Belarus and Ukraine.

The postwar rise in breast and thyroid cancer incidence depicted in these charts illustrates some of the many epidemiological anomalies that we shall review in this chapter, which can only be explained by the predictions of Pauling[21] and Sakharov,[20] which suggest that man-made nuclear fission products, such as radioactive iodine and strontium, would have both immediate and delayed negative effects on human immune and hormonal systems and that these effects would accelerate the onset of immune deficiency diseases, of which AIDS and cancer are prime examples.

WHY THE LINK BETWEEN BREAST CANCER AND RADIATION HAS BEEN CONCEALED

It is only now, with the end of the Cold War, that the Department of Energy under Hazel O'Leary has begun to address publicly the subject of the health effects of low-level nuclear radiation.

We have noted that low-level nuclear radiation does not refer to external or internal background radiation, with which we have lived for millions of years, but rather to the low levels of internal radiation for those who, since 1945, have inhaled or ingested man-made fission products such as radioactive iodine or strontium—some of which stay in the body for the remainder of one's life.

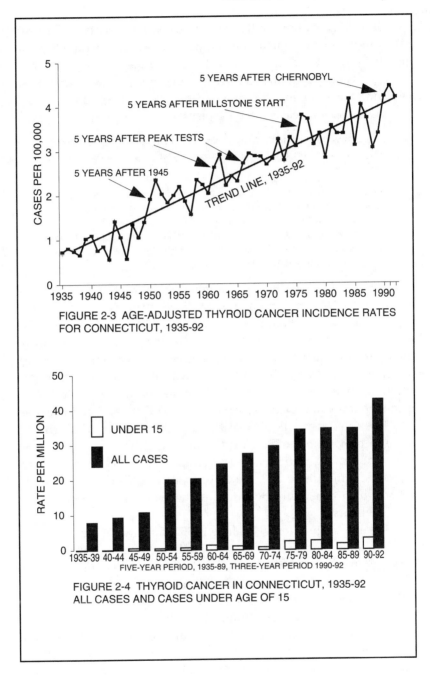

FIGURE 2-3 AGE-ADJUSTED THYROID CANCER INCIDENCE RATES
FOR CONNECTICUT, 1935-92

FIGURE 2-4 THYROID CANCER IN CONNECTICUT, 1935-92
ALL CASES AND CASES UNDER AGE OF 15

Hazel O'Leary has had the courage to reveal the Pentagon's secret use of thousands of human guinea pigs to test the health effects of ingested fission products in the early years of the Cold War. She has also declassified an estimated 2 to 3 billion pages of secret documents, including the following directive issued April 17, 1947, to physicians at the Oak Ridge nuclear weapons plant.

> It is desired that no document be released which refers to experiments with humans and might have adverse effect on public opinion or result in legal suits.
>
> Documents covering such field work should be classified 'secret' . . . It is understood that three documents in this field have been submitted for declassification and are now classified 'restricted'. It is desired that these documents be reclassified 'secret' and that a check be made to insure that no distribution has inadvertently been made to off-project personnel or agencies.[24]

But even O'Leary has yet to admit that millions of Americans—in fact every American alive after 1945—have potentially been exposed to massive volumes of potentially lethal fission products, and that these people must be regarded as the government's unwitting guinea pigs. In fact the DOE during the Bush administration, under pressure from 27,000 plaintiffs who lived downwind of the Hanford nuclear weapons facility (that started operation in 1943), made the following disturbing disclosure: A DOE agency in Seattle (the Dose Reconstruction Project) announced that in 1945, in the haste to provide plutonium for the first atom bombs used in that year, the Hanford plant released a volume of radioactive iodine into a pristine atmosphere as large as that of the 1986 Chernobyl accident—which can easily be rated as the worst single accident in human history.[25]

The exact figure for 1945 alone is 550,000 curies. Nowadays we measure the radioactivity of a liter of milk or water in units of picocuries, with one picocurie equal to one trillionth of a curie. Thus the DOE is now admitting that in 1945, 150 million Americans were unwittingly exposed to 4.5 billion picocuries of radioactive iodine *per capita* that drifted across the nation from Hanford.

Fortunately, despite the cover-up of such secrets, the federal authorities did not "classify" the truly superb American system of gathering and publishing the nation's vital statistics. For this we should be grateful; it enables us to uncover the immediate and delayed effects of radioactive emissions on public health.

Fallout and the Newborn

There is a more immediate indicator of the biological harm of enormous emissions of nuclear fission products than the post-1945 rise in breast cancer incidence rates. It is the emergence that year of the phenomenon of low-birthweight live births—babies born weighing less than 2,500 grams or 5.5 pounds. Figure 2–5 suggests that in the 2 decades, from 1945 to 1965, there was an enormous rise in the low-birthweight percentage so that a considerable portion of the 75 million children who survived birth in those years may have suffered some degree of hormonal and immune system damage that could emerge in later years.

In figure 2–5 we show that New York State began to record the birthweights of live births in 1945, five years before all states were required to follow suit. From 1945 to 1950 the New York rise excluded New York City, but if we allow for the later inclusion of New York City,

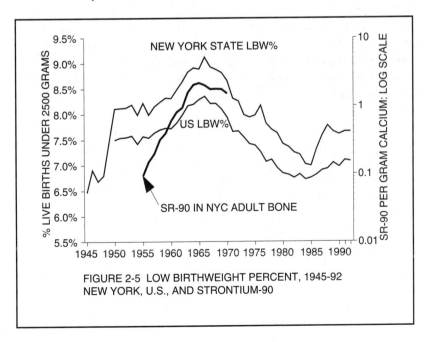

FIGURE 2-5 LOW BIRTHWEIGHT PERCENT, 1945-92
NEW YORK, U.S., AND STRONTIUM-90

we have estimated that in 1945, 6.5 percent of all live births weighed less than 5.5 pounds—the medical designation of an underweight newborn infant.[26] Thereafter, New York low-birthweight live births rose to 8 percent in 1955, when measures of radioactive strontium in the bone of New Yorkers first became evident, and then peaked at 9 percent in 1965 after superpower above-ground tests ceased and the *per capita* levels of strontium in human bone also began to decline.

New York City began measuring birthweights as far back as 1939 and 1940, when its low-birthweight percentages for all races were respectively 7.31 and 7.52. Measurements were suspended during the war years, but were resumed in 1947, when the New York City low-birthweight percentage had risen to 8.24. It is clear, however, that in New York State, the anomalous postwar rise in low birthweights began in 1945.

The rapid rise in the New York low-birthweight percentage starting in 1945 may have occasioned sufficient concern so that in 1948 a Public Health Service conference in Washington, D.C., decreed that as of 1950 every state must record birthweights for white and nonwhite live births, which would be published in annual editions of *US Vital Statistics*.[27]

In the following section we will demonstrate that the radiation-induced postwar rise and fall of low birthweights can serve as a predictor of many otherwise inexplicable epidemiological and socioeconomic anomalies involving the baby boom generation, including the recent rise in breast cancer incidence among young women.

Figure 2–6, taken from the Connecticut Tumor Registry, shows that the incidence of cancers, in children ranging in age from 5 to 9, after declining in the prenuclear years 1935–44, surged upward after 1945. Childhood cancer mortality was extremely rare in 1935—only 2 deaths per 100,000 in the United States. By 1955 it had quadrupled to 8 deaths per 100,000. Its epidemic rise in the 1950s can only be explained as a consequence of the sudden fetal exposure to ingested fission products beginning in 1945.[11]

Another example of the almost immediate adverse impact of ingesting man-made fission products comes from a 1992 article published by Dr. R. K. Whyte, a Canadian professor of pediatrics, in the *British Medical Journal*.[28] In an effort to reexamine the hypothesis that the increase in early infant mortality observed in the 1950s and 1960s

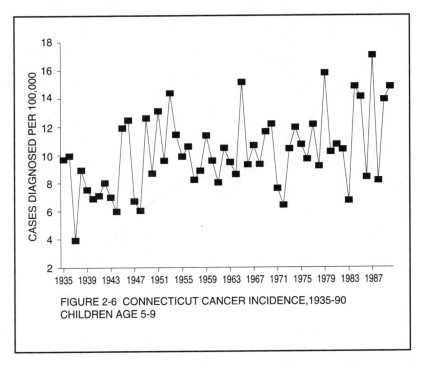

FIGURE 2-6 CONNECTICUT CANCER INCIDENCE, 1935-90 CHILDREN AGE 5-9

was attributable to the early practice of restricting oxygen for sick newborns, Whyte analyzed annual neonatal, first-day infant mortality, and stillbirths in the United States, England, and Wales since 1935.

As shown in figures 2–7 and 2–8 in the case of the United States, Whyte discerned an obviously anomalous upsurge in neonatal and first-day neonatal mortality rates in the peak years of superpower bomb tests. (Neonatal covers newborn deaths under 28 days.)

He found that falling rates of neonatal mortality in both countries were interrupted in the early 1950s, reaching a maximum upward deviation in the mid-1960s. By 1980 rates had returned to the level that would have been expected from the rate of improvement observed in the earlier 1935–1950 period, which was consistent with the end of all atmospheric tests in 1980 and continuing advances in neonatal care. Because a similar pattern was discerned for stillborn rates, he concluded that oxygen restriction for the newborn could not explain the phenomenon, nor could any apparent change in the nutritional management of pregnant women.

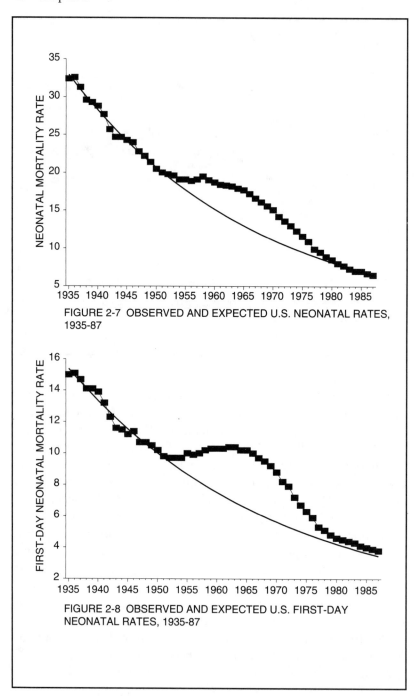

FIGURE 2-7 OBSERVED AND EXPECTED U.S. NEONATAL RATES, 1935-87

FIGURE 2-8 OBSERVED AND EXPECTED U.S. FIRST-DAY NEONATAL RATES, 1935-87

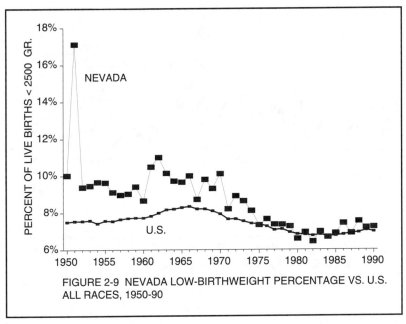

FIGURE 2-9   NEVADA LOW-BIRTHWEIGHT PERCENTAGE VS. U.S. ALL RACES, 1950-90

The observed divergences in neonatal mortality amounted to an excess of 320,000 infant deaths in the United States and the United Kingdom by 1980. Whyte could find no other reason for this epidemiological anomaly other than the atmospheric bomb tests that began in 1945.

FALLOUT AND LOW-BIRTHWEIGHT LIVE BIRTHS

In figures 2–9 and 2–10 we have depicted the annual movement of the low-birthweight percentage of live births, white and nonwhite, since 1950 for the state of Nevada and the United States. These charts, like many of those preceding, also demonstrate the great sensitivity of the newborn to radioactive emissions.

In 1951, the United States shifted some of its atmospheric bomb tests from the Pacific to the newly developed Nevada test site. The circumstances surrounding these initial 1951 Nevada tests are vividly described in Richard Miller's *Under the Cloud: The Decades of Nuclear Testing*.[29] According to Miller, the first two tests occurred on January 27 and 28, 1951. Their radioactive clouds were tracked drifting in a northeasterly direction, finally leaving the United States over New

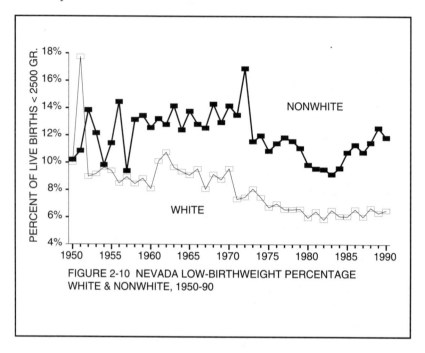

FIGURE 2-10 NEVADA LOW-BIRTHWEIGHT PERCENTAGE
WHITE & NONWHITE, 1950-90

York, New Jersey, Connecticut, and Massachusetts, as did many of the succeeding tests. The third and fourth tests, called *Ranger: Easy* and *Ranger: Baker* were detonated on February 1 and 2 and were tracked drifting to the south and east toward Las Vegas, continuing in a southeasterly direction and finally leaving the U.S. mainland over Florida. These radiation clouds headed in the direction of nearby Las Vegas because of a sudden wind shift that was not anticipated by the inexperienced technicians. These radiation clouds appear to have caused an extraordinary increase in low birthweights in Nevada in 1951, which apparently affected whites in Las Vegas in 1951 more than Native Americans, who in later years, suffered much more as shown by figure 2–10.

It is clear from figures 2–9 and 2–10 that there was an extraordinary increase of nearly 80 percent in the 1951 Nevada low-birthweight percentage for white live births, which was far greater than the corresponding increase for nonwhites. Much of Nevada's white population is concentrated in Las Vegas while nonwhites lived mainly on reservations.

This must have caused great consternation to the test site techni-cians, who had established homes in nearby Las Vegas. They may have then taken pains not to do a test when the wind was blowing toward Las Vegas, for so great an increase in white low birthweights did not occur again.

The biological damage of the Nevada tests was by no means con-fined to Nevada. In figure 2–11 we compare the annual movements of the low-birthweight percentage—for all races—for the 9 states in the Mountain region, closest to the Nevada test site, with that of the United States.

All the Mountain states display the same anomalous rise in 1951. This region, along with all others, reached a final peak level in low birth-weights in 1965, after which, with the cessation of atmospheric tests in 1963, the low-birthweight percentage began a period of rapid improve-ment until 1980. Thereafter, releases from Star Wars nuclear tests in Nevada and accidents such as Three Mile Island in 1979, once again pro-duced a renewed rise. This means there was no way to manage the bio-logical harm from the Nevada tests. Since 1945, U.S. above-ground tests, including the 184 atmospheric bombs detonated at the Nevada

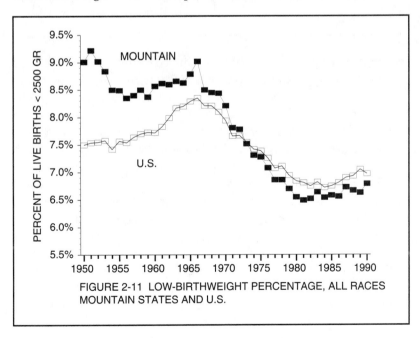

FIGURE 2-11 LOW-BIRTHWEIGHT PERCENTAGE, ALL RACES MOUNTAIN STATES AND U.S.

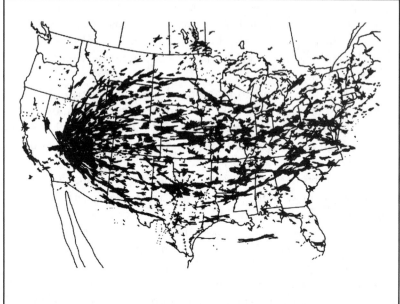

FIGURE 2-12 AREAS OF THE CONTINENTAL UNITED STATES CROSSED BY MORE THAN ONE NUCLEAR CLOUD FROM ABOVE-GROUND DETONATIONS

test site, had a total cumulated yield estimated by the Natural Resources Defense Council to be equal to that of 15,000 Hiroshima bombs.[30]

The consequent biological harm to all areas of the nation was indicated by the rise in the low birthweights that occurred in every state, peaking in the mid-1960s only after the cessation of atmospheric tests in 1963. Richard Miller has tracked the course of the radioactive cloud from each test to show their widespread geographic impact.[29]

Figure 2–12 shows the areas of the continental United States crossed by more than one nuclear cloud from above-ground explosions. Because of the speed with which the radioactive clouds were carried by the prevailing easterly winds and deposited by rain, many large cities, particularly in the Northeast, reported levels of radioactivity as high as those reported close to the test site. Miller offers the following examples of high levels of radioactive fallout from one test called *Upshot Knothole: Annie*, which exploded on

March 17, 1953. The next day the following cities reported over 100,000 units of radioactivity (measured in terms of disintegrations/minute/square foot/day): Knoxville, Tennessee; Fort Worth/Dallas, Texas; New York, New York; Memphis, Tennessee; Philadelphia, Pennsylvania; Nashville, Tennessee; Texarkana, Arkansas; and Washington, D.C.

We shall show that we can find many geographic clusters of counties with high breast cancer rates today that may reflect the harmful effects of both bomb test emissions and emissions from the military reactors that produced the weapons that were tested in the past.

In figure 2–13 we contrast the annual movement of U.S. low-birthweight live births since 1968, when, in the absence of emissions from above-ground tests, the low-birthweight percentage began to improve sharply. But as civilian power reactors began to operate in increasing numbers in the 1970s and major reactor accidents such as Three Mile Island and Chernobyl released fission products into the environment, the U.S. low-birthweight percentage began an omi-

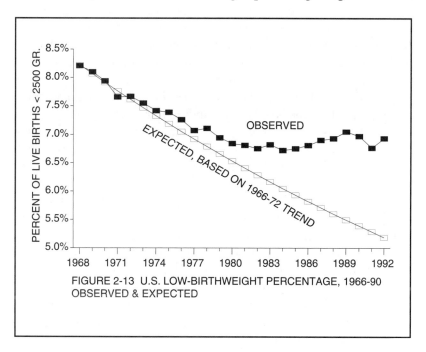

FIGURE 2-13 U.S. LOW-BIRTHWEIGHT PERCENTAGE, 1966-90
OBSERVED & EXPECTED

nous upward divergence from the declining trend established between 1966 and 1972.

RECENT DETERIORATION IN THE QUALITY OF NEWBORN HEALTH

A story on the front page of the June 9, 1995, issue of the *New York Times* stated that "The New York State Health Department has found an unexpectedly high number of deaths among newborns in some of the city's busiest public and private hospitals." No reason was advanced, and the story did not reveal that the observed deterioration among the newborn can be traced back to 1979, the year of the TMI accident, when the percentage of underweight live births, both locally and nationally, began to rise—as it did in the early years of the Nuclear Age.

The rise of the low-birthweight percentage of live births from 1945 to 1965, its subsequent decline until the early 1970s, and its resurgence after 1979 can only be explained in terms of successive waves of ingested fission products—first from bomb-test fallout and then from civilian power reactors. Since we have ascertained that there is a close connection between an increase in low-level radiation and its immediate impact on the immune response affecting both the health of the newborn and the increase in breast cancer incidence, we shall review an alarming set of indicators that suggest ongoing deterioration exists in the health and viability of the newborn.

For the past two decades, the deterioration of the health and viability of the American newborn has been expressed by several sensitive indicators that point to the causal role of low-level radiation associated with increasing emissions from civilian power reactors.

Note that in figure 2–13 we depict the decline in the U.S. low-birthweight percentage in the late 1960s, which diverged upward in the mid-1970s. This increase can be explained. The NRC reported peak-level radioactive iodine and strontium releases in 1974–75 from the Millstone reactors (13 curies), in 1979 from Three Mile Island (14 curies), and in 1985–86 from Indian Point. In addition, in 1985 there were huge but unknown amounts of fission products released from a flawed Star Wars test in Nevada, and in 1986 radiation from Chernobyl arrived in the United States.

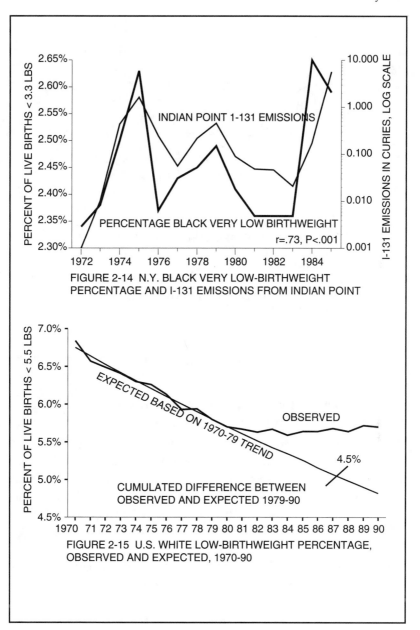

FIGURE 2-14 N.Y. BLACK VERY LOW-BIRTHWEIGHT
PERCENTAGE AND I-131 EMISSIONS FROM INDIAN POINT

FIGURE 2-15 U.S. WHITE LOW-BIRTHWEIGHT PERCENTAGE,
OBSERVED AND EXPECTED, 1970-90

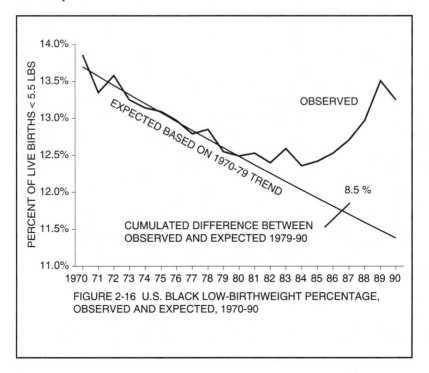

FIGURE 2-16 U.S. BLACK LOW-BIRTHWEIGHT PERCENTAGE,
OBSERVED AND EXPECTED, 1970-90

BLACK NEWBORNS EXPERIENCE GREATER SENSITIVITY TO LOW-LEVEL RADIATION

We can trace the impact of the aforementioned releases on the health of the newborn in both the late 1970s and late 1980s. One of the most sensitive indicators is shown in figure 2–14, in which we see that (allowing for a lag of one year) after each peak release from Indian Point a rise in the percentage of Black live births weighing less than 1,500 grams (3.3 pounds) followed. New medical technology can keep such low-birthweight babies alive but at great cost. Poor nutrition and lack of prenatal care, much more common among Blacks than whites, exacerbates the impact of low-level radiation on Black birthweights.

Even for whites, low-level radiation causes low birthweights. In figure 2–15 the white low-birthweight percentage is seen to diverge upward from the preceding declining trend after the TMI accident of 1979, as measured by the cumulated difference after 1979 between the observed and expected low-birthweight percentages. That cumulated difference for whites is seen to be 4.5 percent.

For Blacks, the upward divergence after 1979 is twice as great, 8.5 percent as measured by the cumulated difference between the observed and expected low-birthweight percentages, as shown in figure 2–16.

Another way to demonstrate that Blacks are more sensitive to low-level radiation is to take note of the fact—reported in *US Vital Statistics*—that for the United States as a whole, the white low-birthweight percentage (*i.e.*, those weighing less than 1,500 grams) remained constant at 1 percent from 1979 to 1988, while for Blacks that percentage rose by 29 percent from 2.5 to 3.2.

In figures 2–17 and 2–18, we show that the upward divergence in the low-birthweight percentage after 1979 was three times greater for Blacks in Pennsylvania where the Three Mile Island accident occurred than it was for whites. Thus for whites in Pennsylvania, the cumulated difference after 1979 was 4.7 percent, just a bit higher than for the United States as a whole. For Blacks, however, the cumulated difference was 14.6 percent.

In figure 2–19, we show that there was a greater upward divergence during the 1980s of the Black low-birthweight percentage in Westchester than in New York City. This may reflect the importance of proximity to Indian Point (close to the Croton water system), which reported large releases of radioactive iodine in 1985 and 1986. Even Long Island may have been affected by drifting radiation clouds from Indian Point.

OTHER MEASURES OF NEWBORN DETERIORATION

Concern about the declining quality of newborn health led public health officials to devise new measures to document more fully the drastic changes that occurred after 1979. Two such measures are the one- and five-minute APGAR scores and the newborn hypothyroid rate.

The APGAR score is a useful measure of newborn health and a predictor of the infant's chances of surviving the first year of life. It is a summary measure of the infant's condition based on heart rate, respiratory effort, muscle tone, reflex irritability, and color. Each of these factors is given a score of zero, one, or two; the sum of these five values is the APGAR score, which ranges from zero to ten.

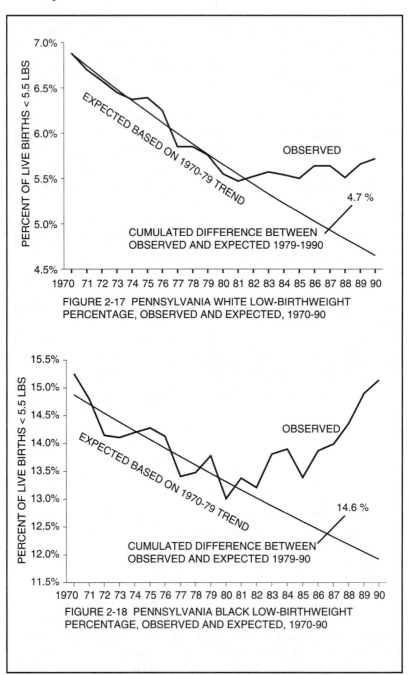

FIGURE 2-17 PENNSYLVANIA WHITE LOW-BIRTHWEIGHT
PERCENTAGE, OBSERVED AND EXPECTED, 1970-90

FIGURE 2-18 PENNSYLVANIA BLACK LOW-BIRTHWEIGHT
PERCENTAGE, OBSERVED AND EXPECTED, 1970-90

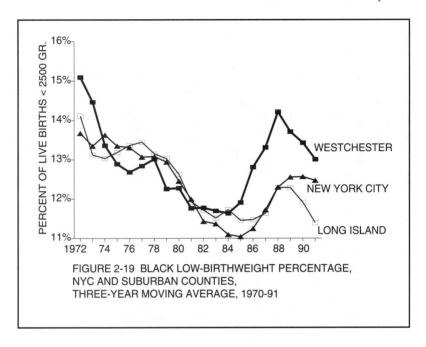

FIGURE 2-19 BLACK LOW-BIRTHWEIGHT PERCENTAGE,
NYC AND SUBURBAN COUNTIES,
THREE-YEAR MOVING AVERAGE, 1970-91

A score of 10 is optimum, and in 1978 when this measure was first reported for all newborn babies in the United States, 38 percent of white live births had a 5-minute optimum APGAR score of 10 and 62 percent did not. By 1992 the percentage failing to attain this optimum score had risen by 39 percent to 82.7. (See figure 2–20). In Pennsylvania the rise was even greater, in 1978 47.5 percent failed to receive an optimum score as compared to 82.7 percent in 1992—a 74 percent increase in the degree of deterioration since the Three Mile Island accident.

Figure 2–21 reveals an equivalent degree of deterioration in APGAR scores after 1979 for Black live births in the United States and Pennsylvania.

Hypothyroidism Among the Newborn

Figure 2–22 records perhaps the most alarming of the newly developed indicators of newborn health, which was first introduced for many states in 1981. For 15 states, accounting for 44 percent of the U.S. population, the number of hypothyroid live births rose from 356 cases in 1986 to 565 in 1992—nearly a 7 percent annual increase. As figure 2–22

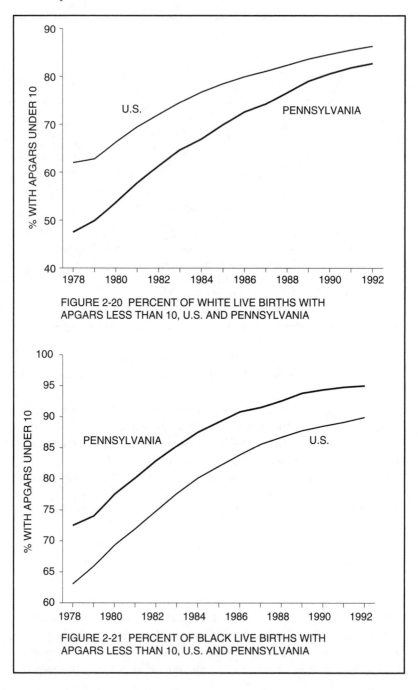

FIGURE 2-20 PERCENT OF WHITE LIVE BIRTHS WITH APGARS LESS THAN 10, U.S. AND PENNSYLVANIA

FIGURE 2-21 PERCENT OF BLACK LIVE BIRTHS WITH APGARS LESS THAN 10, U.S. AND PENNSYLVANIA

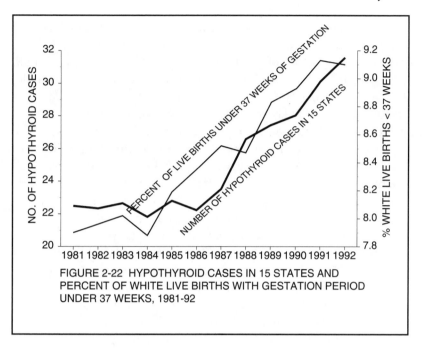

FIGURE 2-22 HYPOTHYROID CASES IN 15 STATES AND
PERCENT OF WHITE LIVE BIRTHS WITH GESTATION PERIOD
UNDER 37 WEEKS, 1981-92

indicates, this increase parallels the rise in premature births—another ominous indicator that the viability of our newborn is seriously at risk, despite the fact that infant mortality rates continue to decline slightly each year.

The connection between the most recent releases of radioactive iodine and strontium into the environment and the sharp rise in premature births and hypothyroidism together with the deterioration of APGAR scores that began in the early 1980s and accelerated greatly after 1985 is further supported by the following recent findings.

First, the incidence of thyroid cancer reported since 1935 in Connecticut rose significantly in the five years following the arrival of fallout from Chernobyl in 1986, paralleling the greater increased incidence in the former Soviet Union.[18]

Second, the incidence of hypothyroidism among newborns in the United States also rose significantly in the two years 1986 and 1987 as compared with the two previous years before the Chernobyl fallout arrived. Hypothyroidism among newborns indicates damage to the fetal thyroid from radioactive iodine (I–131) ingested by the mother.

In 31 states, those for which data was available, the incidence of hypothyroidism rose by a significant 8.4 percent in 1986 and 1987, as did the average levels of I–131 found by the EPA in pasteurized milk. Moreover, in the 5 western and northwestern states of Idaho, Colorado, Kansas, Oregon, and Washington, where in May 1986 the milk contained the highest average levels of radioactive contamination of 85.8 picocuries per liter, the hypothyroid rate increased 21 percent.

The rate declined significantly by 1 percent in the southeastern states of Alabama, Arkansas, Florida, Kentucky, Louisiana, Mississippi, South Carolina, Tennessee, and Virginia, where the average concentrations were less than 5 picocuries per liter, perhaps because of lower rainfall levels just after the Chernobyl radiation arrived.

The correlation between increases of hypothyroidism and I–131 milk readings in the United States after Chernobyl is further supported by the discovery of increased thyroid cancer incidence in Connecticut, Iowa, and Utah five years after arrival of the Chernobyl fallout.[19] Thyroid cancer, like hypothyroidism, can also be acerbated by I–131 concentrating in the thyroid gland.

These findings strongly support earlier findings that show rises in infant mortality correlation with increased levels of I–131 in milk during the summer months after this tragic disaster.[10]

The continuing rise in hypothyroidism and low birthweights after 1986 cannot, however, be associated with Chernobyl fallout alone. Throughout the 1980s the Environmental Protection Agency reported a general rise in the annual average concentration of I–131 in milk,[31] which raises many serious questions about its source, quite apart from Chernobyl.

MEASURING THE RADIOACTIVITY OF MILK SINCE THE BOMB-TEST YEARS

In the mid-1950s, when fallout from Soviet thermonuclear tests began to contaminate our milk and water, the U.S. Public Health Service established milk sampling stations in various cities in each state. Monthly measures of concentrations of radioactive iodine, strontium, and barium were performed for each milk sample at a former Atomic Energy Commission laboratory in Montgomery, Alabama, and published in a series of technical bulletins initially called *Radiation Data and Reports* and after 1975 *Environmental Radiation Data.*[31] Such monthly measures were published for about five dozen stations for nearly four decades, but publication ceased after 1990, with no adequate explanation.

Oddly enough, in 1982 there were some months in which many cities were reported to have large *negative* concentrations of radionuclides in milk, which can have no physical meaning.[11] It is possible to have slight negative readings because of statistical uncertainty in measuring milk with zero levels of radioactivity, but it is not possible for such uncertainty to reach levels greater than -5 picocuries per liter. In 1982, for example, there were large reported releases from a flawed Star Wars test in Nevada, which were followed by large negative barium–140 readings published for June, as high as -42 pCi/l for Nevada and similarly bizarre negative values for Arizona, Utah, California, Colorado, Oregon, Montana, Iowa, and Wyoming, which declined in magnitude with the distance of each station from the Nevada test site. The June measures of I–131 in milk showed a similar concentration of high negative values in each of the New England states. We speculated such high negative values in that month might be associated with two serious radiation releases from the Pilgrim reactor near Boston. These releases were the subject of an investigation conducted by Harvard epidemiologists about subsequent nearby increases in leukemia.[32] We noted:

> The existence of government documents that regularly publish radiation and mortality data would pose a considerable problem to any official who tried to keep such accidents secret.[11]

Radiation Data and Reports were established in 1957 by the Eisenhower administration as a "form of surveillance . . . of radioactivity of food milk and water." These reports proved to be very effective during the years of heavy fallout from thermonuclear tests, when as for example, I–131 readings as high as 990 pCi/l were detected in Salt Lake City in October 1957.

Such measures may have convinced both Presidents Eisenhower and Kennedy of the need for a ban on above-ground tests, although it is difficult to find any direct published evidence of this fact. The recently published memoirs of Anatoly Dobrynin, the Soviet ambassador who was in close touch with Robert Kennedy in the months before the test ban agreement was signed in 1963, quotes the latter as telling him that President Kennedy "had first and foremost a heartfelt desire to conclude a treaty banning all nuclear tests not for himself, but rather for the sake of his children and grandchildren."[33]

Reported increases in monthly radioactive milk readings in 1971 were useful in supporting Senator Glenn's announcement in October 1988 that there had been a previously undisclosed reactor-rod melt-down at the Savannah River nuclear weapons plant in that year, which was immediately followed by anomalous mortality increases in South Carolina.[11]

In 1974, the Nixon administration halted the publication of *Radiation Data and Reports*, citing budgetary limitations. It was replaced by an abbreviated EPA summary with limited circulation within the government and availability to the scientific community only by special request. Since concern about radioactivity in the environment waned with the signing of the atmospheric test ban treaty, there was little interest in the data.

MEANINGLESS NEGATIVE MILK RADIATION MEASURES

As a result, a small and apparently innocuous method of reporting radioactivity in pasteurized milk, which resulted in small negative readings, escaped attention. If a milk sample had little radioactivity, the practice of subtracting unavoidable background radioactivity from the total would occasionally produce a small and spurious negative value, solely as a measure of statistical uncertainty. Normally for such short-lived substances as iodine–131 and barium–140 this would be balanced by as many instances of equally small positive readings, which could be attributed to chance variation. Typically such positive and negative readings would average out to zero over a few months.

Our suspicions were aroused when we encountered incredibly high negative barium–140 measures in the month of June 1982: 57 out of 60 stations reported negative values. The odds that this could happen by chance are equivalent to tossing a coin 60 times and coming up with 57 tails.

When *Deadly Deceit* first became available early in 1990, we were queried by David Evans, a *Chicago Tribune* reporter who had previously written about our finding of increased U.S. mortality just after the arrival of Chernobyl radiation in a story printed May 27, 1988. He expressed interest in doing a story about the little-known EPA Montgomery laboratory responsible for the negative milk radiation measures. I sent him a copy of the data in question, including the following qualification contained in the EPA report:

> When reviewing the data in this report, caution should be exercised in the interpretation of individual negative numbers. Obviously a negative activity value does not have physical significance. Such numbers, however, are significant when taken together with other observations which indicate that the true value of a distribution is near zero. When an average of several measurements produces a result less than zero, this indicates a negative bias in the measurement procedure.

I stressed to Evans that this admission of bias raised several questions that should be answered. If a negative value really means zero, why not substitute zero to avoid the negative bias when an average value is sought for some section of the nation that may be experiencing the kind of exposure that occurred in May of 1986 when extremely high positive radioactivity readings were obtained?

Evans published his story ("Chernobyl Proved Low-Level Radiation May Be Dangerous") in the *Chicago Tribune* on May 4, 1990. He found that the Eastern Environmental Radiation Facility in Montgomery, Alabama, was led by Charles Porter, who had "spent his life monitoring the amount of radiation Americans are exposed to." Porter insisted that in more than three decades, there had never been a milk radiation reading high enough to cause him any worry. Not even the highest single measure of I–131, which peaked at 6,620 picocuries per quart in Seattle on May 12, 1986, worried him; the government safe standard was 15,000 picocuries per liter. He did not offer any source for such high standard, 15 times greater than the highest measure encountered in the peak bomb-test years. When Evans cited our finding of excess mortality in the United States just after Chernobyl, he offered the government safe standard as proof that we were wrong. He didn't offer any explanation for the high negative measures of radioactivity, which had been reported for the months of March and April 1990, just prior to publication of the interview.

Evans apparently was the first reporter to question the way the radioactivity of our milk was being monitored. He may have had some effect—no further negative average readings were published thereafter, and, indeed, no further monthly measures, positive or negative, were published after the December 1990 reading of 1.5 pCi/l for I–131, which was based on only 33 stations as compared to 55 stations for the January 1990 average reading of 4.3 pCi/l, the highest single average measure since the peak Chernobyl measures of May 1986. It is evident that if the laboratory sought to minimize the degree of radioactivity in milk, it could also do so by selecting the stations for which "detectable" levels could be found. But apparently after December 1990, the laboratory decided it could no longer find any detectable levels.

Figure 2–23 records the monthly movement of the average I–131 readings for all stations sending milk samples to the EPA laboratory with detectable levels since January 1983. The monthly averages were generally based on reports for between 50 and 55 stations, so that they can be assumed to be fairly representative of the entire nation. The monthly averages are mainly negative for the years 1981–84, for which we cannot offer explanation because they have no physical meaning. For the years 1985–90, the monthly average for all reporting stations jumped to 2.8 pCi/l with peak values well over 4 pCi/l reached in 1986, presumably because of Chernobyl radiation.

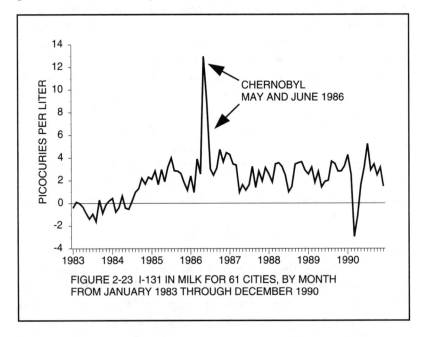

FIGURE 2-23 I-131 IN MILK FOR 61 CITIES, BY MONTH
FROM JANUARY 1983 THROUGH DECEMBER 1990

In addition to Chernobyl, reported increases in 1985 may have been connected with a series of underground tests in Nevada carried out in connection with the Star Wars program as well as leakage from aging nuclear power plants. Thus, I–131 levels in Denver, Colorado, east of the Nevada test site, rose from a daily average of 1 picocurie per liter in 1984 to 5 in 1990, while the milk measured in Hartford, Connecticut, close to several reactors, rose from a daily average of .1 picocuries per liter in 1984 to 4.6 in 1990.

While these measures may not disturb those who believe what the government regards as safe standards, a quick calculation can be made that would worry anybody else. In the course of 9 months during any of the years from 1985 to 1990, a pregnant woman drinking 1 liter of milk per day would have taken in more than 700 picocuries of I–131, an amount that is much larger than what would have been the total intake from the Chernobyl fallout, which persisted for only a few weeks in May 1986 because I–131 has a short half-life of only 8 days. So there must have been considerable amounts of I–131 present in the atmosphere since 1985 that have nothing to do with Chernobyl, but which, nevertheless, could contribute to significant increases in hypothyroidism and other conditions affecting the physical and mental development of the newborn. Yet releases of I–131 from reactors as reported in the 1980s by the Nuclear Regulatory Commission show no increase over the levels reported in the 1970s (see appendix C). Could there be another source of radioactive iodine that could account for the continuing deterioration of newborn health?

Corrosion in Aging Nuclear Reactors

One possible explanation for increased amounts of radioactive iodine in the atmosphere is that in the late 1980s there may have been unreported releases of extremely short-lived fission products due to increasing corrosion of steam generator tubes in pressurized water reactors. This could lead to growing leakage of radioactive water from the primary cooling system into the secondary loop, which contains the steam going to the turbines, which drive the electric generators of the plant. As a result, radioactive elements with half-lives of less than eight days could escape into the environment. Such releases are not regularly monitored and are not required to be reported on a regular basis since under ideal conditions no radioactivity reaches the steam in this type of reactor. The presence of such short-lived fission products cannot be measured by the EPA in milk or water.

This problem is so severe that by 1993, 14 utility companies that operate this type of reactor filed lawsuits against the manufacturer. One plant, the Trojan reactor near Portland, Oregon, was shut down, while four others have been allowed to continue to operate with leaks in their steam generators.[34] By 1994, 13 of the lawsuits were quietly settled without going to trial. The documents were sealed, thus keeping information regarding this serious problem from the public, despite the fact that sudden multiple ruptures of the corroded tubes could lead to a meltdown as serious as that of Chernobyl or Three Mile Island.

Such continuous small releases from nuclear reactors can be more serious than major single episodes, such as from the Chernobyl accident. In 1972 it was discovered that protracted and continuous exposures at low doses are more biologically harmful than short exposures to the same total dose. As will be discussed in greater detail in chapter 5, at these low doses the damage is caused primarily through the creation of so-called "free radicals," which is contrary to the case of high exposures as at Hiroshima or in the case of short medical X rays, where direct damage to the DNA in the cell is the dominant biological mechanism. Low daily exposures to short-lived radioactivity found in the milk are some five to ten times more damaging than the same small dose from a single episode such as the Chernobyl fallout and thousands of times more serious than the same doses from diagnostic use of X rays or from what would be expected from the studies of Hiroshima A-bomb survivors, on which present radiation standards are based.

Thus, the rise in the 1980s of measured amounts of I–131 and other fission products in the milk from underground tests and unmonitored reactor releases could, in the absence of plausible alternative scenarios, explain the rise in hypothyroidism, low birthweight, cancer, and other chronic diseases that rose sharply after 1985. This rise in turn drives up the cost of Medicare, Medicaid, and welfare, which has now produced an enormous fiscal crisis for the nation.

Despite this alarming evidence, beginning in 1991 the EPA stopped publishing the monthly radioactivity measurements in milk.

The public and Congress are therefore deprived of information essential for understanding one of the major causes of the current rise in cancer, low birthweights, and immune deficiency diseases. Nor do we now have independent means to detect radioactivity in our milk and water from another accident of the magnitude of Chernobyl, either from abroad or at home.

When asked why these measures are no longer being published, Charles M. Petko, who has replaced Charles Porter at the Montgomery radiation facility, explained that he was not aware of "any public interest" in such measures.

This is perhaps the most alarming single revelation in this book, which could not have been written if the nation's vital statistics had been similarly concealed. We have only to look at the collapse of the former Soviet Union to see the suicidal consequences of concealing current indicators of the state of public health.

Nuclear Corrosion in the Soviet Union

In 1980, Dr. Murray Feshbach, the foremost American authority on Soviet vital statistics, wrote a classic monograph for the U.S. Census Bureau entitled *Rising Infant Mortality in the USSR*.[35] In it he revealed that for several years the Soviets stopped reporting infant mortality rates to the United Nations. The mortality rates would have indicated an embarrassing rise that was in sharp contrast with the previous decline recorded after World War II. From 1950 to 1970, the Soviet infant mortality rate fell from 80 deaths per 1,000 live births to 23, the most rapid postwar improvement ever recorded for any nation.

Feshbach regards current official infant mortality rates as fictitious, for they exclude Belarus, Ukraine, and Kazakhstan. But it is clear that the rate of deterioration in Soviet infant mortality after 1970 may roughly match the speed of the postwar recovery.

Feshbach was unable to explain the sudden reversal of Soviet infant mortality rates after 1970 in his 1980 monograph, although in two subsequent publications—*Ecocide in the USSR*[36] and *Environmental and Health Atlas of Russia*,[37] he has detailed the extreme carelessness with which the Soviets exposed their people to the lethal effects of ionizing radiation from nuclear power reactors, as well as all other industrial pollutants. The atlas was prepared in Moscow by several dozen

Soviet scientists, who invited Feshbach to direct their efforts. In the foreword, Professor Aleksey Yablockov explained:

> If in the past we suffered from secrecy, in the 1990s our common poverty was the absence of reliable information as such. This occurred for a very simple reason that, with the demise of the Soviet Union, there was a destruction of the whole system of collecting information. There was created a strange and unnatural situation in which my friend Professor Murray Feshbach in Washington, from the stream of newspaper, radio and television could receive more information about us than we could even though we lived here.

The atlas does not cover the heavily stricken republics of the Ukraine and Belarus, but notes that in the Russian republic even as late as 1993 there were "200 violations of operational procedures at Russian reactors" and that "during the last 20 years, the number of newly detected cancer patients among urban dwellers increased 1.7 times," in sharp contrast with the far smaller 26 percent increase in Russia as a whole.

After a *New York Times* story of March 6, 1994, reported that according to Feshbach, Russian mortality rates had increased by 37 percent since 1986, I queried him about how far back such an anomalous trend could be tracked. He replied that from 1970 to 1993, the Russian crude mortality rate had risen by about 63 percent. Thus since 1970, and well before Chernobyl, Russian urban mortality rates had been rising in lockstep with a tenfold increase in the installed capacity of the Soviet civilian nuclear industry, from about 3,000 watts in 1967 to 33,000 watts in 1987.

In the wake of the Chernobyl disaster, we have learned that many Soviet reactors were deliberately placed near large urban centers to make use of centralized steam heating. Thus with the gradual but inevitable corrosion of the steam pipes we can speculate that Soviet urban dwellers were, without any warning, directly exposed at home to unmonitored fission products.

Corrosion may be an unanticipated problem in curtailing the operational lifetimes of all nuclear reactors and may some day be seen as one of the great technological blunders of the twentieth century—similar to the use of lead in the great aqueducts that played a role in inducing the decline of the Roman Empire.

Finally, we should take note that according to a March 25, 1995, story in the *Washington Post*, the rate of thyroid cancer in a region north of the Chernobyl nuclear plant was reported by the World Health Organization to be more than 100 times higher than normal. This was followed by a World Health Organization conference held in Geneva in late November 1995, where, according to a report in the December 15, 1995, issue of *Science*, an expert panel agreed that "the explosive increase in childhood thyroid cancer in Belarus, the Ukraine, and the Russian Federation—the countries most contaminated by the 1986 Chernobyl accident—can be directly linked to the released radiation, and most likely to contamination by radioactive iodine isotopes." It was estimated that "for very young children in the most heavily exposed areas," perhaps 10 percent could eventually contract the disease.

The most authoritative assessment of the significance of the Chernobyl accident has been made by Dr. Yuri M. Shcherbak, an epidemiologist newly appointed as Ukrainian ambassador to the United States. In an article entitled "Ten Years of the Chornobyl Era" published in the April 1996 issue of *Scientific American*, he described it as

> ... the worst technogenic environmental disaster in history.... Indeed it is now clear that the political repercussions from Chornobyl accelerated the collapse of the Soviet empire.... It is a global environmental event of a new kind. It is characterized by the presence of environmental refugees; long-term irreparable damage to ecosystems.... (It) illustrates the great responsibility that falls on the shoulders of scientific and other experts who give advice to politicians on technical matters ... and has taught the nations of the world a dreadful lesson about the necessity for preparedness if we are to rely on nuclear technology.... We have embarked on a new post-Chornobyl era, and we have yet to comprehend all the consequences.

Thus the serious current deterioration in the viability of our own newborn may be paralleling what has been occurring in the former Soviet Union for the past two decades, but greatly accelerated after Chernobyl.

Even though we have better access to the kind of crucial information that was withheld from the Soviet population, Americans are poorly informed about the lethal effects on the newborn of continuing waves of ionizing radiation from nuclear tests and power reactors. The current deterioration in the quality of life for the newborn may be repeating the pattern of the early years of the Nuclear Age.

In the next chapter we will trace the morbidity and mortality consequences of such traumatic exposures to ionizing radiation on those men and women born after 1945, when the Nuclear Age began.

Chapter 3

LOW BIRTHWEIGHTS AND BABY BOOMER IMMUNE DEFICIENCY

An important aspect of the current breast cancer epidemic in the United States is the fact that women are contracting the disease at increasingly earlier ages. In this chapter we shall show that women born after 1945 belong to a generation whose immune response may have been damaged at birth, as suggested by the rise in low birthweights from 1945 to 1965. (See figure 2–5.)

While the natality sections of the *U.S. Annual Vital Statistics* volumes have carried the birthweight data on white and nonwhite live births in each state since 1950, it is only in recent years that the percentage of live births weighing under 2,500 grams (*i.e.*, 5.5 pounds) has been published for each state. Therefore many epidemiological and socioeconomic anomalies affecting the baby boom generation have been concealed for many years. In this chapter we will examine some of the most puzzling delayed manifestations of exposure to low-level radiation by the generation of baby boomers, who were born in the worst possible period in our history—subject to fallout equivalent to exploding 40,000 Hiroshima bombs, according to estimates made by the Natural Resources Defense Council.[30]

Delayed Consequences of Bomb-Test Fallout: 1963-1980

Children born in 1945 reached the age of 18 in 1963, the first year that baby boomers aspiring to go to college began taking SAT exams. This is also the first year of a sudden and unexpected decline of SAT scores that lasted for almost two decades as depicted in figure 3–1. We have added the birth years of those taking the SAT verbal exams from 1952 to 1995, above the mean score recorded by the College Board to show that the decline affected those children born during the bomb-test years 1945 to 1963.

In 1979, Sternglass, who was then professor of Radiology at the University of Pittsburgh Medical School, was the first to predict that the SAT scores would turn up in the 1980s, because the exams would be taken by children born after the cessation of U.S./U.S.S.R. above-ground bomb tests in 1963.

The recently published book, *The Bell Curve*, uses what it calls the "great decline" observed in verbal and mathematical SAT scores from 1963 to 1980 to argue that the genetic inferiority of Blacks is at the heart of our educational problems.[38] Adding the birth years to each annual SAT score in figure 3–1 shows this to be nonsense.

The reason that the SAT scores were highest in the 1950s, declined after 1963, and recovered somewhat after 1980, but never quite reached the previous peaks, can be found by asking when the test takers were

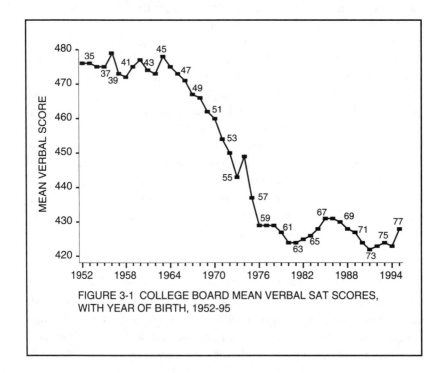

FIGURE 3-1 COLLEGE BOARD MEAN VERBAL SAT SCORES, WITH YEAR OF BIRTH, 1952-95

born and by taking a close look at figure 2–5, which records the rise and fall of the percentage of low-birthweight live births after 1945.

The decline in SAT scores for nearly 2 decades after 1963 merely replicated in inverse fashion the rise in the low-birthweight percentage associated with above-ground bomb tests occurring 18 years earlier, from 1945 to 1963. The nuclear assault on fetal hormonal and immune systems that occurred in those years resulted in physical, mental, and psychological problems that have since continued to plague many of the 75 million baby boomers.

A 1994 U.S. Department of Education Assessment of Educational Progress shows comparable declines in reading, mathematics, and science performances for children born from the 1950s to about 1964, and a slight increase thereafter. Unlike the SAT scores, these exams represent a sample of all 9, 13, and 17 year-olds in the United States.

The authors of *The Bell Curve* assign a different meaning to the "great decline" in SAT scores that began in 1963. They ignore the fact established by Sternglass that each large annual drop in SAT scores appeared to be correlated with large superpower bomb tests that took place 18 years earlier, which allowed him to predict that the SAT scores would improve in the 1980s.[39]

We see the mysterious "great decline" as the result of stunted cognitive development for many children, white and Black, born in the stressful atmospheric bomb-test years. The authors of *The Bell Curve* attribute the falling SAT scores between 1963 and 1980 to inferior education of the disadvantaged and the increasing "democratization" of the pool of test takers. They admit that "throughout most of the white SAT score decline, the white SAT pool was shrinking, not expanding. . . ." They conclude that "rather than democratization, the decline was more probably due to leveling down, or mediocritization: a downward trend of the educational skills of America's most promising youngsters."[33]

Not only is this an inadequate explanation of the reasons for the changing "intelligence and class structure in American life" that the authors are presumably investigating, but it also completely contravenes the authors' argument that the decline in intelligence reflects genetic inferiorities of Blacks. The major observed deterioration of intelligence mainly affected whites aspiring to enter college. And they, of course, cannot explain why the SAT decline stopped after 1980.

Delayed Consequences of Fallout: 1960–1990

There are other socioeconomic anomalies involving baby boomers that have never before been satisfactorily explained. For example, in 1960, when males born after 1945 began to reach the ages of 15 to 24, their mortality rates from acts of violence (accidents, homicide, suicide, and drug abuse) began to rise steadily. These rates reached an all-time peak in 1980 for males born between 1955 and 1964, when above-ground bomb tests had peaked, as shown in figure 3–2.

Thus the same trauma at birth (resulting from exposure to fission products) responsible for impaired cognition and lower SAT scores at the age of 18 also appears to have resulted in peak levels of violent deaths for young male baby boomers when they entered the age group 15 to 24. By 1990, males aged 15 to 24 were born between 1965 and 1974, when above-ground tests had ceased—and their mortality rates came down from the 1980 peak.

These figures support a similar finding by the sociologist Dr. R. M. Pellegrini, who studied an FBI database of *Uniform Crime Reports* and discovered that rates of criminal homicide, forcible rape, and aggravated assault doubled in the 1970s, as compared with previous

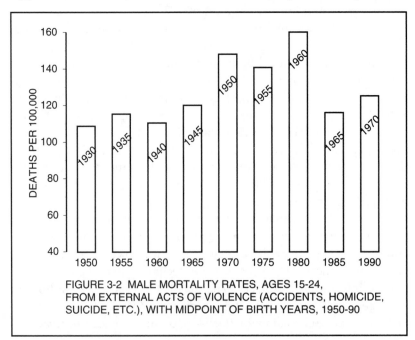

FIGURE 3-2 MALE MORTALITY RATES, AGES 15-24, FROM EXTERNAL ACTS OF VIOLENCE (ACCIDENTS, HOMICIDE, SUICIDE, ETC.), WITH MIDPOINT OF BIRTH YEARS, 1950-90

decades, just as the baby boomers turned ages 15 to 24. Crime rates for those born between 1945 and 1965 are now at all time peak levels, a fact Pellegrini attributes to their exposure to fallout radiation at birth.[40]

Another significant year for socioeconomic anomalies for young male baby boomers was 1970, which marked the start of a 2-decade period in which the increase in the number of males who dropped out of the labor force increased, paralleling the 2-decade increase in low birthweights 25 years earlier.

Figure 3–3 demonstrates that after 1970 there was a steady increase in the number of male baby boomers aged 25 to 44 classified as "not seeking work." The labor force includes those in the armed forces, plus those who are employed or are unemployed but "seeking work." Generally men—if not in school—will be ready to enter the labor force by the time they reach the age of 25. If they are not seeking work by that age, one could presume they are in school, in prison, engaged in crime, or are too sick (or for other reasons unable) to be socially productive.

For each year since 1970, we have included in figure 3–3 the midpoint of the birth years of the 25–44 age cohort to indicate the annual change in the baby boomer composition of men not seeking work.

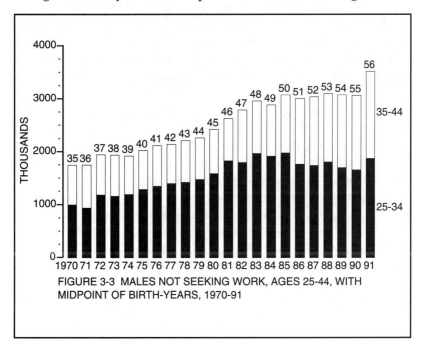

FIGURE 3-3 MALES NOT SEEKING WORK, AGES 25-44, WITH MIDPOINT OF BIRTH-YEARS, 1970-91

In 1970, the 25–44 age-group included those born between 1925 and 1945, with 1935 as the midpoint year of birth. Therefore the 1.6 million labor force dropouts in 1970 can be considered to have been born mainly in prenuclear years. The number of dropouts increases each year so that by 1991, when the age-group 25–44 included men born between 1946 and 1966—almost all baby boomers—the number of dropouts doubled to 3.5 million.[41]

DELAYED CONSEQUENCES OF FALLOUT AFTER 1980

There is also evidence that the health of members of the age-group 25–44 began to decline in the 1970s, as this cohort increasingly included baby boomers. In 1990, the Atlanta Center for Disease Control (CDC) published an article confirming a statement made in *Deadly Deceit* that after 1983 the age-groups 25–34 and 35–44 were increasingly dying of AIDS.[11] [42]

The CDC contrasted the decline in mortality rates for men aged 25–44 in the 1970s with the abrupt upturn in the 1980s and found that the excess in the 1980s nearly equaled the number of AIDS deaths. The CDC article referred to males only, but we have included females in figure 3–4 for they show a similar anomalous mortality increase in the 1980s from disease. Figure 3–4 illustrates the CDC methodology, but instead of using mortality rates for men and women aged 25–44, we use the percentage share of all deaths accounted for by this age-group to emphasize the anomalous nature of the 1980s upturn.

Again, we indicate for each cohort beginning with 1970 the midpoint of the year of birth to show that after 1976 the previous decline began to flatten out as more and more baby boomers were included each year. Thus the sharp upward movement of this percentage after 1983 represents an extraordinarily anomalous increase, reversing a 75-year-long improvement in the capacity of this age-group to resist illness. In an aging population where the number of old people dying each year increases, the 25–44 age-group was so healthy that its share of all deaths steadily declined since 1900, when it accounted for nearly one-third of all deaths.

The increasing degree of immune deficiency that emerged in the early 1980s can be measured by noting that between 1983 and 1988 the U.S. percentage share of all deaths accounted for by those aged 25–44

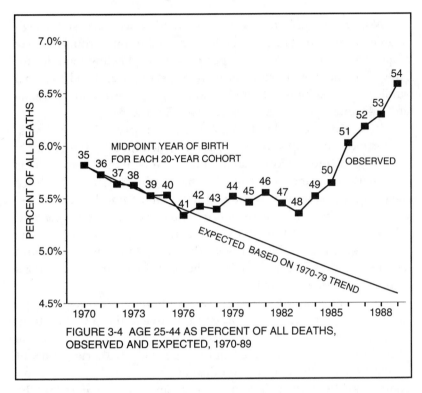

FIGURE 3-4 AGE 25-44 AS PERCENT OF ALL DEATHS,
OBSERVED AND EXPECTED, 1970-89

increased by 18 percent, from 5.35 in 1983 to 6.30 in 1988. We shall call this change an Anomalous Mortality Ratio (AMR).

Mortality breakdowns by age are universally available for all cities, counties, states, and even nations so that we can use the Anomalous Mortality Ratio (the 1988/1983 ratio of the 25–44 age-group's percentage share of all deaths) as a measure of varying degrees of immune deficiency in different areas that may have been exposed to different levels of nuclear fallout, both at birth and thereafter.

Thus in figure 3–5 we can plot the 1988 AMRs for each state against the AIDS mortality rate for that year for each state as calculated by the CDC.[43] The AMR is seen to be a better indicator of immune deficiency of young people than AIDS mortality; AIDS mortality rates can only go down to zero in states with the best performance whereas the AMR can fall below 1.00 in states where the immune response of young people has actually improved between 1983 and 1988, as in the case of Wyoming and Montana.

Note, for example, that even in Texas and Louisiana, despite a high degree of exposure to petrochemicals, mortality rates from AIDS are respectively 6.9 and 5.9 deaths per 100,000, well below the rates for New York and New Jersey, which are respectively 22.3 and 15.0. In a similar fashion, the AMRs are 1.09 and 1.07 for Texas and Louisiana and 1.43 and 1.44 for New York and New Jersey.

In figure 3–6 we plot the state AMRs against the 1984–88 breast cancer mortality rates for each state as calculated by the National Cancer Institute.[44] Note that as in figure 3–5 the correlation is extremely high and could not be the result of chance. All three measures are obviously dealing with the same underlying reality—damage to the immune response. Thus both breast cancer and AIDS are associated with exposure to ionizing radiation. The "best" states are in the relatively dry Mountain and West South Central regions, which have had the least exposure to emissions from civilian power reactors.

Since 1970, the Nuclear Regulatory Commission has kept annual records of the amount of airborne radioactive iodine and strontium emitted from each of the nation's civilian power reactors. For the years 1970–87, such cumulated emissions totaled 370 curies, or about 1.6 curies per million persons for the nation as a whole.[45] There is an enormous difference in the degree of exposure in different parts of the nation.

Civilian reactors are concentrated in the Northeast and Southeast, which have heavy rainfall, as compared with of the relatively dry Mountain and West South Central regions. In figures 3–7 and 3–8 we find in all nine census regions a significant degree of correlation between the AMRs and the age-adjusted breast cancer mortality rates to the varying degrees of regional *per capita* exposure to cumulated *per capita* levels of emissions of radioactive iodine and strontium from 1970 to 1987.[11] [10]

Thus, in regions with high *per capita* exposures to radioactive iodine and strontium, we find high AMRs and high age-adjusted breast cancer mortality rates. In regions with very low exposures to *per capita* reactor emissions of radioactive iodine and strontium, we find very low AMRs and breast cancer mortality rates.

In figure 3–9 we replicate figure 3–8, using a linear rather than a log scale to measure the *per capita* exposure to radioactive fission products

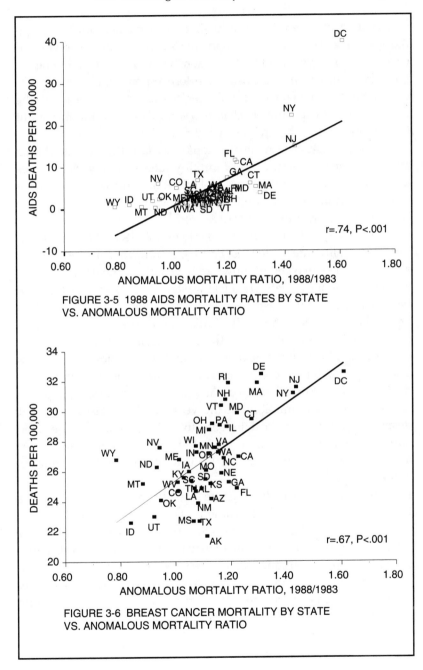

FIGURE 3-5 1988 AIDS MORTALITY RATES BY STATE
VS. ANOMALOUS MORTALITY RATIO

FIGURE 3-6 BREAST CANCER MORTALITY BY STATE
VS. ANOMALOUS MORTALITY RATIO

for each region. Here we see for the first time the logarithmic nature of the dose response to radiation, taking the form of a concave downward curve. As we move from the dry regions with low exposure to heavy rainfall regions with high exposure, the dose response rises most rapidly, then flattens out when we reach the regions of the Northeast with the largest *per capita* exposure. (In chapter 5 we will examine this important logarithmic relationship in much greater detail.)

We can conclude from the previous five charts that both the AMRs and age-adjusted breast cancer mortality rates among various states and regions reflect varying degrees of radiation-induced immune deficiency, from initial exposure at birth, which is then exacerbated by ongoing emissions from nuclear reactors.

Surprisingly, the region with the lowest AMR and lowest breast cancer mortality rate is the West South Central, which includes Texas and Louisiana—two states known to have among the nation's greatest concentrations of petrochemical waste, which are correlated with high male cancer rates.[6] For these states and their major metropolitan areas, the Anomalous Mortality Ratios are also surprisingly low—close to 1.08, significantly below the U.S. average of 1.18.

We shall learn in the next chapter that these states and counties also have age-adjusted breast cancer rates that are significantly below the U.S. average. Since these two states have not been directly exposed to civilian reactor emissions in the years studied, it suggests that despite the occupational carcinogens to which men are exposed, the absence of fission products in the diet represents an offsetting factor at least for women, who are not as likely to be exposed to carcinogens at the workplace.

In the 1980s, when baby boomers reached the age of 35, their cancer incidence rates also rose. According to the National Cancer Institute, cancer incidence rates for the 35–44 age-group registered a 14 percent increase from 1979 to 1988—greater than the increase for any other age-group. Also the breast cancer incidence rates for women under 50 rose by 18 percent in this period, reversing a decline in the previous decade. In the 1980s, women born after 1945 were in their forties and were now contracting breast cancer almost as rapidly as were older women.[39] (See figures 2–1 and 2–2.)

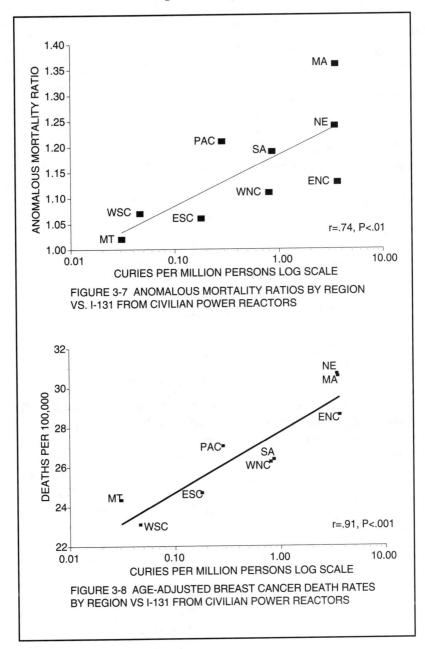

FIGURE 3-7 ANOMALOUS MORTALITY RATIOS BY REGION
VS. I-131 FROM CIVILIAN POWER REACTORS

FIGURE 3-8 AGE-ADJUSTED BREAST CANCER DEATH RATES
BY REGION VS I-131 FROM CIVILIAN POWER REACTORS

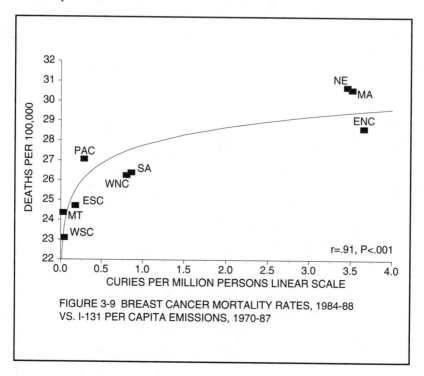

FIGURE 3-9 BREAST CANCER MORTALITY RATES, 1984-88
VS. I-131 PER CAPITA EMISSIONS, 1970-87

Baby Boomer Immune Deficiency and Productivity

Probably the greatest support for our hypothesis that the health and productivity of the baby boomer generation depends on the degree of exposure to man-made fission products comes from recent mortality data broken down by age carried for major nations in the annual *United Nations Demographic Yearbooks.* We show in table 3–1 the Anomalous Mortality Ratios calculated by dividing the 25–44 age-groups percentage share of all deaths for 1988 by the corresponding figure for 1983.[12]

In table 3–1 we have arrayed all reporting nations into three groups according to their presumed exposure to nuclear fallout. We define the major nuclear powers as those making and testing nuclear weapons, including the dangerous reprocessing of used fuel assemblies. We include the former Soviet Union in this group although we have not calculated its AMR. (They did not report an age breakdown of mortality to the United Nations for the year 1983.)

TABLE 3-1 ANOMALOUS MORTALITY RATIOS FOR NUCLEAR AND NONNUCLEAR NATIONS

Nations	Percent of All Deaths Age 25-44 1983	1988	Anomalous Mortality Ratio	
Nations Heavily Exposed to Nuclear Emissions				
Nations making and testing nuclear weapons, including reprocessing				
U.S.S.R.		7.43% (1989)		
U.S.	5.35%	6.30%	1.18	
France	4.25%	4.90%	1.15	
U.K.	2.42%	2.61%	1.08	
Nations not producing nuclear weapons, less heavily exposed				
Switzerland	3.70%	4.10%	1.11	
Hungary	5.65%	6.18%	1.09	
Bulgaria	4.22%	4.56% (1989)	1.09	
Norway	2.82%	3.12% (1989)	1.08	
Poland	5.97%	6.46%	1.08	
Czechoslovakia	4.21%	4.57%	1.08	
Finland	5.18%	5.60% (1987)	1.07	
Nations Least Exposed to Nuclear Emissions				
New Zealand	4.53%	4.88% (1989)	1.08	*
Australia	4.71%	5.02% (1989)	1.07	*
Denmark	3.80%	3.97%	1.04	*
Italy	3.00%	3.05%	1.02	
Cuba	7.88%	8.03%	1.02	*
Sweden	3.04%	3.05%	1.00	
Singapore	8.93%	8.95%	1.00	*
Netherlands	3.53%	3.53% (1989)	1.00	
Canada	5.30%	5.25%	0.99	
German Dem. Republic	3.40%	3.36% (1989)	0.99	
Austria	3.95%	3.62%	0.92	*
West Germany	3.55%	3.10%	0.87	
Japan	5.49%	4.90%	0.80	

* No civilian reactors

Russian mortality rates in 1993 were, however, reported to have increased by 37 percent since the Chernobyl accident of 1986.[46]

There can be no question that the former Soviet Union has suffered most from the lethal health effects of nuclear fallout. The Ukrainian physicist in charge of measuring Chernobyl's radiation, Dr. Vladimir Chernousenko—exiled for revealing the true magnitude of the accident—estimates that perhaps as many as 65 million persons throughout the former Soviet Union have eaten food contaminated by Chernobyl radiation, with a consequent shortening of life expectancy, resulting in about 1 million premature deaths by 1993,[47] a figure recently confirmed by a story in the *New York Times* of August 2, 1995, entitled "Plunging Life Expectancy Puzzles Russia."

Switzerland, Bulgaria, Norway, and Poland, included in the second group in table 3–1, have not produced or tested nuclear weapons but are located close to nations that do. The great surprise in table 3–1 is that there is no mortality deterioration of young people evident for either Germany or Japan.

From the published data on baby boomer mortality in 1983 and 1988 for the major nations we can calculate that the combined AMR for the United States, France, and the United Kingdom is 1.18, which is 40 percent above the combined AMR of .84 for Japan and Germany.

If we take the age-group 25–44 to represent the most productive group of the labor force, then the comparison of the combined AMRs suggests that Japan and Germany now enjoy a 40 percent advantage in productivity over the major nuclear powers. How can this anomaly be explained?

First, wind and rainfall patterns subjected the major nuclear powers to more of the massive atmospheric bomb-test fallout from the Nevada and Siberian test sites than was the case for Germany and Japan. An even more important irony is that these two nations, having lost World War II, were precluded from exposing their progeny to emissions from the manufacture and testing of nuclear weapons and can therefore be said to have won World War III!

Other factors are involved, having to do with the consumption of fresh milk, which if contaminated is the principal vector for the transmission of radioactive iodine to the fetus. Unfortunately in the United States, civilian reactors are often located in rural areas close to dairy farms supplying fresh milk to large cities. A notable example is the case of Washington, D.C. Washington's fresh milk comes from dairy farms in Lancaster County, Pennsylvania, which is close to the infamous Peach Bottom reactors. In April of 1987, the Nuclear Regulatory Commission temporarily closed the Peach Bottom reactors, accusing the operators of "sleeping on the job and taking drugs."

Three months later the infant mortality rate in the District of Columbia fell from an all-time high in April 1987 of 30 deaths per 1,000 live births to 10, reflecting the immediate beneficial effects of removing radioactive iodine from fresh milk.[11]

On the other hand, the Japanese (as well as other Asians) diet includes few dairy products. Even in California, where annual age breakdowns of mortality are available by ethnic origin, the percentage share of all Japanese American deaths accounted for by those aged 25–44 has been declining since 1983, in sharp contrast to a rise for other young Californians.[12]

The rising mortality rates for young people today accompany rising mortality rates of older people, which can also be associated with exposure to man-made fission products. This is revealed by figure 3–10, which traces the annual movements of crude mortality rates in the United States since 1900. There can be no better indicator of the nation's well being than the long-term trend of overall mortality rates, which mainly reflect the mortality of elderly people who account for the bulk of annual deaths.

In 1900 the crude mortality rate was 18 deaths per 1,000 persons, which by 1993 had been cut in half. This cannot be regarded as a good performance. A close examination of figure 3–10 shows that most of the improvement came in the first half of the century, when, by 1950, the mortality rate had fallen to 10 deaths per 1,000 persons.

Thereafter, in the peak bomb-test years of the 1950s, the rates flattened out. Had the prenuclear rate of decline continued to 1993 there would have been 16 million fewer premature deaths after 1950, and the rate in 1993 would have been 6 deaths per 1,000—equal to the current Japanese mortality rate. Note that the mortality rate has been slowly increasing since 1982, when it reached its lowest level of 8.5 deaths per 1,000. The rate in 1994 was 8.7 deaths per 1,000.

The special vulnerability of the elderly to fallout is indicated by figure 3–11, which traces the mortality rates of those over 85 since 1933. Note the upsurge during peak bomb-test years, similar to the upsurge in low birthweights shown in figure 2–5. Note, too, the fact that there has been no improvement in the mortality rates of the old since 1979. This is similar to the renewed rise in low birthweights since 1979 depicted in figure 2–13 and suggests that routine and accidental releases from civilian reactors have replaced bomb tests as the continuing and exacerbating source of harm to the human immune response.

That the immune response of old people was affected by bomb-test fallout, much like that of the newborn, is indicated by figure 3–12, which traces the extraordinary rise in mortality rates from septicemia among those over the age of 55. Septicemia, popularly known as blood poisoning, is mainly a disease of old age and signals the growing inability of the immune response of those over 55 to resist to disease. The twelvefold increase since 1950 depicted in figure 3–12 exceeds the growth rate of AIDS mortality in the 1980s as the fastest growing cause of death. Thus, we can regard the post-1950 increase in septicemia as the Acquired Immune Deficiency Syndrome of old people.

If we take a closer look at the annual movements of crude mortality rates since 1970, as in figure 3–13, we see that an extraordinary upturn occurred in the 1980s, in sharp contrast to the declining trend registered in the 1970s. An even closer look reveals anomalous upturns in 1972, after a fuel meltdown at one of the Savannah River nuclear weapons reactors, after the TMI accident of 1979, and after the 1986 Chernobyl accident, similar to the corresponding anomalous increases in low birthweights after 1979 shown in figure 2–13.

The same anomalous upturns occurred during those years in the airborne release of radioactive iodine and strontium from U.S. civilian power reactors, as shown in figure 3–14, which, of course, does not reflect the Chernobyl radiation reaching the United States in 1986. The releases from civilian power reactors must be assigned a causal role when considering the correlation with the anomalous changes in morbidity and mortality of both the young and old, as well as the increasing immune deficiency of baby boomers that began in the 1970s.

As shown in figure 3–15 the anomalous mortality increases after 1974, 1979, and 1986 are highly correlated with the increases in those years in annual U.S. medical expenses and, in turn, with the annual U.S. budget deficit. The exponential increase in health costs, now fast approaching the trillion dollar level, was not anticipated

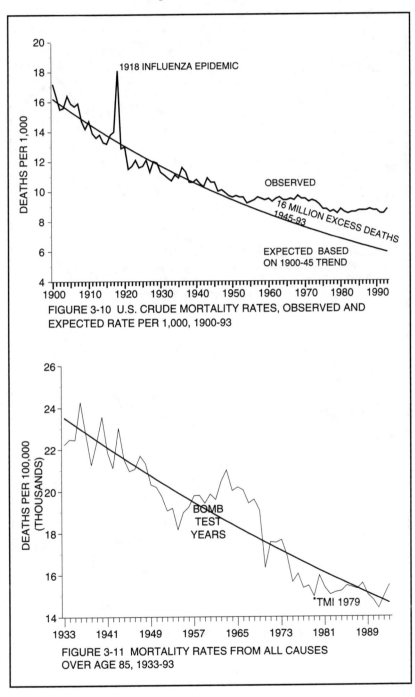

FIGURE 3-10 U.S. CRUDE MORTALITY RATES, OBSERVED AND
EXPECTED RATE PER 1,000, 1900-93

FIGURE 3-11 MORTALITY RATES FROM ALL CAUSES
OVER AGE 85, 1933-93

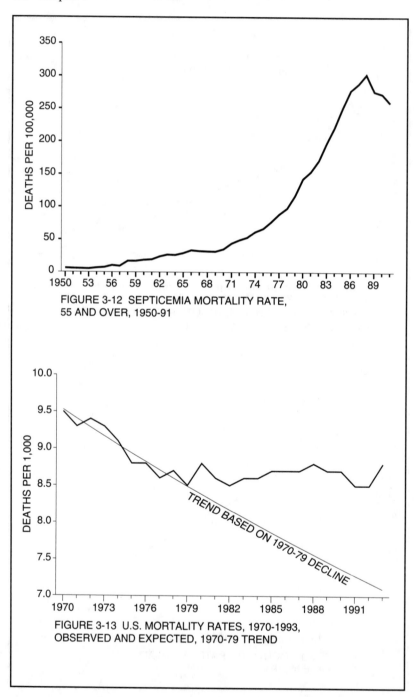

FIGURE 3-12 SEPTICEMIA MORTALITY RATE,
55 AND OVER, 1950-91

FIGURE 3-13 U.S. MORTALITY RATES, 1970-1993,
OBSERVED AND EXPECTED, 1970-79 TREND

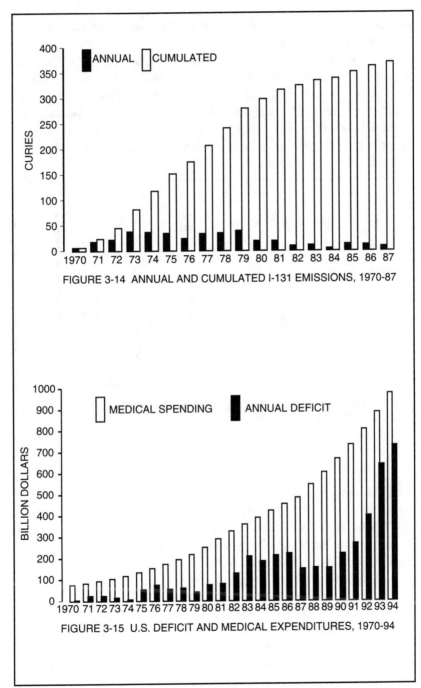

FIGURE 3-14 ANNUAL AND CUMULATED I-131 EMISSIONS, 1970-87

FIGURE 3-15 U.S. DEFICIT AND MEDICAL EXPENDITURES, 1970-94

and contributed greatly to the exponential rise of federal spending on Medicare and Medicaid.

As shown by figure 3–16, the exponential increase in all medical expenditures of about 10 percent each year was exacerbated by much higher increases immediately after 1974, 1979, and 1986. It is clear that another accident of the magnitude of TMI or Chernobyl would only compound current growth rates in illness and health costs and would contribute to the budget deficits at both state and federal levels.

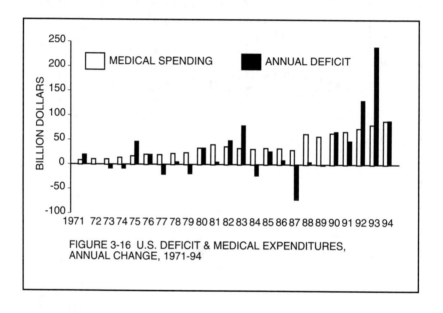

FIGURE 3-16 U.S. DEFICIT & MEDICAL EXPENDITURES, ANNUAL CHANGE, 1971-94

The temporal anomalies reviewed in this chapter concerning breast cancer and AIDS, along with the deterioration in the health of the newborn and the elderly show that there has been an overall decline in the health of all age-groups, which underlies our current health crisis. In the chapters to follow we shall focus on the combined impact of nuclear radiation interacting with all other environmental pollutants, which affects the food we eat and the air we breathe.

Thus the breast cancer epidemic must be seen as part of a general health crisis that cannot be explained without taking into consideration the great environmental changes produced by the Nuclear Age, which were kept from the public by the nuclear nations fighting the Cold War.

Chapter 4

BREAST CANCER MORTALITY AND EMISSIONS FROM NUCLEAR REACTORS

Joseph Mangano, an epidemiologist working with other members of the Radiation and Public Health Project, recently published a ground-breaking article demonstrating that since 1950 there were significant cancer mortality increases in the 94 counties surrounding the Oak Ridge, Tennessee, nuclear weapons plant.[14] In so doing, Mangano exposed some critical flaws in the methodology employed by the National Cancer Institute in their three-volume 1990 study of *Cancer in Populations Living Near Nuclear Facilities*,[9] which we will discuss in detail later.

How to Define Proximity to a Reactor

The Oak Ridge plant along with the Hanford plant in Washington State are the nation's two oldest nuclear facilities, both of which have been in operation since 1943. The plants have long histories of generating large amounts of radioactive gases and liquid and solid wastes. In its study of cancer near reactors, the National Cancer Institute decided to confine its Oak Ridge investigation to the two counties—Anderson and Rowe—in which the plant is located. Thus, they completely ignored the fact that the rural counties downwind of the plant to the north and northeast) are most directly exposed to emissions. NCI did find an above average increase in cancer mortality in these two counties since 1950, but there were too few cancer deaths involved in this limited definition of the exposed population for the increase to be statistically significant.

A change in mortality in any county cannot be considered significant if it can be shown to be the product of chance variation. Most of the 3,000-odd counties in the United States are small rural counties. Any single county would have to register an extremely high above average mortality increase to be judged statistically significant, simply because there would be too few deaths involved.

Knowing this, Mangano chose to look at the change from 1950–52 to 1987–89 in the aggregated age-adjusted cancer mortality rates (from all types of cancer) of 94 contiguous counties roughly within 100 miles of the Oak Ridge plant, an area that accounted for nearly 20,000 cancer deaths in the final period. The gain in the combined cancer mortality rates for all these counties proved to be 34 percent, as compared to a corresponding 5 percent increase for the United States as a whole. The probability that so great a divergence over a 37-year period could be the result of chance is less than 1 in 10,000 cases. Proximity to the plant must be a factor involved in this epidemiological anomaly.

Mangano also found significantly greater combined cancer mortality risk for counties located downwind (to the north and northeast of the plant) as compared to those located upwind (to the south and southwest). Additionally, he found that residents of the elevated Mountain counties with higher rainfall levels were at a greater than average risk as opposed to those in the lowland counties with less precipitation.

In the absence of a plausible alternative explanation, it is evident that some malevolent force of mortality has been emanating from the Oak Ridge reactors for a long enough time to have a much wider geographic impact than would be shown by merely the two counties chosen by NCI for study.

BREAST CANCER MORTALITY NEAR OAK RIDGE

We can best illustrate the significance of Mangano's finding by replicating his procedure with the aid of our age-adjusted county breast cancer database. (The main findings of this database are discussed in the next chapter. For our present discussion, it is sufficient to know that for the United States as a whole, the increase in age-adjusted white female breast cancer mortality is quite moderate—only 1 percent for the period from 1950–54 to 1985–89.)

In figure 4–1, we have mapped the counties within a 100-mile radius of Oak Ridge, each identified with the 5-digit state and county FIPS code, which accords with the alphabetical sequence of the county name. Excluding counties that were only partially in the 100-mile radius, we found there were 71 counties that were wholly within this arbitrarily defined circle. For these counties, we found, as did Mangano, that the combined age-adjusted breast cancer mortality rose by 29 percent compared with the corresponding national increase of 1 percent, and that for the large number of deaths involved (1,652 in 1985–89) so great a divergence could hardly occur by chance. We shall indicate the probability that any divergence could not be due to chance as $P < .001$, meaning the chance probability is less than 1 in 10,000 cases. We must therefore conclude that there is some malevolent force of mortality operating in the area around Oak Ridge, as is reflected in the significant increase in deaths from breast cancer.

Can we attribute this great divergence to Oak Ridge alone? Probably not. For one thing, there are five other reactor sites (Brunswick, McGuire, Hatch, Oconee, and Savannah River) in the states of North Carolina, South Carolina, and Georgia, which may be at least partly responsible. There may also be other sources of toxic discharge in the area that should also be investigated.

In order to focus on the role that emissions from Oak Ridge may have played. We will examine those counties closest to Oak Ridge that are most directly exposed to emissions because of the topographical characteristics that Mangano found to be important.

Following Mangano's suggestion, we have chosen 20 contiguous rural counties to the north and northeast of Oak Ridge. Because the aggregated breast cancer mortality rates here show an even more significant increase since 1950–54 than the 71 counties—a gain of 38 percent—there is an equally infinitesimal probability that the divergence from the national norm could be due to chance. The data for these 20 counties are shown in table 4–1, and the 20 counties are shaded in figure 4–1, which also displays the 71 counties, all of which are within 100 miles of Oak Ridge.

In table 4–1 we show for each identified county the age-adjusted white female breast cancer mortality rates in three five-year periods:

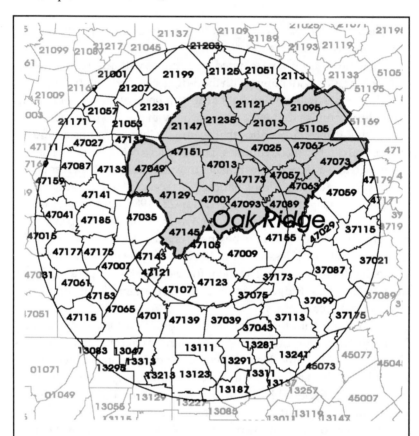

FIGURE 4-1 This map uses age-adjusted breast cancer mortality rates since 1950–54 in counties within 100 miles of Oak Ridge to illustrate the major points made by Joseph Mangano. The circles indicate counties falling within 50 and 100 miles of Oak Ridge. The shaded counties are those contiguous downwind counties closest to Oak Ridge whose combined age-adjusted rate is seen to have risen by 38 percent since 1950–54, as contrasted to the moderate 1 percent increase for the United States. The probability that so great a difference could be due to chance is less than 1 in 1 million cases (P<.0000001).

The 8 upwind counties within 50 miles of Oak Ridge have registered a decline of 4 percent since 1950–54, suggesting the importance of prevailing wind patterns in evaluating the impact of emissions from any one reactor. There are too few deaths in these small upwind rural counties for any upward or downward trend to achieve statistical significance.

For all 71 counties within 100 miles of Oak Ridge the overall 29 percent increase in breast cancer mortality is also highly significant. It is more difficult to pinpoint this increase to Oak Ridge alone. Many of these counties are also close to the Savannah River Plant and other nearby reactors.

TABLE 4-1 WHITE FEMALE BREAST CANCER MORTALITY
AGE-ADJUSTED RATES 1950-89
71 COUNTIES WITHIN 100 MILES OF OAK RIDGE
Deaths per 100,000 Women

FIPS Code	County	ST	Age-Adjusted Mortality Rates			Percent Change 80-84/ 50-54	85-89/ 50-54	Number of Deaths		
			1950-54	80-84	85-89			50-54	80-84	85-89
20 DOWNWIND COUNTIES WITHIN 50 MILES OF OAK RIDGE										
47001	ANDERSON	TN	18.7	21.6	23.9	16%	28%	17	50	58
47013	CAMPBELL	TN	14.6	28.8	20.4	97%	40%	9	35	29
47025	CLAIBORNE	TN	21.9	20.9	15.1	-5%	-31%	10	15	12
47049	FENTRESS	TN	4.1	23.2	6.4	458%	54%	1	10	4
47057	GRAINGER	TN	20.6	13.9	16.8	-33%	-18%	6	7	9
47063	HAMBLEN	TN	3.8	17.3	22.7	351%	492%	2	24	39
47067	HANCOCK	TN	22.3	7.3	44.4	-68%	99%	4	1	9
47073	HAWKINS	TN	20.6	22.0	21.7	7%	5%	13	30	30
47089	JEFFERSON	TN	15.7	21.5	25.3	36%	60%	7	23	28
47093	KNOX	TN	19.1	22.8	22.1	19%	16%	95	225	231
47129	MORGAN	TN	3.5	12.8	16.4	266%	368%	1	7	9
47145	ROANE	TN	21.6	16.9	16.5	-22%	-24%	14	27	30
47151	SCOTT	TN	10.7	15.1	12.2	40%	14%	3	7	7
47173	UNION	TN	10.7	13.1	28.2	22%	162%	2	5	11
21013	BELL	KY	5.1	23.1	21.5	350%	318%	4	24	22
21095	HARLAN	KY	11.0	15.8	22.1	43%	100%	11	21	28
21121	KNOX	KY	15.3	19.9	27.6	31%	81%	9	18	29
21147	MC CREARY	KY	3.5	17.7	23.3	405%	564%	1	7	10
21235	WHITLEY	KY	19.3	18.4	21.7	-5%	12%	13	21	25
51105	LEE	VA	6.3	24.2	18.5	284%	194%	4	20	18
TOTAL 20 COUNTIES			**15.5**	**20.8**	**21.4**	**34%**	**38%***	**226**	**577**	**638**
8 UPWIND COUNTIES WITHIN 50 MILES OF OAK RIDGE										
47009	BLOUNT	TN	25.4	16.9	20.0	-33%	-21%	25	44	56
47035	CUMBERLAND	TN	25.0	24.2	22.8	-3%	-9%	9	23	31
47105	LOUDON	TN	16.2	16.4	13.6	1%	-16%	8	16	15
47107	MC MINN	TN	18.0	18.8	20.2	4%	12%	13	28	30
47121	MEIGS	TN	18.6	17.9	13.4	-4%	-28%	2	4	3
47123	MONROE	TN	12.5	13.0	15.9	4%	27%	6	13	15
47143	RHEA	TN	11.4	14.4	18.0	27%	58%	4	10	15
47155	SEVIER	TN	16.8	19.7	15.5	17%	-8%	8	28	26
TOTAL 8 COUNTIES			**19.0**	**17.8**	**18.3**	**-6%**	**-4%**	**75**	**166**	**191**
TOTAL 28 COUNTIES			**16.3**	**20.1**	**20.6**	**23%**	**26%***	**301**	**743**	**829**
TOTAL 71 COUNTIES			**15.8**	**20.6**	**20.4**	**30%**	**29%***	**578**	**1522**	**1652**
CONTINENTAL US			**24.4**	**24.9**	**24.6**	**2%**	**1%**	**91392**	**167803**	**178868**

* P<.0001

1950–54, 1980–84, and 1985–89, along with the number of breast cancer deaths in each period and percent changes in the rates since
1950–54. The number of deaths is included because it is necessary for
testing the statistical significance of any given change. (A similar map
and table will be found in appendix B for each of the 60 reactor sites
examined in this book.) The information provided in this table will
generally be sufficient to make judgments as to which counties closest to the reactor site may represent a breast cancer problem area.

THE MEANING OF AGE-ADJUSTMENT

To appreciate the true meaning of these tables and maps we should first
probe more deeply into the purpose of using age-adjusted mortality
rates and how to judge whether a given increase in such rates can be
judged to be statistically significant.

An age-adjusted mortality rate for any county or group of counties reflects what the rate would be if the county or counties had the
same proportion of young and old people that the nation had in the
year 1950. This means that any difference in county age-adjusted rates
over time or from one county to another cannot be attributed to differences or changes in the age mix in the counties involved. This is necessary in any exploration of environmental effects, otherwise a county
with a large proportion of old people would display high cancer rates
due solely to its disproportionate number of old people. (We offer a
more detailed explanation of how we secure age-adjusted mortality
rates in appendix A.)

A detailed examination of each of the 71 counties within 100
miles of Oak Ridge would reveal an extremely wide range of variation in the percentage changes, from an overall increase of 314 percent for Carroll County, Tennessee, to a decline of 100 percent for
Sequatchie, Tennessee, both representing chance variation because
these counties are so small. There is no single county shown in figure
4–1 large enough, *i.e.*, with enough breast cancer deaths, for any single percentage change to be significant in a statistical sense.

This is why the National Cancer Institute's decision to limit its
investigation of the Oak Ridge cancer risk to the two counties in which
Oak Ridge is located was disingenuous. There is no way that any sta-

tistically significant change could emerge from so limited a definition of an exposed county.

As discussed in detail in appendix A, there is a way in which several contiguous counties can be combined into a single aggregate with enough deaths for its statistical significance to be tested—in effect by eliminating the essentially artificial boundaries of each county. For Oak Ridge, we have isolated 20 downwind counties as a significant breast cancer problem area. In appendix B we have treated 60 reactor sites in the same way.

The task of defining clusters of problem counties is greatly facilitated by our having a county database that permits us to secure age-adjusted mortality rates for any desired combination of counties and to determine the statistical significance of the observed change in rates.

For example, consider the eight counties in table 4–1, which are located to the south (upwind) of Oak Ridge. They are within 50 miles and display a 4 percent decline in mortality since 1950–54, in sharp contrast to the 38 percent increase shown for the 20 downwind counties north of Oak Ridge. While the 4 percent decline is not large enough to be judged statistically significant, it suggests that the risk of living near a reactor site is reinforced by topographical characteristics such as living downwind of the reactor site.

What we have done in the case of Oak Ridge and the other 59 reactor sites studied here is to begin with the "home" county or counties in which the reactor is located and add contiguous rural counties generally located to the north and northeast, in accordance with the prevailing pattern of wind. After reaching a distance of about 50 miles, we have usually accounted for a number of breast cancer deaths large enough so that the upward divergence of the aggregated breast cancer mortality trend from that of the United States can be shown to be statistically significant.

All in all, for 55 out of 60 reactor sites we have been able to define some 346 contiguous mainly rural counties that adjoin one or more reactor sites that have registered aggregated increases in current breast cancer mortality rates significantly higher than the corresponding national increase. Our sole purpose here is to demonstrate the limitations of the NCI definition of proximity to nuclear reactors, which in almost all cases resulted in too small a number of deaths to achieve statistical significance.

The Concept of Statistical Significance

The concept of statistical significance plays so great a role in any inferences to be drawn from our database that we shall now consider how such tests of statistical significance are performed and what they really mean. The next few pages may be familiar to readers who have taken courses in statistics, but a basic understanding of the characteristics of the bell-shaped normal curve is essential for anyone wishing to understand the world we live in. (Some readers may want to supplement these pages with a statistics text; others may want to skip to the next chapter.)

First let us consider how we can evaluate the fact that the 20 counties downwind of Oak Ridge registered a 38 percent increase in the combined mortality rate since 1950–54, as compared to 1 percent increase registered by the United States.

What is crucial to any test of statistical significance is the number of deaths involved, which in this case is 638 in 1985–89 (obtained by adding the deaths in each of the 20 counties). Any divergence in the trend of a set of observed mortality rates from the national trend can be evaluated with respect to the probability that it could be due to chance by referring to the well-known bell-shaped normal curve. The normal curve describes the dispersion or expected variation around some central tendency produced in nature by chance.

For example, imagine that a group of marksmen are shooting at a target. After each shot, the shot's distance to the right or left of the target is measured and recorded. After hundreds of thousands of shots, a frequency distribution can be created by counting the number of shots that hit the target, how many fell within one inch to the left or right of the target, how many fell two inches to the left or right, etc. This distribution will show that the greatest number did hit the target, a somewhat smaller number fell one inch to the left, and a fairly equal number fell one inch to the right. An equal but smaller number will be found to fall two inches to the left and right of the target and so forth. In the long run, the shots to the left will be balanced by those to the right, yielding zero as the average distance from the target.

Rarely will any one shot fall several yards away from the target, representing, perhaps, when one of the marksmen was momentarily disturbed. It will be found that the dispersion of all shots from the target is measured by the standard deviation, in which within one standard deviation on either side of the target will be found about two-thirds of all shots, and within two standard deviations 95 percent of all shots will be found. Any result falling more than two standard deviations away from the target is usually regarded by statisticians as statistically improbable and could not be the result of a normal degree of chance variation. A result falling three standard deviations to the right of the zero value will occur less than one time in one thousand cases.

We can now engage in a thought experiment. First, we keep drawing samples of counties with a total of about 638 breast cancer deaths in 1985–89 and note their rate as O (for observed), then we calculate the difference from the expected rate, which we shall call E. For groups of counties drawn at random with about 638 breast cancer deaths, for each time we observed the rate O and calculated its percentage increase from 1950–54, we would expect in the long run to find that on average the samples drawn would reflect the 1 percent increase in breast cancer mortality that characterizes all counties in the United States. It may require many such drawings for this average to emerge, but in a thought experiment there is no limit to the number of times we can draw a sample.

What would be the expected rate for 1985–89 for each sample? It would be the 1950–54 rate multiplied by 1 percent, which is the overall national increase. If for each sample we record the difference between the samples O and E (imagine we do this thousands of times), we could make a frequency distribution of the differences, which would resemble the bell-shaped normal curve for the distribution of the marksmen. The average of all differences would be zero, but on either side of the zero there would be positive and negative differences grouped around the mean value in the same way that we found most of the marksmen's efforts grouped around the target. How do we calculate the standard deviation of the distribution of sample differences?

If we can do this, then we can calculate the probability that any single sample result could be due to chance. If, for example, the marksmen's shots fell too far to the right or left of the zero value (equivalent to three or more standard deviations), we can say that the shots cannot be regarded as a chance result and that some positive or negative bias has affected that particular sample.

So the question to be answered for the 20 counties downwind of Oak Ridge is as follows: How often can we expect to find a sample of this size that shows a rate increase that differs from the expected 1 percent increase as great as 38 percent?

The expected rate (E) would be (15.5)(1.01) = 15.7, which is obtained by multiplying the observed 1950–54 rate by the 1 percent national increase from 1950–54 to 1985–89. Thus the difference (O-E) that we want to test is the difference between the observed value in 1985–89, which is 21.4, and the expected value of 15.7, which is 5.7 deaths per 100,000. Is this difference too large to be due to chance?

As in the case of the marksmen, we can conceive that by recording the O-E difference for each sample drawn we can create a bell-shaped normal distribution for which in the long run the average O-E difference would be zero, since in the long run all samples of this size should show a 1 percent increase. How many standard deviations would be represented by a difference as large as 5.7 in such a normal distribution?

Fortunately, there is a simple formula that yields the standard deviation of the normal curve describing the frequency distribution of all such sample differences:

$$\text{SQUARE ROOT } ((O^2 + E^2)/N)$$

where O is the observed sample mortality rate, E is the expected mortality rate and N is the number of deaths in the sample. Substituting these values in the formula yields a standard deviation of 1.05, and the difference 5.7 when divided by 1.05 equals 5.4 standard deviations. Is this a statistically probable result?

Here are the probabilities that statisticians have calculated for observations that fall too far to one side of the mean value of a normal distribution:

2 standard deviations, P is less than 1 out of 100

3 "   "   "   1,000

4 "   "   "   10,000

5 "   "   "   1,000,000

Clearly, the probability of finding by chance a cluster of counties as large as the 20 downwind Oak Ridge counties that registered an increase in breast cancer rates of 38 percent is less than 1 in 1 million cases. We must conclude that these 20 counties as a group have been exposed to some malignant force of mortality that strongly supports our suspicion that wind-borne emissions from Oak Ridge are at fault.

What about the 8 upwind counties that registered a 4 percent decline in rates as against a national gain of 1 percent? Here O=18.3 and E=19.2, and the difference to be tested is -0.9. Applying the formula above tells us that this difference is associated with only -.5 standard deviations because of the small number of deaths involved (191 in 1985–89).

Thus we can say this sample is too small for any result to be regarded as statistically meaningful. In other words, the upwind counties may have been affected by the Oak Ridge emissions, but if so, such damage was much less than the damage sustained by the downwind counties. We shade the 20 downwind counties to indicate that they share topographical characteristics that appear to make their residents most vulnerable to the Oak Ridge emissions.

Thus we now have the means to test whether the change in age-adjusted breast cancer rates over time for any combination of counties is too great to be due to chance. If yes, we must try to find an environmental factor that may explain what must be regarded as an epidemiological anomaly.

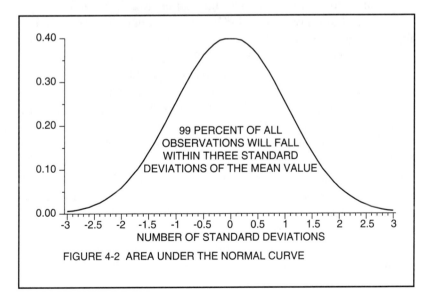

99 PERCENT OF ALL OBSERVATIONS WILL FALL WITHIN THREE STANDARD DEVIATIONS OF THE MEAN VALUE

NUMBER OF STANDARD DEVIATIONS

FIGURE 4-2 AREA UNDER THE NORMAL CURVE

In a later chapter we show the changes in breast cancer mortality in Kentucky and Virginia—both located downwind of Oak Ridge, with far greater mortality increases than Tennessee—suggest that the downwind effects of Oak Ridge emissions may extend considerably further than 50 or even 100 miles.

We have first centered our attention on the cluster of contiguous counties within 50 miles of the reactor site, in particular those that appear to share enough topographical characteristics to be most vulnerable to wind-borne emissions. We have not tried to find all such counties but to obtain a large enough sample to permit a statistically significant conclusion to be drawn concerning the connection between breast cancer mortality and the exacerbating effect of wind-borne emissions from nuclear reactors.

A NOTE ON THE HUMAN SIDE OF THE OAK RIDGE TRAGEDY

It is difficult for the statistics on the significant increase in cancer near Oak Ridge and other reactor sites to fully portray the human tragedies behind them. This was brought home to me when, on the occasion of the publication of Mangano's paper in July of 1994, I was invited, as director of the Radiation and Public Health Project that had sponsored his research, to address an Oak Ridge audience on its significance.

The invitation was extended by Dr. William Reid, a remarkable and courageous Oak Ridge oncologist who was the subject of an article in *Time* magazine (May 11, 1992) entitled "Living Happily Near a Nuclear Trash Heap." The article's subtitle was "The Frogs and the Trees Are Radioactive, You Can't Catch the Fish or Wade in the Streams, and a Doctor warns of Cancer Risks, but That Doesn't Ruffle the People of Oak Ridge."

Reid had been invited to join the staff of the Oak Ridge Methodist Medical Center in early 1991 and immediately found himself treating many patients with rare types of kidney cancer and unusual kinds of immune deficiency diseases, which appeared to be related to the huge concentrations of radioactive waste that had accumulated in Oak Ridge over the past 50 years. As soon as he reported these concerns to the Martin Marietta Co., which had assumed management of the Oak Ridge facility from Union Carbide in 1984, the

Oak Ridge Methodist Medical Center began a disciplinary process that eventually forced him off the staff.

According to the article, the public response to Reid's charges "was strangely muted. Residents long ago learned to live with radioactivity and risk. . . . The federal complex is still the largest employer of the population of 30,000." No health studies of women had ever been carried out, and so great was the "culture of secrecy and concern about job security" that the head of the Oak Ridge Atomic Trades and Labor Council was quoted as saying: "One thing that kept people from coming forward is that they were afraid they might jeopardize their security clearance by talking about something that was classified."

Reid's patients, most of whom appeared to be women, were appreciative of his efforts on their behalf, so much so that they formed an Oak Ridge Concerned Citizens Group. This group made up about half of the audience of about 100 that I addressed in the Oak Ridge Public Library—the other half was obviously suspicious and hostile.

Before speaking I was driven around the facility with a Geiger counter and could hear the clicking when we approached areas with withered trees and signs with the ominous warning "No Water Contact." I was told that if we left the main road that circles around the facility, alarms would go off and the car would be immediately subject to seizure.

I am sad to report that most of the men in the audience hotly disputed my presentation of the Oak Ridge breast cancer data, but I was greatly moved by the expressions of gratitude on the part of the women. Reid told me as I left for the airport, that the *Time* magazine article had resulted from the intercession of women involved in the filming of the Karen Silkwood story. Someday, perhaps, the history of Oak Ridge will be portrayed in a manner that would do justice to this truly heartbreaking American tragedy.

Chapter 5

GEOGRAPHIC DIFFERENCES IN BREAST CANCER MORTALITY SINCE 1950

A rmed with an understanding of what we mean by age-adjusted cancer mortality rates and how to test the significance of changes in mortality rates over time, we begin our analysis of the geographic changes in breast cancer mortality with table 5–1, in which we show the age-adjusted breast cancer mortality rates for the United States and for each state and census region for three different five-year time periods.

The first period, 1950–54, represents the baseline period for which the earliest age-adjusted data are available. The period 1980–84 corresponds to the latest five-year period used in the National Cancer Institute's study of cancer mortality near nuclear facilities. We use this period to compare our results with those obtained by the NCI. The 1985–89 period enables us to update the NCI study, although both studies make use of the same basic data. We have a vastly different interpretation of what the data means. We will let the reader evaluate the different interpretations, but we think it noteworthy that the NCI cancer study did not publish a tabulation of age-adjusted state cancer mortality rates for each time period, which we think should precede any analysis of changes in cancer mortality at the county level.

The reader's attention should be directed to several interesting facts about this tabulation of age-adjusted breast cancer mortality rates by states. The only similar table ever published by the NCI was one for age-adjusted breast cancer rates for the years 1984–88,[44] and in that

TABLE 5-1 AGE-ADJUSTED BREAST CANCER MORTALITY RATES, WHITE WOMEN, 48 STATES AND DC, 1950-89
Age-adjustment to 1950 Standard Population

State	Deaths per 100,000 Women			Percent Change			No. of Breast Cancer Deaths		
	1950-54	80-84	85-89	80-84/ 1950-54	85-89/ 80-84	85-89/ 1950-54	1950-54	80-84	85-89
Maine	24.5	24.6	24.1	0%	-2%	-2%	661	993	1040
New Hampshire	25.8	26.0	27.6	1%	6%	7%	437	820	948
Vermont	24.2	25.8	26.2	7%	2%	8%	270	441	480
Massachusetts	28.1	29.2	28.5	4%	-3%	1%	4238	6089	6164
Rhode Island	27.3	27.1	29.4	-1%	9%	8%	644	952	1081
Connecticut	28.0	27.3	26.6	-3%	-3%	-5%	1669	2937	3068
Total N. England	**27.4**	**27.8**	**27.5**	**1%**	**-1%**	**0%**	**7919**	**12232**	**12781**
New York	30.4	29.2	29.3	-4%	0%	-3%	12912	16292	16604
New Jersey	29.4	29.3	29.3	-0%	-0%	-0%	3999	7007	7446
Pennsylvania	25.1	26.5	26.5	5%	0%	5%	7005	10987	11522
Total Mid Atlantic	**28.5**	**28.3**	**28.3**	**-1%**	**0%**	**-0%**	**23916**	**34286**	**35572**
Ohio	25.0	26.8	26.4	7%	-1%	6%	5382	8724	9126
Indiana	22.7	24.7	24.2	9%	-2%	7%	2418	4093	4252
Illinois	26.6	26.8	26.2	1%	-2%	-2%	6320	8900	8981
Michigan	26.0	26.2	25.4	1%	-3%	-2%	3932	6492	6723
Wisconsin	26.9	25.7	24.3	-4%	-5%	-10%	2554	3991	4055
Total E. No. Central	**25.6**	**26.3**	**25.6**	**3%**	**-3%**	**0%**	**20606**	**32200**	**33137**
Minnesota	26.3	24.1	24.1	-8%	0%	-8%	2165	3236	3431
Iowa	24.2	23.0	22.3	-5%	-3%	-8%	1877	2452	2443
Missouri	23.3	23.8	23.0	2%	-3%	-1%	2666	3816	4022
North Dakota	23.0	24.3	21.4	5%	-12%	-7%	311	507	479
South Dakota	22.6	23.6	22.8	4%	-3%	1%	358	542	547
Nebraska	23.7	24.4	23.3	3%	-5%	-2%	894	1276	1295
Kansas	21.9	22.3	22.2	2%	-1%	1%	1188	1783	1862
Total W. No. Central	**23.9**	**23.6**	**23.0**	**-1%**	**-3%**	**-4%**	**9459**	**13612**	**14079**
Delaware	22.3	28.6	28.3	29%	-1%	27%	179	470	522
Maryland	26.4	26.9	26.3	2%	-2%	-0%	1397	2893	3086
District of Columbia	29.9	28.8	28.2	-4%	-2%	-6%	492	228	212
Virginia	19.7	24.0	24.5	22%	2%	24%	1205	3226	3675
West Virginia	18.6	22.1	21.9	19%	-1%	18%	764	1408	1468
North Carolina	17.7	22.1	23.3	25%	6%	32%	1158	3330	3982
South Carolina	18.4	22.7	22.2	24%	-2%	21%	518	1577	1751
Georgia	18.3	20.6	21.8	13%	6%	19%	1033	2599	3061
Florida	18.4	22.8	22.8	24%	0%	24%	1354	9070	10783
Total So. Atlantic	**20.1**	**23.1**	**23.3**	**15%**	**1%**	**16%**	**8100**	**24801**	**28540**
Kentucky	19.2	23.0	21.6	20%	-6%	12%	1268	2515	2507
Tennessee	18.1	20.8	21.1	15%	1%	17%	1186	2706	2998
Alabama	17.1	22.3	20.8	31%	-7%	22%	812	2167	2186
Mississippi	17.8	19.2	18.7	8%	-3%	5%	506	1074	1083
Total E. So. Central	**18.2**	**21.6**	**20.8**	**18%**	**-4%**	**14%**	**3772**	**8462**	**8774**

TABLE 5-1 CONTINUED
AGE-ADJUSTED BREAST CANCER MORTALITY RATES,
WHITE WOMEN, 48 STATES AND DC, 1950-89
Age-adjustment to 1950 Standard Population

State	Deaths per 100,000 Women			Percent Change			No. of Breast Cancer Deaths		
	1950-54	80-84	85-89	80-84/ 1950-54	85-89/ 80-84	85-89/ 1950-54	1950-54	80-84	85-89
Arkansas	15.4	19.1	19.5	24%	2%	27%	545	1288	1466
Louisiana	19.0	21.0	20.5	10%	-3%	7%	822	1927	2010
Oklahoma	17.8	21.9	21.7	23%	-1%	22%	954	2075	2086
Texas	18.0	20.1	20.0	12%	-0%	11%	2911	7536	8408
Total W. So. Central	**17.8**	**20.3**	**20.2**	**14%**	**-0%**	**14%**	**5232**	**12826**	**13970**
Montana	20.1	23.9	20.9	19%	-12%	4%	279	567	531
Idaho	18.9	22.3	18.9	18%	-15%	0%	243	585	571
Wyoming	20.1	21.3	19.9	6%	-7%	-1%	118	253	267
Colorado	23.9	21.8	21.5	-9%	-1%	-10%	849	1742	1929
New Mexico	16.3	22.7	21.3	39%	-6%	31%	192	766	845
Arizona	18.0	23.3	22.1	29%	-5%	23%	287	1972	2334
Utah	17.1	21.4	20.4	25%	-4%	19%	249	704	780
Nevada	20.7	24.1	23.8	16%	-1%	15%	73	521	655
Total Mountain	**20.1**	**22.6**	**21.4**	**13%**	**-5%**	**7%**	**2290**	**7110**	**7912**
Washington	23.8	24.2	24.6	2%	2%	3%	1489	2999	3411
Oregon	23.3	23.9	23.2	3%	-3%	-0%	956	2038	2151
California	25.5	26.1	25.9	2%	-1%	1%	7653	17237	18541
Total Pacific	**25.0**	**25.7**	**25.4**	**3%**	**-1%**	**2%**	**10098**	**22274**	**24103**
Total Above states	**24.4**	**24.9**	**24.6**	**2%**	**-1%**	**1%**	**91392**	**167803**	**178868**

tabulation the states were arranged in alphabetic sequence. When the states are arranged in geographic sequence, by region, as in table 5–1, many striking geographic patterns are immediately apparent, which point to the importance of environmental factors.

KEY GEOGRAPHIC DIFFERENCES IN BREAST CANCER MORTALITY

First note that both in the earlier and later periods the breast cancer mortality rates are significantly above the U.S. average of about 25 deaths per 100,000 in New England and the Middle Atlantic and East North Central regions—a fact that is obscured by an alphabetic arrangement by states. This geographic difference could not possibly be due to a difference in genetic factors and therefore is clearly environmental in origin. Note, too, that in the southern and Mountain regions, the mortality rates have been rising since 1950–54 far more rapidly than in the nation as a whole. One would think that with all the concern expressed about the origins of the breast cancer epidemic, these two geographic indicators of varying degrees of breast cancer risk would be of sufficient interest to warrant exploration by the NCI. In table 5–1 we have the first important glimpse of what we can learn from an objective epidemiological investigation of the geographic characteristics of breast cancer mortality in the United States.

At first glance of table 5–1, the great geographic variation in breast cancer mortality trends over time is puzzling. The three northeast regions with the highest breast cancer mortality rates show very little change over time, as is true for the age-adjusted rates for the United States as a whole, which are dominated by these three densely populated northeast regions. We must also ask why have some states, such as New Mexico and North Carolina, registered increases as great as 30 percent since 1950, compared with the moderate increases shown for the United States as a whole—only 2 percent since 1980–84 and 1 percent since 1985–89.

This last figure (1 percent), however, is slightly understated. For the years 1985–89—unlike prior periods—the NCI chose to treat all reports of one or two breast cancer deaths in any age-group of any given county with the same code to avoid possible privacy disclosures for that county. In our tabulations of the county data, we were thus forced to treat all such instances as equivalent to one death since that was the most likely choice. This means that all of our county mortality rates for 1985–89 are slightly understated but by no more than about 2.5 percent.

According to the latest data from the National Center for Health Statistics, the total number of white female breast cancer deaths in the United States (excluding Hawaii and Alaska) in the years 1985–89 was 183,339—2.5 percent higher than the total figure of 178,868 carried in table 5–1. Had we used 2 deaths rather than 1 for all ambiguous cases, our national total for the 1985–89 period would have been 191,147 breast cancer deaths, which would have yielded a 4.3 percent overestimate.

It is therefore likely that the true U.S. age-adjusted breast cancer mortality rate for 1985–89 may be close to 25.2 deaths per 100,000, an increase of 3 percent from 1950–54 rather than an increase of only 1 percent. This remains a moderate overall increase over the past 4 decades, equivalent to 0.1 percent each year. This is in sharp contrast to the corresponding average annual increase in breast cancer incidence since 1950, which is about 20 times greater, as suggested by figure 2–1. (From 1985 to 1991 the number of white female breast cancer deaths rose by 6.6 percent, more than 1 percent each year, which is 10 times greater than the postwar annual increase.)

INCIDENCE RATES INCREASE MORE THAN MORTALITY

The popular perception that we are in the grip of a breast cancer epidemic is based on incidence rather than mortality data. For example, the NCI has estimated the 1990 age-adjusted white female breast cancer incidence rate to have risen by 34 percent since 1973 for the United States as a whole—representing an annual increase of 2 percent.[44] The corresponding average annual increase according to the Connecticut Tumor Registry is 3 percent in the state of Connecticut.

The slight underestimation of age-adjusted breast cancer mortality rates for 1985–89 in our breast cancer database affects the U.S. total and all counties and combinations of counties to the same degree, so we did not attempt any upward adjustment of the 1985–89 county breast cancer mortality rates. In light of the relatively slight long-term increase in national breast cancer mortality since 1950, we shall find that the corresponding large increases displayed by "nuclear" counties, no matter how they are defined, are extraordinarily significant indeed.

Turning first to the rates shown in table 5–1 for the first period of 1950–54, 5 to 10 years after nuclear tests began in 1945, we see that they differed widely, with the lowest rates existing in the rural east and west south central regions, with Arkansas as low as 15.4 deaths per 100,000 women, compared with rates twice as high in such northern states as New York.

One conclusion that can be drawn immediately is that genetic or heredity factors cannot possibly account for such large differences. The population in the south central states is essentially the same as in the northern states of the United States due to the high rate of migration. Thus it is clear that environmental factors dominate, as has been found in numerous studies in the past and most recently for the case of Australian and Canadian immigrants.[48] Moreover, the fact that the greatest single rise of 39 percent by 1980–84 occurred in the rural mountain state of New Mexico, where the first Trinity nuclear test occurred in 1945, followed by comparable rises of 29 percent in other states near the Nevada test site, such as Arizona and Utah respectively, shows that the dominant factor could not be genetic but has to be the short-lived fission products that came down rapidly from these relatively low-yield bomb tests.

Another highly significant fact emerges from a close inspection of table 5–1. The West South Central states of Arkansas, Louisiana, Texas, and Oklahoma as a group had throughout the period 1950–89 the lowest breast cancer mortality rates of all the nine census regions in the nation, despite the fact that they had the largest petrochemical manufacturing facilities and were large users of DDT and other chlorine-based pesticides and herbicides. Thus, petrochemicals, pesticides, and herbicides, *by themselves*, cannot be responsible for the epidemic rise of breast cancer throughout the years of the great expansion of petrochemicals and the rising use of pesticides and herbicides.

Further examination of table 5–1 reveals that following the end of above-ground nuclear tests in 1963, the enormous increase in breast cancer rates in the rural states of the Mountain region, closest to the Nevada test site, not only ceased, but mortality rates actually declined significantly between 1980–84 and 1985–89, exactly as expected if fallout in the diet is the single most important environmental factor. Thus breast cancer mortality in the region declined from its high of 22.6 deaths per 100,000 to 21.4 by 1985–89, with Idaho, directly north of Nevada declining most strongly of all, by 15 percent as compared with a 5 percent decline for the whole region.

In sharp contrast, equally rural southern states along the Atlantic coast from Delaware to Florida continued to show rising breast cancer mortality rates with continuing releases from numerous civilian power reactors and those of the Oak Ridge and Savannah River nuclear weapons plants, in the southern states of Tennessee and South Carolina. This contrasting pattern with the Mountain region accords with the fact that no civilian power reactor was established there in the period under review.

Yet while all but one of the 9 southern states along the Atlantic coast with nuclear plants registered continuing increases in breast cancer mortality from 1980–84 to 1985–89, this was not the case for equally rural and high rainfall states like Louisiana, Kentucky, and Mississippi, which had no reactors operating before 1982; they registered declines of 3, 6, and 3 percent respectively in the 1980s.

The rural states of the South Atlantic region with their high rainfall levels did not escape bomb-test fallout. Since 90 percent of fallout comes down in the rain, it is not surprising that as a group breast cancer mortality rose even more—by 15 percent between 1950–54 and 1980–84 as compared to 13 percent for the dry Mountain states.

Along with organochlorine compounds and other chemicals, the past overuse of medical X rays or other forms of medical radiation cannot play a dominant role in explaining these temporal increases (and declines) in breast cancer mortality in these poor rural states that can least afford the past overuse of such expensive therapies.

Turning now to the other more urban and industrialized census regions we can affirm again that their high mortality rates in 1950–54 cannot have a genetic origin, nor could these high rainfall states have escaped the widespread fallout from bomb tests and power reactors. As shown by figure 2–1, the great rise in breast cancer incidence rates in Connecticut occurred after the onset of nuclear testing and was exacerbated by large airborne emissions of I–131 and strontium-90 from the nearby Haddam Neck and Millstone reactors. Thus for the case of breast cancer incidence in Connecticut, there was a 17 percent rise already for the period 1948–53 that would contribute to an increase of mortality rates by 1954 above the rates for the prenuclear period 1935–44.

As for New York State, we will learn from figures 8–2 and 8–3 in chapter 8 that New York City, only 30 miles from Indian Point, registered sharp rises in breast cancer mortality throughout the postwar period prior to the start-up of Indian Point in 1962, when bomb-test fallout came down in the rain and snow of the Appalachian Mountains, contaminating the lakes and rivers that serve drinking water to the large metropolitan areas of the Northeast. As we shall see in chapter 8, New York City breast cancer mortality rates rose from a low of 16.9 deaths per 100,000 men and women in 1943 just before the first large releases from

Hanford and the New Mexico trinity test in 1945 to 19.0 deaths for the period 1950–54, a sudden increase of 19 percent, similar to the corresponding rise in incidence in nearby Connecticut. Moreover, as the data for largely rural upstate New York shown in figure 8–2 shows, New York City, with all its air, automobile, and chemical pollution had a lower breast cancer mortality rate than rural areas of New York between 1940–43 before fallout arrived, again supporting the conclusion that neither ordinary chemicals nor the medical uses of radiation can explain the temporal and geographical patterns of breast cancer changes since the onset of the Nuclear Age.

The contamination by fallout of the drinking water supplies derived from rivers and stored in lakes or reservoirs for the large urban populations such as that in New York City explains why the breast cancer rates for New York City rose so much faster than for rural areas after 1945 than in rural New York State shown in figure 8–2. Rural areas depend largely on well water, so that initially drinking water from deep wells was not contaminated by fallout from relatively low-yield nuclear bombs. Such bombs, prior to the later thermonuclear bombs used after 1954, produced heavy contamination from short-lived isotopes that came down in a matter of hours, unlike the fallout from hydrogen bombs that produced high altitude clouds that did not rain out for months or years, so that the short-lived activity like that of I–131 largely died out, leaving the long-lived strontium-90, cesium-137 and others to become dominant, reaching the aquifers typically after five to ten years.

The key role of drinking water sources also explains why there was no large decline in breast cancer rates in the heavily populated areas of high rainfall urban areas of the northeast and Great Lakes states after the end of atmospheric tests that took place in Nevada and in other dry Mountain states using mainly deep well water. After the Partial Test Ban Treaty of 1963, large nuclear plants began to operate near the large metropolitan areas of the North. As in the case of New York City, the reservoirs and lakes from which the drinking water originated were frequently located near nuclear reactors as in the case of Indian Point, only four miles from the Croton system serving both New York City and the county of Westchester. But note in both figures 8–2 and 8–3 that after 1970, New York City breast cancer rates dropped sharply, reflecting the city's ability, after many decades of development, to shift its chief drinking water supply to the Catskill water shed area far from the Croton reservoirs so close to Indian Point. Westchester breast cancer mortality rates, still dependent on the vulnerable Croton system, are seen to continue to rise steeply throughout the 1970s and 1980s.

LOGARITHMIC CANCER DOSE RESPONSE TO IONIZING RADIATION

Since the permissible releases or dose to the internal organs were based on data from extrapolations of short high-dose exposures to the flash of the bombs or to brief medical exposures to external sources of radiation, the standards for permissible routine daily releases of fission products destined to be ingested and that would then emit internal low-level radiation, can be shown to be too large by factors of hundreds to thousands of times. Moreover, since the standards were set in the late 1950s to allow the continuation of nuclear testing deemed essential for national security, these releases were not questioned, and the warnings expressed by Pauling and Sakharov in 1958 were ignored.

As a result breast cancer mortality rates continued to climb in the 1980s, as shown particularly for the case of Rhode Island, downwind of four large reactors in Connecticut and two smaller reactors at the Brookhaven National Laboratory in Suffolk County just 12 miles to the south. Of all the states listed in table 5–1, Rhode Island experienced the largest increase in breast cancer mortality in the 1980s, while the increase in Suffolk County from 1950–54, when BNL began operations, to 1985–89, we shall show was 40 times greater than the national increase in the corresponding age-adjusted rate for white females.

Thus the state-by-state data in table 5–1 strongly support the regional correlation of age-adjusted breast cancer mortality rates with cumulated releases from commercial nuclear power plants and identify fission products in the diet and drinking water as the principal new environmental factor affecting cancer rates introduced since World War II. This conclusion is further strengthened by a recent study of the geographical distribution of organochlorine residues in tree bark, which show that the western plains and southwest mountain states with the lowest breast cancer mortality rates have the highest concentration of pesticide residues. Similarly, China has very low breast cancer rates and the highest tree-bark concentrations of chlorine-based pesticides, while the United Kingdom has very high breast cancer mortality and low pesticide levels. Thus, for the age group 45–54, the breast cancer mortality rate in rural China as reported to the World Health Organization for 1990–92 was only 6.8 deaths per 100,000, with DDT levels of 10–1,000 nanograms per gram of lipid, while the United Kingdom had a breast cancer mortality rate of 55.8 with only 0–100 nanograms of DDT. [49]

The above analysis of the differential urban/rural trend among states can be generalized in figure 5–1, in which we have plotted for each state its ratio of mortality increase from 1950–54 to 1985–89 against its Standardized Breast Cancer Mortality Ratio in 1950–54.

It is clear that in general such rural states as North Carolina and New Mexico, which initially had rates far below that of the United States had by 1985–89 registered the greatest increases, as compared with more moderate changes for highly urban states like New York and Connecticut. This relationship is seen to be consistent and significant, as indicated by a line of regression fitted to the observations, which yields a negative correlation value of .74, for which the chance probability is less than 1 in 1,000 cases.

In figure 5–2, we have carried out the same correlation analysis at the county level. We have taken all counties in each of the nine census

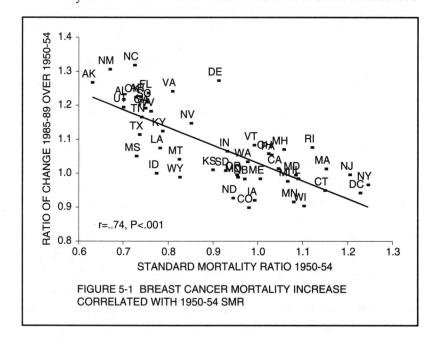

FIGURE 5-1 BREAST CANCER MORTALITY INCREASE CORRELATED WITH 1950-54 SMR

FIGURE 5-2 REGIONAL CORRELATIONS SHOWING THAT COUNTIES WITH
LOWEST BREAST CANCER MORTALITY RATES IN 1950-54 REGISTERED
THE HIGHEST PERCENT INCREASES IN 1985-89

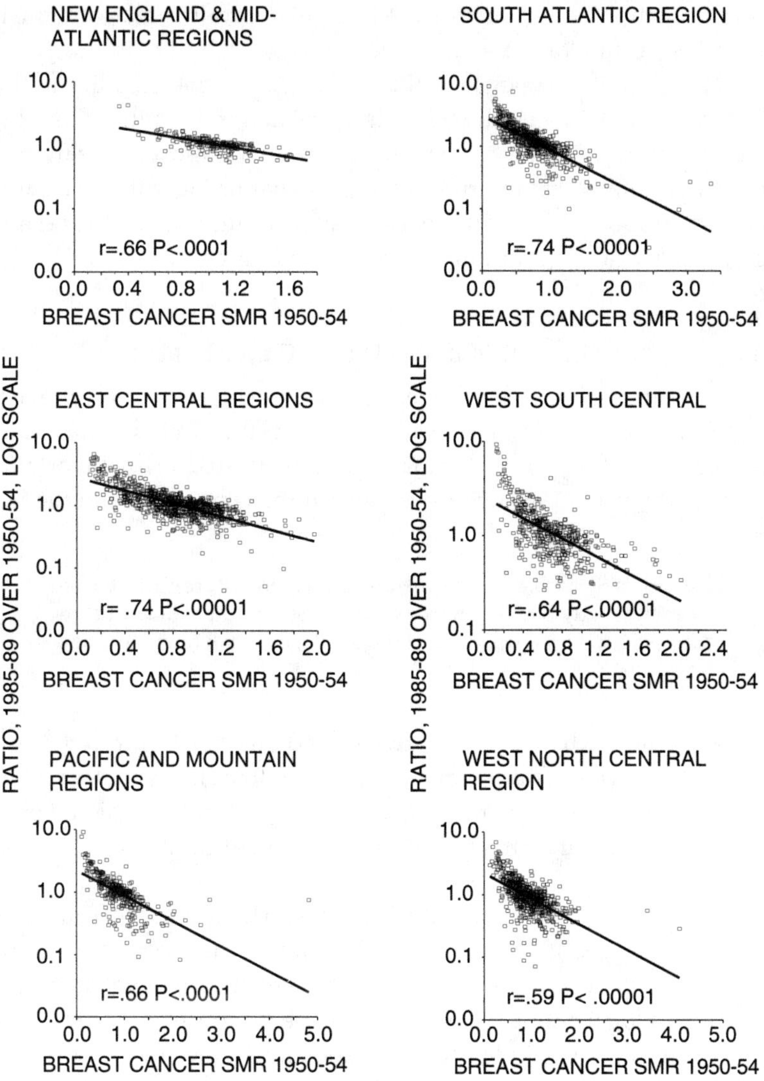

NEW ENGLAND & MID-ATLANTIC REGIONS

r=.66 P<.0001

BREAST CANCER SMR 1950-54

SOUTH ATLANTIC REGION

r=.74 P<.00001

BREAST CANCER SMR 1950-54

EAST CENTRAL REGIONS

r= .74 P<.00001

BREAST CANCER SMR 1950-54

WEST SOUTH CENTRAL

r=..64 P<.00001

BREAST CANCER SMR 1950-54

PACIFIC AND MOUNTAIN REGIONS

r=.66 P<.0001

BREAST CANCER SMR 1950-54

WEST NORTH CENTRAL REGION

r=.59 P< .00001

BREAST CANCER SMR 1950-54

RATIO, 1985-89 OVER 1950-54, LOG SCALE

regions (eliminating only those with no breast cancer deaths in either period) and found this negative correlation to be universal for all counties in the nation. Those counties with age-adjusted 1950–54 mortality rates that were extremely low—because they were small rural counties in a relatively pristine state—appeared to have experienced the worst effects of some malignant force of mortality that obviously spared no section of the nation.

Note that the response of these initially pristine counties to this malignant force is seen to be inversely related to its initial mortality rate, and thus inversely to the amount of early exposure to environmental pollutants, giving rise to a supralinear or logarithmic form to the dose response. This differential response suggests that rural and urban breast cancer mortality rates are converging.

THE CONVERGENCE OF RURAL AND URBAN CANCER TRENDS

The epidemiologist Michael Greenberg was the first to observe the convergence of rural and urban cancer rates in the United States in an examination of a county database of age-adjusted cancer mortality rates for the years 1950–75. He attributed the convergence to the fact that:

> the United States has become an urban-oriented culture characterized by increasingly similar smoking, drinking, and nutritional habits, occupational and other risk factors in villages, small towns and suburbs as well as cities.[50]

Rural and urban counties have shared one risk factor in the past half century, which is not mentioned here: fallout from nuclear bomb tests and from military and civilian reactors, acting in a biologically more deadly manner than high doses of radiation given in a short burst.

Dr. Abram Petkau, a biophysicist working for the Canadian Atomic Energy Commission, was the first to discover in 1972—by accident—a biochemical mechanism by which low-level radiation can cause a logarithmic increase in the dose response of cancer to low levels of radiation. He found that exposure to low radiation levels promotes the formation of free radicals, which are dangerous to the cells that constitute the immune system.[51] [52]

Petkau subjected animal cell membranes immersed in water to various levels of X ray radiation and observed that it takes as much as 400 or 500 rads to rupture the cell. (A rad is a measure of the impact of radiation on the human body; about 400 rads was the level that instantly killed the Hiroshima victims.) He was amazed to find that cells that withstood extremely high radiation levels had ruptured when he added a small amount of radioactive sodium salt, which measured less than one-tenth of a rad, to the water surrounding the cell membrane. He finally deduced that over time the low-level radiation promoted the formation of so-called free radicals.

A free radical is an oxygen molecule with an extra negative charge. Free radicals are drawn by the force of electrical attraction to destroy a cell by initiating a chain reaction that unravels the fatty membrane structure. At low levels of radiation intensity a free radical can efficiently find a cell to destroy, but at high levels free radicals tend to negate or neutralize each other.

Consequently the dose response to low-level radiation would be logarithmic, which is to say that at very low levels of radiation the dose response (as in the form of cancer) would rise most rapidly but would tend to flatten out at higher radiation levels.

Therefore in accordance with the logarithmic relationship characteristic of the dose response to varying levels of radiation exposure found by Petkau and others, the convergence of rural and urban cancer rates can be seen to demonstrate that the greater percentage increase of the relatively pristine rural states corresponds to the initial stages of the rapidly rising dose response curve, while the smaller increase of the urban areas, with above average initial cancer rates, reflects that portion of the dose-response curve where the dose response flattens out. The urban county rates in 1950–54 were already higher than average and were consequently at that stage of the dose-response curve where the response can be expected to flatten out.

This is truly an extraordinary finding. It effectively disposes of the assumption that the nuclear scientists had hoped would govern the dose response of cancer to low-level radiation—that it would be linear and that there would be some level low enough to be safe. Figure 5–3 illustrates the difference in the dose response to radiation from the two assumptions about the shape of the curve in reaching a given percent increase in cancer as the radiation level rises.

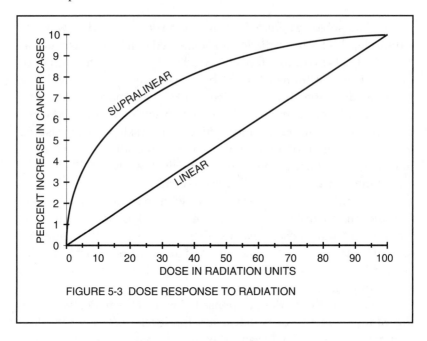

FIGURE 5-3 DOSE RESPONSE TO RADIATION

The supralinear curve represents the type of a logarithmic response in which the most rapid rise occurs at low radiation levels, while the straight line represents a linear response, in which a constant given increase in radiation would produce a constant increase in cancer risk. This assumption was based on the hope that if the dose were low enough the response would be negligible. This is not possible if the response is logarithmic—the slope becomes steeper and steeper the smaller the dose is.

We found in figure 3–8 an example of a logarithmic response to radiation at the regional level, between the most recent breast cancer mortality rates to airborne *per capita* levels of cumulated emissions of radioactive iodine and strontium from civilian power reactors. In figure 3–8 we saw that recent age-adjusted mortality rates for the nine census regions were significantly correlated with the log values for each region of the *per capita* emission levels. In figure 3–9, we show the same relationship when the mortality rates are plotted against the linear values of the *per capita* emission levels. As we move from the dry regions of the Mountain and West South Central regions exposed to low radiation levels to the more heavily exposed regions, the dose-response curve assumes the downward concave or supralinear shape that Petkau first noted in 1972.

Unlike the DOE nuclear facilities engaged in the production of nuclear weapons, civilian power reactors are required by the Nuclear Regulatory Commission to report the annual airborne and liquid emissions of radioactive iodine, strontium, and other fission products. We have summarized these annual reports for each reactor, arranged by state and region since 1970, in appendix C and have used them to create figures 3–7, 3–8, and 3–9.

Figure 5–2 demonstrates in another way that a logarithmic relationship between radiation exposure and breast cancer mortality increase is supported by the fact that, in general, rural counties that initially had the lowest breast cancer rates registered the highest percentage increases since 1950–54. In figure 5–2 we show that this pattern applies to all counties in each of the 9 census regions of the nation and is perhaps the most powerful indicator that there is no level of radiation low enough to be considered safe.

Even rural counties in dry regions like the Mountain and West South Central states, furthest away from the exacerbating effects of

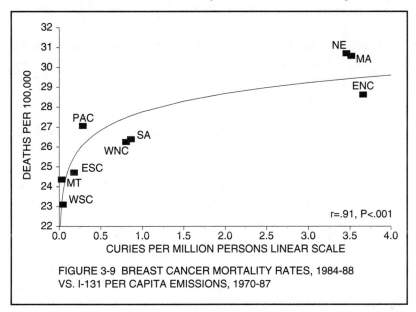

FIGURE 3-9 BREAST CANCER MORTALITY RATES, 1984-88
VS. I-131 PER CAPITA EMISSIONS, 1970-87

civilian reactor emissions, registered large percentage increases in breast cancer mortality as a result of exposure from bomb-test fallout.

Surprisingly the Mountain states, which were initially adversely affected by bomb-test radiation from the Nevada test site, registered a significant 5 percent improvement from 1980–84 to 1985–89 according to table 5–1. We shall show that this improvement can be linked to the relative absence of civilian reactors in this region, an important subject that we will treat in greater detail in chapter 8.

Table 5–1 also permits us to evaluate the relative importance of low-level radiation versus the widespread use of pesticides and chemical pollutants and the past overuse of X rays among the environmental causes of the geographic variations in breast cancer mortality.

From 1950–54 to 1980–84 only 9 of the 49 states failed to register increases in breast cancer mortality. This alone is a significant fact ignored by the NCI study. Along with the relatively high increases registered by most rural counties, can we say then that all three factors were contributing equally to the observed overall increase? The answer is no, for the following reasons.

Past overuse of X rays could be viewed as contributing to the high breast cancer rates in the affluent urban states but not to the above average increase in the mortality rates of the far less affluent rural states.

There are significantly different trends among the rural states, indicating that low-level radiation outranks exposure to pesticides and other chemical pollutants. For example, almost every rural state registered increased mortality from 1950–54 to 1980–84, mainly as a result of exposure to bomb-test radiation. That is not true for the percentage increases shown in table 5–1 for the period 1980–84 to 1985–89, when emissions from civilian reactors replaced bomb-test fallout as a causal factor.

Note that for this final period there were generally declines in mortality in rural states that had no operating reactors, such as in North and South Dakota, Kansas, West Virginia, Kentucky, Louisiana, Oklahoma, Texas, Montana, Wyoming, Colorado, New Mexico, Arizona, Utah, and Nevada. Since all of these rural states had similar exposures to pesticides and other chemical pollutants, we may conclude that exposure to bomb-test radiation was the principal cause of their overall increased mortality since 1950–54.

Chapter 6

WHY THE NATIONAL CANCER INSTITUTE FAILED TO FIND INCREASED CANCER RISK NEAR NUCLEAR REACTORS

Now that we understand some of the basic principles governing the change in breast cancer mortality rates over time, we can replicate the 1990 NCI study, entitled *Cancer Mortality in Populations Near Nuclear Facilities*, which found no increased cancer risk near nuclear facilities.[9] To do so, we shall use our database of age-adjusted county breast cancer mortality rates, which we secured from the NCI.

How The NCI Defined Exposed Counties

The primary flaw in the NCI methodology lies in their limited definition of counties most likely to be affected by emission from a nearby reactor. This led to so few cases of cancer that no statistically significant changes resulted. For the 62 nuclear facilities they chose to study, they identified only 107 exposed counties, occasionally adding 1 additional adjoining county for an average total of less than 2 counties per facility. While the NCI included data on breast cancer mortality from 1950 to 1984 in each county in which the facility was located, they did not publish any age-adjusted cancer mortality rates for the various states and regions.

In table 6–1 we have applied our age-adjusted breast cancer rates for the 3 indicated 5-year periods to the NCI definition of the counties

TABLE 6-1 WHITE FEMALE BREAST CANCER RATES, 1950-89
IN 107 NUCLEAR COUNTIES AS DEFINED BY THE NCI
Deaths per 100,000 Women

Start Date	Name of Facility	Age-Adjusted Mortality Rates			Percent Change		Number of Deaths		
		1950-54	80-84	85-89	80-84/ 1950-54	85-89/ 1950-54	1950-54	80-84	85-89
	US ex AK, HI	24.4	24.9	24.5	2%	1%	91392	167803	178868
1943	Hanford	13.2	19.8	21.7	50%	64%	19	96	118
1943	Oak Ridge	19.9	19.8	20.8	-1%	4%	31	77	88
1947	Mound	26.5	26.5	26.2	-0%	-1%	383	671	730
1949	INEL	4.8	20.6	20.1	333%	322%	3	26	31
1950	Paducah	22.6	18.9	19.2	-17%	-15%	34	49	57
1950	Savannah River	18.5	20.5	19.4	11%	5%	22	64	72
1951	Fernald	29.6	28.4	28.4	-4%	-4%	715	931	1,005
1952	Portsmouth	19.5	6.5	10.9	-67%	-44%	7	6	9
1953	Rocky Flats	23.6	25.5	22.5	8%	-5%	71	351	366
1957	Shippingport/Beaver	22.1	24.7	23.2	12%	5%	103	209	209
1960	Dresden	20.4	25.8	28.0	27%	37%	85	222	258
1960	Yankee Rowe	27.0	28.7	28.8	6%	7%	161	244	255
1962	Big Rock Point	25.0	20.3	18.6	-19%	-25%	25	34	31
1962	Hallam	26.0	24.3	30.0	-7%	15%	122	164	213
1962	Indian Point	29.9	30.7	32.2	3%	8%	655	1163	1276
1963	Fermi	23.0	23.0	30.6	-0%	33%	41	86	120
1963	Humboldt Bay	25.6	24.2	27.3	-6%	6%	42	72	96
1964	Pathfinder	24.6	23.1	25.1	-6%	2%	55	101	108
1966	Nuclear Fuel Services	29.3	32.4	25.8	10%	-12%	63	98	78
1967	Haddam Neck	22.7	23.7	24.7	4%	9%	49	107	119
1967	La Crosse	16.9	17.5	15.2	4%	-10%	13	21	15
1967	San Onofre	23.7	27.1	26.2	14%	10%	555	2894	3167
1969	Ginna	27.4	24.2	29.7	-11%	8%	53	67	81
1969	Nine Mile Point	25.6	23.9	28.9	-7%	13%	59	79	95
1969	Oyster Creek	27.4	28.9	28.7	6%	5%	56	479	608
1970	Millstone	22.4	26.8	28.2	19%	26%	97	197	223
1970	Point Beach	28.0	31.2	28.1	12%	0%	63	113	102
1970	Robinson	15.5	19.4	22.4	25%	45%	16	44	50
1971	Monticello	31.4	27.1	22.0	-14%	-30%	32	60	58
1971	Palisades	22.8	22.3	23.7	-2%	4%	28	47	51
1972	Maine Yankee	28.9	33.3	21.8	15%	-25%	38	66	56
1972	Pilgrim	23.2	32.0	28.3	38%	22%	154	409	374
1972	Quad Cities	23.1	23.4	24.5	1%	6%	119	177	189
1972	Surry	32.0	22.6	24.7	-29%	-23%	9	11	16
1972	Turkey Point	20.1	24.0	23.3	20%	16%	3021	447	1474
1972	Vermont Yankee	26.1	24.3	23.0	-7%	-12%	107	145	143
1972	Zion	34.0	26.3	27.6	-23%	-19%	218	377	455
1973	Browns Ferry	19.6	28.0	18.5	43%	-6%	19	55	37
1973	Fort Calhoun	20.3	26.0	15.5	28%	-23%	20	29	21
1973	Kewaunee	28.0	31.2	28.1	12%	0%	63	113	102
1973	Oconee	10.8	21.3	18.3	97%	69%	15	73	81
1973	Prairie Island	25.6	26.1	28.5	2%	11%	41	63	77

TABLE 6-1 CONTINUED
WHITE FEMALE BREAST CANCER RATES, 1950-89
IN 107 NUCLEAR COUNTIES AS DEFINED BY THE NCI
Deaths per 100,000 Women

Start Date	Name of Facility	Age-Adjusted Mortality Rates			Percent Change		Number of Deaths		
		1950-54	80-84	85-89	80-84/ 1950-54	85-89/ 1950-54	1950-54	80-84	85-89
1974	Arkansas	16.3	22.5	17.1	38%	5%	9	26	23
1974	Calvert Cliffs	38.8	15.8	18.8	-59%	-52%	7	13	20
1974	Cooper Station	27.1	23.5	17.9	-13%	-34%	32	30	21
1974	Duane Arnold	19.1	22.5	25.4	17%	33%	81	139	151
1974	Hatch	8.6	12.1	16.1	41%	87%	4	13	18
1974	Peach Bottom	25.5	27.5	25.6	8%	0%	325	645	665
1974	Rancho Seco	21.3	25.6	25.7	20%	21%	254	850	959
1974	Three Mile Island	25.2	27.0	26.4	7%	5%	466	857	905
1975	Brunswick	16.3	24.8	13.9	52%	-15%	4	25	21
1975	Cook	24.1	22.9	24.3	-5%	1%	72	110	125
1975	Trojan	28.6	26.5	20.8	-7%	-27%	48	93	79
1976	Fort St. Vrain	21.9	21.5	22.4	-2%	3%	95	253	305
1976	Salem	23.3	28.0	28.2	20%	21%	156	362	400
1976	St. Lucie	6.5	20.7	23.5	221%	263%	3	74	112
1977	Crystal River	11.7	25.8	21.0	120%	79%	2	86	111
1977	Davis Besse	25.5	18.7	19.6	-27%	-23%	21	31	32
1977	Farley	17.6	13.5	17.3	-23%	-2%	17	32	40
1978	North Anna	18.6	21.2	19.1	14%	3%	15	43	48
1980	Sequoyah	19.5	25.7	22.0	32%	13%	81	207	190
1981	McGuire	16.9	22.5	26.4	33%	57%	98	342	459
	All sites combined	24.6	26.0	25.8	6%	5%	5988	14873	16245

near each of the installations, involving 107 selected counties. This allows us to examine the trends since 1950, when compared with the corresponding national trends.

We have therefore calculated the combined age-adjusted rates for each nuclear installation and also for all 107 counties taken as an aggregate for each of the 3 time periods.

Of the 62 facilities in the NCI study with 107 exposed counties, only 36 registered increases from 1950–54 to 1980–84 (the final time period in the NCI study) that were greater than the corresponding 2 percent national increase. Twenty-six sites did not register an increase. This does not suggest that exposure represented a significant added cancer risk. The fact that in the aggregate all 107 "nuclear" counties registered a 6 percent increase—based on 14,873 deaths in 1980–84 as against 5,988 in 1950–54—does represent a significant upward divergence, equivalent to more than 3 standard deviations (according to the formula discussed in chapter 3), with a chance probability of less than .001. The NCI study, oddly enough, did not mention this fact, although they did publish the supporting data.

Our conclusion—that in the aggregate the 107 "nuclear" counties chosen for study by the NCI show a statistically significant increased breast cancer risk—is fully supported on page 118 of volume 1 of the NCI report. Here the authors show that for all 107 counties, taken as an aggregate, there are significant increases in cancer mortality of all types (including breast cancer) if the rates after start-up are compared with those before start-up. The authors neglected to acknowledge this fact.

SIGNIFICANCE OF THE INCREASE IN AGGREGATED MORTALITY RATES

In table 6–2, we have reproduced the data included in the NCI tabulation but have added the tests of significance that the NCI neglected to include, which would indicate which changes could be attributed to chance variation. The absence of such measures from this NCI table can be regarded as a "smoking gun" for what it reveals about the lengths to which the NCI would go to misrepresent their own data.

Let us state in detail what this table reveals. First, for all 107 study (*i.e.*, what the NCI considers to be possible "nuclear") counties, the NCI has assembled all cancer deaths, broken down by 15 different types of cancer, both before and after start-up of each of the 62 facilities.

The authors do not show the before and after cancer mortality rates, but show instead the before and after Standardized Mortality Ratio, which can be viewed as the ratio between the observed age-adjusted cancer mortality rate and the corresponding age-adjusted U.S. mortality rate. Note that for breast cancer, for example, the SMR was 1.00 before start-up but rose by 6 percent in the years after start-up. This is equivalent to stating that prior to start-up the 107 "nuclear" counties had the same degree of breast cancer mortality as the United States, but in the years after start-up the breast cancer mortality was 6 percent greater than that of the United States. Note: the number of deaths involved after start-up is so large (48,371) that it is possible to calculate the probability that so great a divergence between the change in the observed rate and the U.S. rate is equiva-

**TABLE 6-2 NCI CANCER MORTALITY CHANGES
BEFORE AND AFTER START-UP
ALL AGES, ALL FACILITIES COMBINED
107 STUDY COUNTIES AND 292 CONTROL COUNTIES
WITHIN 100 MILES**

Disease	Before No. of Deaths	SMR	After No. of Deaths	SMR	Change in SMRs	Standard Deviations
107 Study Counties						
Leukemia, Aleukemia	16007	0.99	21176	0.98	0.99	
All Cancer, exc. Leuk.	334200	0.99	504293	1.02	1.03	15.0
Hodgkin's Disease	3841	0.96	3678	0.98	1.02	
Other Lymphoma	10008	1.05	16173	1.04	0.99	
Multiple Myeloma	3844	1.00	7448	1.01	1.01	
Digestive Organs	113804	0.97	148054	1.02	1.05	13.4
Stomach	23141	0.92	21014	0.96	1.04	4.0
Colon & Rectum	52043	1.00	73051	1.06	1.06	11.2
Liver	11202	0.94	9049	0.98	1.04	2.7
Trachea, Bronchus, Lung	53646	0.99	117746	1.03	1.04	9.6
Breast, Female	31843	1.00	48731	1.06	1.06	9.2
Thyroid	1206	0.93	1477	1.05	1.13	3.3
Bones, Joints	2349	0.96	2217	0.99	1.03	
Bladder	10584	1.06	13752	1.07	1.01	
Brain, etc.	8450	1.01	12970	1.00	0.99	
Benign, unspec. Neoplasms	949	1.02	3403	0.98	0.96	
292 Control Counties						
Leukemia, Aleukemia	35971	0.97	42574	1.01	1.04	5.7
All Cancer, exc. Leuk.	796510	1.01	997794	1.02	1.01	7.2
Hodgkin's Disease	9578	1.04	7712	1.06	1.02	
Other Lymphoma	21246	0.97	31063	1.01	1.04	4.9
Multiple Myeloma	8805	1.00	14634	1.02	1.02	
Digestive Organs	280537	1.03	297004	1.04	1.01	3.9
Stomach	60266	1.03	44646	1.03	1.00	
Colon & Rectum	126812	1.05	144620	1.06	1.01	2.7
Liver	28059	1.01	17636	0.96	0.95	
Trachea, Bronchus, Lung	123851	0.99	227766	1.00	1.01	3.4
Breast, Female	75053	1.02	94992	1.05	1.03	6.5
Thyroid	3020	1.00	2886	1.04	1.04	
Bones, Joints	5720	1.01	4221	0.96	0.95	
Bladder	25307	1.09	27298	1.07	0.99	
Brain, etc.	18638	0.97	2551	1.00	1.03	
Benign, unspec. Neoplasms	2306	1.05	6957	1.05	1.00	

lent to 9.2 standard deviations. The probability of getting such a result by chance is less than 1 in several trillion, a fact not acknowledged by the NCI authors.

As we learned in chapter 4, the statistical significance of any divergence over time of county cancer mortality rates from that of the United States increases inversely with the square root of the number of deaths in the final period. The NCI methodology attempted to minimize this divergence by extending the period after start-up as long as possible, instead of using the more direct method employed by Mangano and the Radiation and Health Project of simply comparing the initial period with the final period. Extending the period of study also increases the number of deaths and therefore also increases the significance of any observed divergence from the national change.

It is important that we understand just how the National Cancer Institute, mandated by President Nixon in 1971 to guide the War on Cancer, has misled the public in this study with regard to the risk of living near reactor sites. If such a divergent trend cannot be due to chance variation, then some plausible explanation for the divergence must be sought. The absence of such an explanation can justify a charge of negligence on the part of the National Cancer Institute for failing to warn the public of the increased risk in the counties chosen by NCI for study.

Note that according to table 6–2, the NCI has determined that for the 107 "nuclear" counties (before start-up), the overall age-adjusted mortality rate for all cancers (except leukemia) was 1 percent less than that of the United States—for this is the meaning of a prestart-up SMR of .99. After start-up—based on 504,293 deaths—the total cancer SMR for these counties rose to 1.02, meaning that after start-up cancer mortality was now higher than in the United States. The question to be answered is whether this change is statistically significant.

The number of poststart-up deaths is now so large that the chance probability of this change is equivalent to 15 standard deviations, according to the formula discussed in chapter 4, where we noted that for a result equivalent to 5 standard deviations the chance probability was less than 1 out of 1 million. Nobody has ever tried to calculate the chance probability associated with 15 standard deviations, but it is of the order of 1 out of a number as large as the number of atoms in the earth!

For anyone to imply that such a great change could be due to chance is equivalent to saying it is possible that the moon is made of green cheese! For the NCI to publish the figures in table 6–2 without any indication of the statistical significance of the recorded changes in cancer mortality after start-up represents a scandalous degree of deception.

Table 6–2 shows that equally significant increases in other kinds of cancer mortality occurred after start-up, particularly for those forms of cancer described on page three of the NCI report as "known to be especially susceptible to induction by radiation (*i.e.*, leukemia, female breast cancer and lung cancer)."

A STRANGE CHOICE OF CONTROL COUNTIES

The NCI may have hoped to divert attention from these embarrassingly significant increases in cancer risk after start-up—by choosing a truly bizarre method of comparing the increase in the cancer mortality rates of the 107 "nuclear" counties to 292 carefully selected "control" counties, rather than to the change in the national rates.

Here we come to the second flagrant flaw in the methodology used by the NCI authors. They based their decision, as to whether or not an increased cancer risk in a "nuclear" county could be attributed to the operation of the facility, solely on a comparison with a set of 3 control counties generally located within 50 to 100 miles of the facility and frequently adjacent to it or within 100 miles of another nuclear plant.

According to Mangano's Oak Ridge findings, counties as far as 100 miles away can be exposed to the airborne releases with subsequent increased cancer risk. Moreover, according to page 19 of volume 1 of the NCI report, one of the criteria used to select control counties was that in addition to the usual demographic characteristics, they were chosen for comparable infant mortality rates. There is extensive evidence in scientific literature that infant mortality, just like childhood leukemia, is highly sensitive to low-level radiation exposure as produced by fission products in the milk and diet.[53][54] It is clear that the choice of "control" counties alone virtually guarantees that there would be little or no difference in cancer rates. This permitted the misleading conclusion that "there is no evidence that an excess occurrence of cancer has resulted from living near a nuclear facility."

For each "nuclear" county chosen by the NCI for study, the results were to be judged by three control counties, which were often fairly close to counties already designated by NCI as "nuclear." For example, for the Ginna, Nine Mile Point, and West Valley facilities in New York State, 7 control counties were chosen (Cayuga, Ontario, Wyoming, Genessee, Steuben, Livingston, and Jefferson), all of which are within 50 miles of 1 or more of the 3 counties studied (Wayne, Oswego, and Cattaraugus).

In fact, the bias shown by the NCI in its choice of control counties is best illustrated by the fact that for three-quarters of all nuclear facilities studied by the NCI, one or more control counties were chosen that were adjacent to a study county.

The NCI methodology chosen assumed, in effect, that if reactor emissions represented a risk, that risk would not extend any further than the borders of the county in which the reactor was located. But table 6–2 shows that even for the 292 control counties chosen by the NCI to offset the increases found in the 107 "nuclear" counties, they were apparently close enough to the "nuclear" counties so that the increases in the control county cancer SMRs after start-up were also highly significant. This increase of 4 percent for all cancers is equivalent to 7.2 standard deviations, and the 3 percent increase for breast cancer is equivalent to 6.5 standard deviations. These results warrant our belief that since the control counties were generally within 100 miles or closer to the reactor sites, these counties, too, should have been included in any definition of counties exposed to reactor emissions.

In the case of the Oak Ridge plant, which began to operate in 1943, the NCI defined the study, or exposed, counties as consisting of only Anderson and Roane. The NCI omitted consideration of any downwind county to the north of the Oak Ridge reactors, and as we saw in chapter 4, these counties were most directly affected.

The NCI found that cancer mortality in Anderson and Roane Counties increased from 1950–54 to 1979–83 by 2 percent more than the corresponding U.S. change. Because these 2 counties reported only 991 cancer deaths in the final 1979–83 period, this increase could not be regarded as statistically significant. However, by extending the area examined to include nearby contiguous downwind counties, it is easy to expand the number of deaths involved to demonstrate that some malevolent force of mortality has been coming out of Oak Ridge.

For the case of Oak Ridge, the authors of the NCI study chose 6 control counties, 3 of which (Blount, Jefferson, and Hamblen) are located between 10 and 75 miles from Oak Ridge or well within the 100-mile circle of counties for which Mangano found a highly significant increase in cancer rates. The 3 remaining control counties chosen are located between 75 and 110 miles from Oak Ridge. In areas that are close to three large civilian nuclear power plants. Thus Bradley County is a mere 5 to 25 miles east of the Sequoya nuclear power plant, Coffee County is located some 70 miles northeast of the Browns Ferry plant in northern Alabama, and Henderson County, in North Carolina, is located between 40 and 60 miles northeast of the Oconee plant in South Carolina.

It is worth repeating that despite this bizarre method of selecting control counties, an examination of the aggregated NCI data for all 107 study or "nuclear" counties and for all 292 selected control counties combined for the periods before and after start-up, as taken from page 118 of volume 1 of the NCI report, all show significant increases in cancer risk relative to that for the United States as a whole, which is in direct contradiction to the ultimate conclusion reached by the NCI.

Finally, we demonstrate in appendix D that the NCI was perfectly aware that counties within 50 miles of each reactor in the aggregate had breast cancer rates that were significantly above average and were thus unsuitable to be chosen as control counties.

Chapter 7

THE NATURE OF INCREASED CANCER RISK NEAR REACTORS

Despite flaws in the NCI methodology, the information they culled provides a useful frame of reference to study the factors that enhance the cancer risk near reactor sites. Of particular interest is the way the NCI organized its study of installations by start-up date. It turns out that women living near the oldest DOE reactor sites, built in the first decade of the Nuclear Age, have registered by far the highest long-term increases in breast cancer mortality of any group of counties in the nation. Thus the results of our analysis of breast cancer near the Oak Ridge plant can be replicated for all the old DOE nuclear facilities that had reactor operations. There are, however, three DOE nuclear reactor sites built before 1950 that were inexplicably omitted from the NCI study, which we have added: the Los Alamos and Sandia Labs in New Mexico and the Brookhaven National Lab in Suffolk County, New York. For all such facilities, we can still use the limited NCI definition of counties at risk, but by aggregating all such counties we can easily achieve the statistical significance necessary to show the adverse effects of long-term exposure to nuclear emissions.

RISK HIGHEST NEAR OLD DOE REACTORS

In table 7–1, using the limited NCI definition of "nuclear" home counties, we have compared 7 DOE facilities, which had reactors located in 14 counties with 5 other DOE facilities that did not include reactors located in 9 counties. The comparison of the aggregated rates of counties with reactors versus those without yields a remarkable discovery.

Women living in the 14 counties exposed to reactor emissions registered an extraordinary and significant increase in breast cancer mortality. This was in striking contrast to the experience of women living in counties with DOE facilities engaged in weapons manufacture and processing, which are not associated with the release of reactor fission products into the surrounding environment.

The five other DOE facilities were mainly concerned with uranium enrichment or weapons manufacture and did not involve the potential exposure of nearby residents to reactor emissions of radioactive iodine and strontium. Note that we have included in the first group three DOE reactor sites that the NCI study omitted. The Los Alamos Laboratory was, of course, the birthplace of the atomic bomb in 1945. The Sandia and Brookhaven laboratories began operations in 1950. All three of these DOE laboratories have long been operating so-called experimental reactors, with a consequent build-up of radioactive wastes that are associated with significant increases in breast cancer in the counties in which the reactors are located.

The Brookhaven National Laboratory reported its emissions of reactor fission products for the years 1950–66—which we have associated with anomalous increases in infant mortality in the 1960s and in breast cancer incidence in the 1980s.[22]

In table 7–1, for the 14 counties in which the 7 DOE facilities with reactors are located, the combined age-adjusted breast cancer rate increased by 37 percent from 1950–54 to 1985–89, in sharp contrast to the 6 percent decline recorded for the counties defining the 5 facilities without reactor emissions. Again, the number of deaths involved for both groups of facilities is too large for this divergence to be attributed to chance: that probability is equivalent to five standard deviations, with a chance probability of less than one in one million cases. Women living in the counties with DOE nuclear facilities without reactors are evidently not at as great risk as those living near facilities that include reactors.

This is a key finding, enabling us to focus our search for increased breast cancer risk on only those nuclear facilities with reactor emissions. It clearly shows the difference in undesirable health effects produced by fission products created by reactors as compared to natural sources of radiation such as radium and uranium.

TABLE 7-1 WHITE FEMALE BREAST CANCER MORTALITY RATES IN 23 COUNTIES WITH DOE FACILITIES
Deaths per 100,000 Women

County	ST	Age-Adjusted Mortality Rates			Percent Change		Number of Deaths		
		1950-54	80-84	85-89	80-84/ 1950-54	85-89/ 1950-54	1950-54	80-84	85-89
DOE FACILITIES WITH REACTORS									
HANFORD (1943)									
BENTON	WA	8.6	17.9	25.7	109%	200%	7	47	77
FRANKLIN	WA	8.2	13.1	19.9	59%	142%	2	12	18
GRANT	WA	25.6	26.9	15.3	5%	-40%	10	37	23
OAK RIDGE (1943)									
ANDERSON	TN	18.7	21.6	23.9	16%	28%	17	50	58
ROANE	TN	21.6	16.9	16.5	-22%	-24%	14	27	30
INEL (1949)									
BINGHAM	ID	7.0	17.7	21.9	153%	213%	3	14	21
BUTTE	ID	0.0	20.6	7.7			0	2	1
JEFFERSON	ID	0.0	26.9	19.1			0	10	9
SAVANNAH RIVER (1950)									
BURKE	GA	6.9	19.7	10.9	184%	57%	1	5	4
AIKEN	SC	18.9	20.0	21.8	6%	15%	16	50	64
BARNWELL	SC	28.7	25.2	8.8	-12%	-69%	5	9	4
LOS ALAMOS/SANDIA (1943, 1950)									
LOS ALAMOS	NM	63.1	49.9	18.9	-21%	-70%	2	21	10
BERNALILLO	NM	22.3	25.6	26.7	15%	20%	62	285	342
BROOKHAVEN (1950)									
SUFFOLK	NY	23.2	31.3	32.4	35%	40%	232	1140	1285
ABOVE 14 COUNTIES		**20.9**	**27.9**	**28.6**	**33%**	**37%**	**371**	**1709**	**1946**
DOE FACILITIES WITHOUT REACTORS									
MOUND (1947)									
BUTLER	OH	27.9	24.1	24.9	-14%	-11%	100	172	202
MONTGOMERY	OH	27.1	28.3	27.0	5%	-0%	265	442	451
WARREN	OH	16.5	21.3	25.0	29%	51%	18	57	77
FERNALD (1951)									
HAMILTON	OH	30.0	29.7	29.5	-1%	-2%	615	759	803
PORTSMOUTH (1952)									
PIKE	OH	19.5	6.5	10.9	-67%	-44%	7	6	9
ROCKY FLATS (1953)									
BOULDER	CO	22.0	24.6	20.8	12%	-6%	34	113	108
JEFFERSON	CO	25.0	26.0	23.4	4%	-6%	37	238	258
PADUCAH (1950)									
BALLARD	KY	21.5	25.4	9.2	18%	-57%	5	7	3
MC CRACKEN	KY	23.0	17.9	20.7	-22%	-10%	29	42	54
ABOVE 9 COUNTIES		**27.9**	**26.8**	**26.1**	**-4%**	**-6%**	**1110**	**1836**	**1965**

Fission products, such as strontium-90, which concentrate in the bone like calcium, emit beta rays that can travel many millimeters and can reach the bone marrow where the cells of the immune system originate. Alpha particles emitted by radium and uranium can travel only a few thousandths of a millimeter and are therefore unable to affect immune system function to the same degree, which is not to say that they do not have other detrimental effects. Alpha particles can do serious damage when deposited in the lung or digestive organs.

In fact, that is precisely what the NCI data show for Fernald and Portsmouth in the NCI tables I–8.7 and I–8.8 in volume 1 of the NCI study.[9] In these tables, no significant increases are shown for the Standardized Mortality Ratios for breast cancer after start-up, but extraordinarily significant increases are shown for cancer mortality of the digestive organs and for lung cancer as indicated by the number of standard deviations associated with each increase as follows:

	SMR Before Start-up	SMR After Start-up	Deaths After Start-up	Ratio of Gain	No. of St. Dev.
Portsmouth					
Digestive Organs	.77	.95	316	1.23	2.6
Lung	.60	.91	200	1.51	4.0
Fernald					
Digestive Organs	1.07	1.16	20756	1.08	7.7
Lung	1.12	1.31	14165	1.17	13.0

"NUCLEAR" COUNTIES WITHIN 50 MILES OF REACTOR SITES

In table 7–2, in accordance with Mangano's findings, we have extended the definition of "nuclear" counties to include contiguous rural counties within 50 miles of each installation to show that those living that close, especially if downwind, are at greater risk than is suggested by table 6–1, where the limited NCI definition of a "nuclear" county was used. Our choice of 50 miles was guided by the fact that the Nuclear Regulatory Commission uses a 50-mile definition to calculate population doses in connection with nuclear plant licensing procedures.

In table 7–2 we have summarized the results of extending the definition of "nuclear" counties for each reactor site to include a total of 346 exposed rural counties within roughly 50 miles of each reactor.

TABLE 7-2 AGE-ADJUSTED WHITE FEMALE BREAST CANCER RATES 1950-89 IN 346 NUCLEAR COUNTIES WITHIN 50 MILES OF EACH SITE
Deaths per 100,000

No. of Counties	Reactor Site	Age-Adjusted Mortality Rates			Percent Change 80-84/50-54	85-89/50-54	Breast Cancer Deaths			St. Dev.	
		1950-54	80-84	85-89	50-54	50-54	50-54	80-84	85-89	80-84	85-89
11	Hanford (1943)	19.6	21.7	23.8	11%	21%	144	316	369		2.6
20	Oak Ridge (1943)	15.5	20.8	21.4	34%	38%	261	672	687	5.3	5.8
14	Savannah River (1950)	17.7	21.3	18.9	20%	7%	86	237	227	2.0	
3	Idaho Natl. Eng. (1949)	4.8	20.6	20.1	333%	322%	3	26	31	3.8	4.1
11	Los Alamos/Sandia (1943)	17.7	24.4	24.0	38%	36%	101	476	563	4.8	5.0
1	Brookhaven (1950)	22.9	30.0	31.0	31%	36%	378	1444	1627	7.1	8.5
6	Beaver Valley (1957)	21.4	25.7	25.3	20%	18%	436	817	828	3.6	3.4
6	Dresden (1960)	21.9	27.5	27.1	26%	24%	243	504	513	3.5	3.4
2	Yankee Rowe (1960)	27.0	28.7	28.8	6%	7%	161	244	255		
6	Big Rock Point (1962)	19.7	20.4	20.4	4%	4%	39	78	88		
5	Indian Point (1962)	28.3	30.1	30.7	6%	8%	912	1659	1803	1.8	2.4
4	West Valley (1963)	25.3	30.6	28.8	21%	14%	228	350	331	2.5	1.6
8	Fermi/Davis Besse (1963)	25.1	25.8	26.6	3%	6%	558	846	948		
6	Humboldt Bay (1963)	21.5	25.4	24.7	18%	14%	77	212	235		
5	Pathfinder (1963)	23.7	22.9	25.2	-3%	6%	72	125	136		
2	Haddam Neck/Millstone (67-70)	22.5	25.6	26.8	14%	19%	146	304	342		2.3
11	La Crosse (1967)	21.6	21.9	21.2	1%	-2%	197	301	301		
4	San Onofre (1967)	23.0	26.5	25.5	15%	11%	680	3530	3885	5.8	4.4
15	Ginna/Nine Mile/Fitzpat. (1969)	28.2	27.3	28.6	-3%	1%	1426	1987	2108		
6	Oyster Creek (1969)	28.0	29.6	29.7	6%	6%	781	2254	2577	1.8	2.1
5	Point Beach/Kewaunee (1970)	25.6	27.3	26.1	7%	2%	196	364	374		
15	Robinson (1970)	17.4	22.1	22.1	27%	27%	119	325	373	3.0	3.2
5	Monticello (1970)	24.3	22.9	25.4	-6%	5%	62	109	132		
4	Palisades/Cook (1971-75)	21.9	25.1	24.5	15%	12%	199	386	394	1.9	
8	Maine Yankee (1972)	23.9	27.3	24.8	14%	4%	262	427	429	1.9	
3	Pilgrim (1972)	28.1	30.6	30.6	9%	9%	1315	1716	1721	2.5	2.5
3	Quad Cities (1972)	24.8	24.8	24.6	-0%	-1%	202	294	309		
3	Surry (1972)	23.2	25.9	29.4	12%	27%	62	185	238		2.5
5	Turkey Point (1972)	18.7	23.6	23.6	26%	26%	422	3391	3881	9.3	10.2
3	Vermont Yankee (1972)	22.5	24.4	27.9	8%	24%	66	119	140		1.8
3	Zion (1972)	32.1	27.3	27.9	-15%	-13%	257	503	590		
10	Browns Ferry (1973)	17.5	23.8	21.9	36%	25%	109	368	376	4.1	3.0
2	Fort Calhoun (1973)	18.2	32.9	17.3	80%	-5%	19	35	24	2.3	
5	Oconee (1973)	16.3	22.7	25.5	39%	56%	88	339	435	4.1	6.3
7	Prairie Island (1973)	24.1	24.5	27.9	2%	16%	119	247	314		1.8
12	Arkansas One 1 & 2 (1974)	14.4	17.9	20.0	24%	39%	51	138	185	1.8	3.1
2	Calvert Cliffs (1974)	23.9	28.3	26.8	18%	12%	87	329	326	2.1	
3	Cooper Station (1974)	24.9	27.8	21.6	12%	-13%	28	28	21		
10	Duane Arnold (1974)	21.7	24.2	24.1	12%	11%	246	412	397		
14	Hatch 1 & 2 (1974)	12.0	16.2	18.2	35%	52%	29	78	93	1.8	2.7

TABLE 7-2 CONTINUED
AGE-ADJUSTED WHITE FEMALE BREAST CANCER RATES 1950-89 IN 346 NUCLEAR COUNTIES WITHIN 50 MILES OF EACH SITE
Deaths per 100,000

No. of Counties	Reactor Site	Age-Adjusted Mortality Rates			Percent Change 80-84/ 85-89/		Breast Cancer Deaths			St. Dev.	
		1950-54	80-84	85-89	50-54	50-54	50-54	80-84	85-89	80-84	85-89
7	Peach Bottom (1974)	24.6	26.2	26.8	7%	9%	593	1643	1869	1.8	2.6
6	Rancho Seco (1974)	20.8	25.3	26.5	21%	27%	211	827	1010	3.9	5.3
9	Three Mile Island (1974)	23.3	25.6	27.2	10%	17%	740	1183	1258	2.2	3.8
6	Brunswick (1975)	18.0	19.5	21.1	8%	18%	54	145	189		
7	Trojan (1975)	23.8	24.0	25.1	1%	5%	183	456	532		
2	Fort St. Vrain (1976)	21.7	19.7	23.2	-9%	7%	61	140	197		
3	Salem (1976)	26.9	30.1	30.1	12%	12%	663	1338	1408	2.9	3.0
5	St. Lucie (1976)	16.0	23.3	24.8	46%	55%	37	479	649	5.6	7.6
7	Farley (1977)	16.1	17.4	20.8	8%	29%	37	84	105		1.8
4	Crystal River (1977)	16.6	23.3	23.8	40%	43%	21	223	333	3.5	4.5
10	North Anna (1978)	13.0	20.5	22.5	58%	73%	34	108	132	3.2	4.2
6	Sequoya (1980)	18.0	22.3	20.9	24%	16%	104	268	269	2.5	
6	McGuire (1981)	18.0	21.7	26.3	21%	46%	164	501	663	2.9	6.7
346	Total, all sites	24.1	26.1	26.4	8%	10%	13769	33570	37220	10.2	12.4
	Continental US	24.4	24.9	24.5	2%	1%	91392	167803	178868		

(See appendix B.) Since the size of each county varies greatly, some-times only 3 or 4 counties were required for the aggregated mortality trend to achieve statistical significance. Sometimes many more were needed. On average, for the 60 reactor sites 7 or 8 counties were required. (Later we shall consider the results of extending the definition of proximity to include all counties within a radius of 50 miles and then 100 miles.)

Appendix B includes maps and basic breast cancer mortality data for the contiguous "nuclear" counties within 50 and 100 miles of 60 reactor sites. We include the three DOE reactor sites that were omitted from the NCI study. Since we are testing the effects of such reactor emissions as radioactive iodine and strontium on breast can-cer risk, we have excluded the five DOE nuclear installations that do not have operating reactors (Mound, Portsmouth, Paducah, Fernald, and Rocky Flats). This brings the total number of reactor sites examined in table 7–2 to 60.

Table 7–2 shows a far greater divergence in breast cancer mortality trends than the NCI counterpart (table 6–1) does. Only 5 of the 60 sites failed to show an overall increase greater than the national increase within 50 miles of the reactor, and only 17 failed to show a statistically significant increase, for which the increase was equivalent to less than 1.8 standard deviations. (In this table we only show the number of standard deviations over 1.8, which can be regarded as the minimum number to denote significant change.) This is in sharp contrast to the results of table 6–1, where using the NCI definition of "nuclear" counties, only about one-half of all facilities studied by the NCI registered increased breast cancer risk over time—and almost no change achieved statistical significance. In the aggregate, the rates for the 346 rural "nuclear" counties increased by 8 and 10 percent from 1950–54 to 1980–84 and to 1985–89, a divergence from the national change equivalent to more than 10 standard deviations. Therefore there can be no question that these 346 mainly rural counties within 50 miles of reactor sites represent problem areas in which the risk of dying of breast cancer has increased significantly over time.

Another way to dramatize the epidemiological anomaly of the extent to which the breast cancer mortality risk is heightened in these 346 "nuclear" rural counties is as follows: in 1950–54 they accounted for 15 percent of all breast cancer deaths, but by 1985–89 they accounted for 21 percent of the total, although representing only 11 percent of all counties.

It bears repeating that the upward divergence of breast cancer trends among the aggregated counties downwind of reactors, as compared with the United States, could not possibly be due to chance. The divergence from the national trend is equivalent to more than 10 standard deviations, for which the chance probability is infinitesimal.

The upward divergence of breast cancer rates for these counties also cannot be regarded as an assurance for those living further away, beyond suggesting that over time some malevolent force associated with reactor emissions is making downwind proximity to operating reactors an increasingly important risk factor. Aside from the consumption of milk, dairy products, meat, and vegetables produced near nuclear plants and shipped over large distances, there are several additional factors to be considered in assessing such risk.

Breast Cancer Mortality Trends and Rainfall

Mangano also found a far more significant increase in white cancer mortality trends in 20 high-altitude counties (with elevations exceeding 1,500 feet above sea level) near Oak Ridge than in 20 equally close low-altitude counties, which suggests that high precipitation levels also play a role in the direct exposure of residents of neighboring counties to the ingestion of nuclear fission products.[14] We have already noted in chapter 5 that the flat low-rainfall states between the Rocky Mountain range and the Mississippi River have the lowest exposure to fallout and accordingly have the lowest breast cancer mortality rates.

Thus a more precise definition of contiguous "nuclear" counties, which may be more directly exposed to fission products from each individual reactor site, should include nearby high-altitude counties with high rainfall levels. Counties that are downstream of reactor sites are also more likely to be directly exposed over time to radioactive run-off than people living upstream.

Unfortunately, most of the nation's civilian reactors have been built in states with precipitation levels of over 30 inches per year. There are only five civilian reactors (Pathfinder, Cooper Station, Fort Calhoun, Fort St. Vrain, and Quad Cities) in states with annual precipitation levels below 15 inches. These are the only reactor sites in appendix B that fail to show a significant upward divergence in breast cancer mortality near the reactor sites.

The Convergence of Rural and Urban Cancer Rates

The 346 "nuclear" counties within 50 miles of each reactor site act as another example to demonstrate the convergence of rural and urban cancer mortality rates, which can be taken as a characteristic of the logarithmic dose response to radiation.

We illustrate this convergence in figure 7–1, in which, for each of the 346 counties within 50 miles of 60 reactor sites, we have plotted the ratio of change in the breast cancer rates from 1950–54 to 1985–89 against the corresponding rate in 1950–54. The lower right quadrant is dominated by the more urban and industrial counties that had above-average cancer mortality rates in 1950–54 and had lower than average ratios of increase. There are few observations in the upper

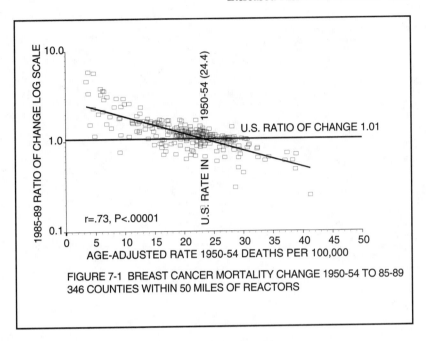

FIGURE 7-1 BREAST CANCER MORTALITY CHANGE 1950-54 TO 85-89
346 COUNTIES WITHIN 50 MILES OF REACTORS

right quadrant for urban counties with above average rates that had greater than average ratios of increase, and relatively few observations in the lower left quadrant for rural counties with less than average ratios of increase. The correlation ratio of .73 for the 346 counties is very close to the correlation of .74 accounted for by the corresponding analysis of the logarithmic increase in mortality rates observed for all rural counties in chapter 5.

The universal tendency for rural and urban cancer rates to converge over time means that there will some day be very little difference between them. All areas will ultimately achieve the same high levels of cancer mortality. This is especially true if other nuclear plants are built, and the contamination of drinking water and milk is allowed to continue, not to speak of further accidents like TMI and Chernobyl. Thus it becomes all the more important to understand the historical context in which this great change occurred, which we will review in the next chapter.

Chapter 8

FALLOUT AND BREAST CANCER

We have learned that large urban states and counties had the nation's highest breast cancer mortality rates in 1950–54, the earliest period for which age-adjusted rates are available. We see from the convergence of rural and urban cancer mortality rates that urban rates have not advanced percentage wise as much as the rates for rural counties have. In many cases, urban rates have declined slightly. This does not mean that urban rates have improved in any significant sense; their breast cancer rates remain significantly above the national average.

Along with nearby rural counties, the large urban counties are vulnerable to neighboring reactor emissions in addition to all the other stresses of urban life and greater exposure to environmental toxins of all kinds. It is probable that urban/rural differences existed well before the Nuclear Age began. We shall see that the earliest biological impact of nuclear fallout affected large cities like New York, dependent as they are on surface water reservoirs rather than underground wells. Large cities were also first to be exposed to the adverse consequences of nuclear fallout acting synergistically with exposure to industrial chemicals and air pollution.

MILK CONSUMPTION IN LARGE CITIES

Another explanation for the greater adverse biological impact of low-level radiation in the large urban centers has to do with the quality of the milk consumed there, which all too often comes from dairy farms located close to civilian power reactors. This story is told in chapter 8 of *Deadly Deceit* (entitled "Infant Mortality and Milk") and is particularly applicable to residents of large urban counties in the northeast with the heaviest concentration of nuclear reactors.

We offered as a chilling example the case of the troublesome Peach Bottom reactors located in Lancaster County, Pennsylvania, one of the nation's leading milk production centers. On April 30, 1987, the Nuclear Regulatory Commission closed the Peach Bottom reactors, accusing the plant operators of "taking drugs and sleeping on the job." In that month infant mortality in Washington, D.C., a major consumer of milk from Lancaster County, had reached an all-time peak level of 35 deaths per 1,000 births. Three months later the rate declined sharply to 10 infant deaths per 1,000 births—the national average—implicating radioactive iodine in the milk available to mothers in the nation's capital.[11]

PAST OVERUSE OF X RAYS IN AFFLUENT URBAN AREAS

There are other ways in which breast cancer may have been promoted in large urban areas by ionizing radiation. It is the opinion of Dr. John Gofman that many of the current high breast cancer incidence rates can be attributed to unnecessarily high doses from early X rays and fluoroscopy. Ironically, the less affluent rural counties probably could not afford such overexposure.

In this matter, there may be no greater authority than Gofman, a former director of biomedical research at the Lawrence Livermore National Laboratory, who was fired in 1959 when he predicted that emissions from the new generations of civilian power reactors would cause future cancer epidemics. He recently announced his belief that past applications of radiation in nuclear medicine have been overlooked. Even the widespread use of mobile X ray units for mass screening of tuberculosis, frequent irradiation of breasts in the treatment of tuberculosis, and irradiation for thyroid enlargement in infants, may be involved. He cites the fact that in 1950 New York City hospitals had a maximum dose of 100 rads per chest examination. Today's mammograms expose highly sensitive breast tissue to no more than 0.4 rads.[55]

New York City also has the best statistical records of breast cancer mortality prior to 1950. Before we examine them it is worth reviewing some of the early effects of the initial introduction of fission products into the pristine atmosphere in 1945, before our county breast cancer mortality data became available in 1950. Because of the logarithmic nature of the dose response to low-level radiation, it is likely that the greatest damage occurred in the years 1945–50, not covered by our breast cancer mortality database.

THE TRAUMATIC IMPACT OF NUCLEAR EMISSIONS IN 1945

We now know that 1945 may have been by far the worst year in our history with respect to the subsequent epidemiological anomalies uncovered in this book. Recapping material in chapter 2, in that year the following events occurred:

1. According to recent DOE reports, enormous emissions from Hanford and Oak Ridge, equaling the magnitude of Chernobyl emissions, exposed the American population to per capita emissions of more than 4 billion picocuries of radioactive iodine.

2. The first atomic bomb, developed at Los Alamos, was set off in New Mexico on July 19, 1945.

3. In 1945 the percentage of underweight live births began to rise in New York State to reach an all-time peak just after the cessation of above-ground testing. New York City began recording the postwar rise in low-birthweight live births in 1948—New York was the first city to do so.

4. Breast cancer incidence started to rise in Connecticut in 1945, after a decline from 1935 to 1944, and has continued to rise ever since.

The ultimate impact of the introduction of man-made fission products into a once pristine atmosphere are revealed by the extraordinary increase in the age-adjusted breast cancer mortality rates in the counties most directly affected by the earliest emissions. For example, the greatest increases occurred in the counties in which the first DOE reactor sites were built in 1943—Hanford, Oak Ridge, and Los Alamos. In table 7–1 we included some additional DOE reactor sites built a few years later—INEL, Sandia, Savannah River, and Brookhaven—in order to secure a total of 14 counties with sufficient current deaths to achieve statistical significance.

In table 7–1 we noted that women in these 14 counties registered an increase of 37 percent in the aggregated age-adjusted breast cancer mortality rate over the 35-year period. This represents the highest significant increase we have found for any group of counties linked by a common early exposure to nuclear fission products.

In table 5–1 we listed North Carolina and New Mexico as states with the greatest percentages of overall increase in breast cancer mortality since 1950–54. These increases, about 30 percent, fall short of the record of the 14 counties in which the DOE reactors are located.

Breast Cancer and Los Alamos

North Carolina can be viewed as a rural state equally exposed to emissions from Oak Ridge and Savannah River, but the New Mexico breast cancer mortality rise was initially puzzling to us; New Mexico has no civilian reactors. The National Cancer Institute had not included the Sandia/Los Alamos laboratories among the DOE nuclear facilities selected for study, despite the fact that these two laboratories had recorded the generation and on-site burial of large amounts of radioactive wastes.[56]

While the NCI appeared not to regard radiation from the Los Alamos Nuclear Laboratory (LANL) as a problem, local residents have long been apprehensive. A communication from Susan Hirshberg of Santa Fe Concerned Citizens for Nuclear Safety, states these fears, with supporting references from official LANL documents:

> Los Alamos purposely released large amounts of radioactivity into the air through a series of test explosions that were performed in Bayo Canyon between 1944 and 1961. There were over 250 explosions each of which released 100 to 1,000 curies of lanthanum-140 and strontium-90 into the air. The Bayo Canyon tests were known to have caused extensive exposure to fallout in Los Alamos County, particularly in the years prior to 1950. A 1949 document from the lab's health division tersely states, "It was formerly felt that little or no significant radioactivity was being deposited in the surrounding country as a result of these (Bayo Canyon) operations." More recent observations have shown that this is not the case.
>
> Tens of thousands of curies of tritium were released into the air from at least one test explosion in the 1950s. Other sources such as waste dumps and day-to-day LANL operations also released large amounts of tritium. . . . LANL continued to release many thousands of curies of tritium into the air well into the 1980s. In 1974 alone, over 38,000 curies of tritium were released. . . .

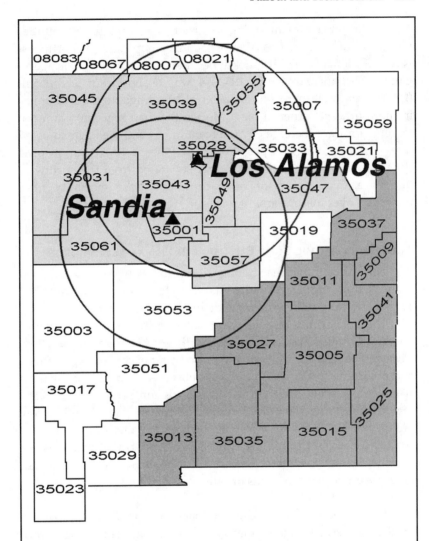

FIGURE 8-1 NEW MEXICO BREAST CANCER INCREASES
In this county map of New Mexico, the counties are divided into three sectors. The northwestern tier of shaded counties are those roughly within 50 miles of the Sandia and Los Alamos laboratories. The southwestern tier (also shaded) includes those counties directly affected by the first Trinity test of 1945. These two sectors contribute to the extraordinary increase in New Mexico's age-adjusted breast cancer rates since 1950–54 shown in table 8–1. The circles represent areas within 50 miles of Los Alamos and Sandia. The Trinity test site is located just west of Lincoln County (35027) in the lower right corner of Socorro County (35053).

In the process of mapping a cluster of 11 contiguous counties within 50 miles of the Los Alamos/Sandia complex in the northwest sector of New Mexico, it quickly became apparent that their aggregate overall increase since 1950–54 was a significant 36 percent (P<.001), but that there was a cluster of 10 contiguous rural counties in the southeast corner of New Mexico that had registered an even larger significant increase of 72 percent in its combined age-adjusted rates—from 12.1 deaths per 100,000 in 1950–54 to 20.9 in 1980–84 (P<.001). These counties were clearly separated from the northwest tier by a third group of rural counties whose mortality rates improved over these years.

THE TRINITY ATOMIC BOMB EXPLOSION IN 1945 AT ALAMOGORDO

We soon realized that the southeastern counties were those exposed to the well-recorded and totally unanticipated impact of the very first Trinity nuclear bomb, which was detonated July 19, 1945.

The 1945 Trinity test site was located in the southeast corner of Socorro County, about 30 miles north of Alamogordo in Otero County. The resulting radioactive cloud by far exceeded expectations and according to *Day of Trinity*[57] was observed to drift "northeast at 10 miles per hour, dropping its trail of fission products across the region, measuring 100 miles long and 30 miles wide." Within a few hours, the radioactivity in towns such as Coyote, Carrizozo, and Ancho in Lincoln County were measured at 35 to 100 roentgens per hour. (A roentgen, similar to a rad, is a measure of radiation intensity; exposure to 400 roentgens or rads was sufficient to kill Hiroshima victims instantly.)

The northeastern drift of the radioactive cloud did not stop at the borders of New Mexico. Humankind's first exposure to fission products from a nuclear bomb explosion was found to produce X ray film imperfections at the Eastman Kodak labs in Rochester, New York, in the fall of 1945. This in turn was traced to the presence of radioactive cerium in strawboard produced for Eastman Kodak in Indiana from water taken from the Wabash and Iowa Rivers. The Kodak radiation specialists finally came up with the explanation:

> The tiny white dots on their film were the footprints of the atomic explosion that occurred in July in New Mexico. Neutron bombard-

ment from the detonation had transformed the stable cerium–140 found in the soil into radioactive cerium–141. . . .

Closer to the test site, the atomic radiation had already manifested its presence in a variety of unusual ways . . . the Herefords in the immediate vicinity of the Trinity were losing their hair. . . .[57]

A more ominous indication of the immediate direct impact of the Trinity explosion was the fact that white infant mortality in New Mexico rose by 11 percent from 1944 to 1945, compared with a corresponding 4 percent decline in the United States. The fact that a peak in breast cancer mortality occurred in New Mexico 35 years later takes on additional significance in light of the fact that the Trinity explosion had a yield of only 12 kilotons. It was completely dwarfed by the yield of U.S. and Soviet atmospheric bomb tests in the period 1951–62, which was estimated by the Natural Resources Council to total some 580,000 kilotons.[30]

The effect of the Trinity explosion is seen most clearly by an inspection of table 8–1, where 9 out of the 10 counties in the southeast corner of New Mexico are seen to have registered increases in breast cancer mortality rates between 1950–54 and 1980–84, for an average of a 72 percent increase for this group. During this same period, the 11 counties spared by the releases from Los Alamos, Sandia, and Trinity improved their mortality rates by an average of 16 percent. This last group showed a remarkably consistent overall decline of 25 percent from 1950–54 to 1985–89, suggesting again that pesticides and herbicides by themselves cannot explain the rise in breast cancer mortality in rural counties.

Thus, in the absence of a plausible alternative explanation, it appears what was a pristine rural area in the southeast sector of New Mexico registered its largest percentage increase in breast cancer mortality from 1950–54 to 1980–84 as a result of an event that occurred 40 years earlier. If that is true, we may well wonder about the effects of the 100 or more atmospheric bombs tested at the Nevada test site beginning in 1951. Figure 2–12 tracks the Nevada above-ground tests and suggests how widespread the consequent damage must be.

This is indeed a sobering thought 50 years after birth of the Nuclear Age, and serves as a warning of the delayed health effects of low-level radiation from the making and testing of nuclear bombs.

TABLE 8-1 NEW MEXICO WHITE FEMALE BREAST CANCER MORTALITY RATES 1950-89
Deaths per 100,000 Women

FIPS Code	County	ST	Age-Adjusted Mortality Rates			Percent Change 80-84/ 85-89/		Number of Deaths		
			1950-54	80-84	85-89	50-54	50-54	50-54	80-84	85-89
COUNTIES WITHIN 50 MILES OF SANDIA AND LOS ALAMOS										
35001	BERNALILLO	NM	22.3	25.6	26.7	15%	20%	62	285	342
35028	LOS ALAMOS	NM	63.1	49.9	18.9	-21%	-70%	2	21	10
35031	MC KINLEY	NM	4.5	30.3	12.3	575%	175%	1	12	6
35039	RIO ARRIBA	NM	7.3	17.3	21.9	136%	200%	3	11	16
35043	SANDOVAL	NM	0.0	24.7	24.2			0	20	30
35045	SAN JUAN	NM	10.3	18.1	23.0	76%	123%	3	24	36
35047	SAN MIGUEL	NM	12.3	20.7	23.4	68%	90%	6	12	18
35049	SANTA FE	NM	26.9	24.2	24.2	-10%	-10%	18	53	68
35055	TAOS	NM	7.4	9.8	11.7	32%	59%	2	5	8
35057	TORRANCE	NM	13.2	14.9	17.1	13%	29%	2	3	4
35061	VALENCIA	NM	4.6	25.4	16.4	457%	259%	2	30	25
TOTAL	**ABOVE 11**		**17.7**	**24.4**	**24.0**	**38%**	**36%**	**101**	**476**	**563**
COUNTIES TRACKING 1945 TRINITY TEST										
35005	CHAVES	NM	14.9	23.0	23.3	55%	57%	10	39	45
35009	CURRY	NM	4.7	19.8	19.5	319%	311%	2	21	25
35011	DE BACA	NM	13.3	27.7	18.3	109%	38%	1	3	2
35013	DONA ANA	NM	13.0	20.4	20.0	57%	53%	9	44	57
35015	EDDY	NM	18.8	13.9	14.9	-26%	-21%	13	26	29
35025	LEA	NM	8.2	17.2	17.5	110%	113%	5	30	28
35027	LINCOLN	NM	0.0	23.0	6.9			0	8	4
35035	OTERO	NM	13.0	29.2	15.0	124%	15%	3	28	18
35037	QUAY	NM	22.3	28.0	4.7	26%	-79%	6	11	2
35041	ROOSEVELT	NM	2.7	24.7	21.3	798%	674%	1	13	10
TOTAL	**ABOVE 10**		**12.1**	**20.9**	**17.9**	**72%**	**47%**	**50**	**223**	**220**
ALL OTHER COUNTIES IN NEW MEXICO										
35003	CATRON	NM	20.2	0.0	15.6	-100%	-23%	1	0	2
35007	COLFAX	NM	23.4	12.4	14.1	-47%	-40%	8	6	9
35017	GRANT	NM	19.4	19.4	16.3	-0%	-16%	8	17	17
35019	GUADALUPE	NM	9.2	6.3	3.1	-32%	-66%	1	1	1
35021	HARDING	NM	67.6	0.0	51.4	-100%	-24%	4	0	1
35023	HIDALGO	NM	0.0	16.4	44.5			0	4	7
35029	LUNA	NM	36.5	22.4	19.9	-39%	-45%	6	15	12
35033	MORA	NM	5.8	17.7	0.0	204%	-100%	1	2	0
35051	SIERRA	NM	18.9	20.4	16.3	8%	-14%	4	11	5
35053	SOCORRO	NM	22.8	14.2	19.1	-37%	-16%	4	5	7
35059	UNION	NM	25.7	33.2	4.0	29%	-85%	4	6	1
TOTAL	**ABOVE 11**		**21.4**	**18.0**	**16.1**	**-16%**	**-25%**	**41**	**67**	**62**
TOTAL	**NEW MEXICO**		**16.3**	**22.7**	**21.3**	**39%**	**31%**	**192**	**766**	**845**
TOTAL	**UNITED STATES**		**24.4**	**24.9**	**24.6**	**2%**	**1%**	**91392**	**167803**	**178868**

These results also illustrate the logarithmic nature of the dose response of breast cancer to radiation. While that response is greatest for pristine rural areas with initial low exposures to carcinogens, all other areas are adversely affected, too. The logarithmic nature of the dose response suggests that the greatest radiation-induced harm to the immune response may have come from the earliest bomb tests, in spite of their low yields compared to the enormous emissions from the later thermonuclear tests, which produced worldwide contamination of the atmosphere, primarily in the form of rain.

A secondary conclusion is that—in the absence of further exposure from the manufacture and testing of nuclear weapons—because of continuing exposure to emissions from civilian power reactors, the convergence of rural and urban cancer mortality rates in the United States may increasingly obscure the historical causes for that convergence. New Mexico, now least affected by emissions from civilian power reactors, illustrates how persistent the delayed health effects of exposure are to man-made fission products. It is only in the most recent five-year period that breast cancer mortality in New Mexico, clearly a product of early exposure to nuclear radiation, has begun to decline. The greatest percentage declines in recent years occurred in the area downwind of the Trinity explosion, but the current combined rate remains 47 percent above the original very low 1950–54 mortality rate. As we saw in table 5–1, that is true for all the states comprising the Mountain region. Despite the fact that they were the first states to be adversely affected by emissions from the Nevada explosions, in the absence of emissions from civilian reactors they are now beginning to improve their mortality rates—a hopeful sign indeed.

The case of New Mexico illustrates the fact that for a full explanation of the causal factors behind each cluster of the worst breast cancer counties, an intimate knowledge of a host of local environmental factors is required.

BREAST CANCER MORTALITY IN THE NEW YORK METROPOLITAN AREA

The nation's greatest concentration of breast cancer mortality can be found in the New York metropolitan area. This area, with 3.9 percent of the white female population, accounts for 5.4 percent of all breast cancer deaths. Because this area represents the nation's single worst breast cancer problem, we have chosen it for a detailed epidemiological examination.

We begin with table 8–2, in which we summarize the change since 1950 in the age-adjusted breast cancer mortality rates of the combined eight counties making up the New York metropolitan area. (No further breakdown of the five counties of New York City is available in the NCI cancer data files.)

TABLE 8-2   WHITE FEMALE BREAST CANCER MORTALITY RATES 1950-89 NEW YORK METROPOLITAN COUNTIES
Deaths per 100,000 Women

County	ST	Age-Adjusted Mortality Rates			Percent Change		Number of Deaths		
		1950-54	80-84	85-89	80-84/ 1950-54	85-89/ 1950-54	1950-54	80-84	85-89
NEW YORK CITY	NY	31.8	29.4	28.3	0.92	0.89	6817	6102	5755
WESTCHESTER	NY	30.7	30.7	32.0	1.00	1.04	586	943	1011
NASSAU	NY	34.8	33.0	32.8	0.95	0.94	646	1522	1541
SUFFOLK	NY	23.2	31.3	32.4	1.35	1.40	232	1140	1285
TOTAL		31.6	30.2	29.8	0.96	0.95	8281	9707	9592
U.S. TOTAL		24.4	24.9	24.6	1.02	1.01	91392	167803	178868

We note that the combined breast cancer mortality rate is far above the national average. In fact, despite some improvement over the 35-year span, that improvement is meaningless in the face of the fact that the 1985–89 aggregated rate of 29.8 deaths per 100,000 women is the highest in the nation for such a concentrated urban area—equivalent to 15 standard deviations, for which the chance probability is too small to be calculated.

What this means is that for densely populated urban areas subject to reactor emissions, we can judge the degree to which breast cancer mortality has been affected over time, not by the significant increase in rates, but by the degree to which mortality rates have remained in excess of the national average.

The reason for the improvement, such as it is, which mainly affected New York City, actually demonstrates that most of the radiation-induced biological damage occurred in the period 1945–70 (See figures 8–2 and 8–3) and is based on annual breast cancer mortality movements in both New York City and State since 1940.

With the start-up of Indian Point in Westchester in 1962, breast cancer mortality there kept pace with the city until the city shifted most of its water supply away from the Croton system. Thereafter a startling divergence became evident.

Figure 8–2 contrasts the sharp upward annual movement of breast cancer mortality rates (not age-adjusted) in New York City that began at a low point of only 16 deaths per 100,000 persons (men and women) in 1943 and increased to an initial peak of about 21 deaths in the early 1960s. In the same 17-year period there was a highly divergent downward movement in the rest of the state—from about 18 deaths per 100,000 to 16. (New York State breast cancer mortality rates cover men and women. Since male breast cancer deaths are only about 1 percent of female deaths, the trends shown in figures 8–2 to 8–5 depict mainly those of female breast cancer.)

This is the period during which the atmospheric bomb test fallout of the years 1945–62 affected surface drinking water used by New York City sooner than drinking water drawn from underground wells

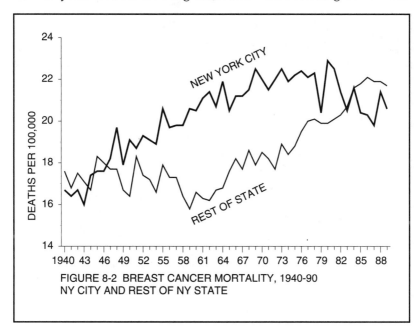

FIGURE 8-2 BREAST CANCER MORTALITY, 1940-90
NY CITY AND REST OF NY STATE

found in the rest of the state. After 1962, with the start-up of the first Indian Point reactor, mortality rates rose in tandem for both the city and the balance of the state, except for the years after 1970, when an abrupt change took place, which is best illustrated by figure 8–3.

BREAST CANCER IN WESTCHESTER

In figure 8–3 we contrast breast cancer mortality trends since 1960 in New York City with that of Westchester County to dramatize the enormous change that has taken place in recent years. This change has to do with the start-up of the Indian Point reactors in Westchester county in 1962 and 1973–76. The start-up of the Indian Point reactor, close to the Croton Reservoir, was soon followed by a rise in the Westchester breast cancer mortality rate. This was also true for New York City, since both shared Croton drinking water in the late 1960s. After many decades of development, about 1969, the city was able to shift the bulk of its water requirements to two new sources of water in the Catskill Mountains and the headwaters of the Delaware River, more than 100 miles from the Croton system. Large pipelines were built to bring the water into the city, and by 1967 the gigantic water supply system was completed.[51]

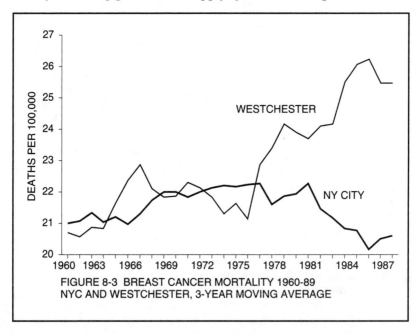

FIGURE 8-3 BREAST CANCER MORTALITY 1960-89
NYC AND WESTCHESTER, 3-YEAR MOVING AVERAGE

Thus, under normal conditions about 90 percent of New York City's water has come, since 1970, from the new distant reservoirs and only 10 percent is still obtained from the Croton watershed, located just 5 miles downwind (northeast) of the Indian Point nuclear reactors. New York City's rate stopped rising in the early 1970s and actually began to decline, but with the start-up of two more large reactors at Indian Point in the early 1970s, the Westchester rate rose sharply until it exceeded New York City's.

In appendix C, we show that the Indian Point reactors #1 and #2, according to reports submitted to the NRC in 1989, released more than 14 curies of airborne radioactive iodine and strontium in 1985 and 1986—equal to 14 trillion picocuries. (This enormous release, equivalent to what the NRC reported to have been released from the stricken Three Mile Island reactor in 1979, was later revised downward to 2 trillion picocuries, which is still a worrisome release.)

We drew this to the attention of a reporter of New York's *Village Voice* who wrote a story published on September 1, 1992, entitled "Reservoirs at Risk." It revealed that New York City environmental officials did not know of this release and did not have access to radioactivity measurements of Croton water.[59]

The Millstone reactors on Connecticut's Long Island Sound (only 12 miles from Long Island) released enormous amounts of airborne and liquid radioactive fission products in the early 1970s, as shown by figure 8–4. Data shown in appendix C indicate that since 1970s, the #1 Millstone reactor released 32.6 trillion picocuries of airborne radioactive iodine and strontium. As a result, in 1975 highly radioactive readings (26 picocuries per liter) were found in milk at the closest sampling station, which is 5 miles northwest of the plant—these readings were higher than the previous peak of 23 reported for Connecticut in 1962—the final year of superpower above-ground tests.[11]

Although airborne emissions from Indian Point could also affect Nassau County, which is well within the 50 mile range, Long Island is far more threatened by the huge amounts of airborne and liquid fission products discharged from the Millstone plant. (See figure 8–5) According to data in appendix C, airborne releases from both Indian Point and Millstone come to 50 curies since 1970s, which means that the 6.8 million residents of Connecticut, Westchester County, and Long Island have been exposed at the rate of 7.6 million picocuries per per-

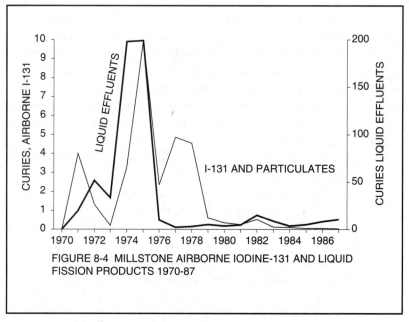

FIGURE 8-4 MILLSTONE AIRBORNE IODINE-131 AND LIQUID
FISSION PRODUCTS 1970-87

son—nearly 5 times the national *per capita* average of 1.64 million picocuries (alternatively expressed as 1.64 curies per million persons).

These are incredibly large amounts—sufficient to make the Long
Island Sound a highly radioactive body of water—and far exceed
reported releases from the Three Mile Island accident of 1979. They
help explain the sharp breast cancer mortality rises since 1970s for
Westchester (figure 8–3), Long Island (figure 8–5), and, as we shall soon
see, in Connecticut, too.

BROOKHAVEN AND BREAST CANCER IN SUFFOLK

The data supporting figures 8–2 through 8–5 were assembled by members of the Radiation and Public Health Project in 1993 in response to
a request by a Long Island breast cancer survivors coalition One in
Nine. We were asked to serve as their scientific advisors because of
their frustration with the explanations offered by public officials for the
Long Island breast cancer epidemic. They were particularly angered
by being initially told by the National Cancer Institute that there were
no environmental factors involved and that the epidemic was due to
the dominating presence of "affluent Jewish women."

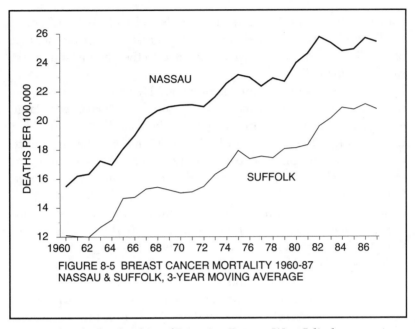

FIGURE 8-5 BREAST CANCER MORTALITY 1960-87
NASSAU & SUFFOLK, 3-YEAR MOVING AVERAGE

Under the leadership of Lorraine Pace, a West Islip breast cancer survivor, the One in Nine women undertook a door-to-door survey and found some blue collar (and non-Jewish) neighborhoods where almost every other household reported a recent breast cancer case or death. They prepared colored maps (red for deaths, yellow for incidence) of their results, which were featured on several national television shows. This publicity forced the New York State Tumor Registry to release—for the first time—age-adjusted breast cancer incidence rates for every community in Long Island.

We were first shown this data at an Adelphi College conference in the fall of 1993. After mapping the data, my colleague Dr. Sternglass, immediately noticed that the highest rates were within 15 miles of the Brookhaven National Laboratory (BNL). He speculated that these high rates may be delayed manifestations of radioactive discharges from BNL in the 1950s and 1960s, which, in an article published in 1972, he had associated with anomalous increases in Long Island infant mortality in the 1960s.[54]

We then sought to bring our suspicions to the attention of the mainstream press without much success. This changed after an accidental reported release of radioactivity from an experimental BNL reactor in March 1994 moved the Long Island University School of Public Service to ask that we prepare a paper assembling evidence that past BNL emissions may have contributed to the Long Island breast cancer epidemic.[22]

The paper made the simple point that BNL emissions of radioactive strontium—recorded in the 1950s and early 1960s, were large enough that sufficient traces might still be found in the drinking water of those towns close to BNL whose breast cancer incidence rates were significantly above the county average. We noted, too, that in the past elevated levels of tritium, a reactor product, had been found in homes near BNL and that a *New York Times* story about the March 1994 accidental release had referred to "a plume of contaminated underground water flowing in a southerly direction." We thought this might explain why the town of Brookhaven, located southwest of BNL, had reported the single highest breast cancer incidence rate in all of Long Island.

The paper, which was published by the Long Island University School of Public Service in December 1994,[22] produced a furious response from "concerned BNL scientists," along with a request that we debate the issue at a public meeting at the LIU campus. At this meeting, Dr. Sue Davis, the BNL associate director of Radiological Safety, characterized our findings as "unsupported and unfounded, incoherent and confusing." She cited the "numerous reputable scientists," including two dozen Brookhaven engineers, physicists, and physicians, who found our methodology "scientifically deficient and consisting of selected evidence."

She admitted that BNL had been cited by the EPA as a Superfund waste site but denied any responsibility for consequent possible health problems in the immediate area, saying "the causes of cancer are not known nor simplistic," but offered no advice on how to pursue an investigation of the possible environmental causes. Nor did she explain why no measurements of the radioactivity of drinking water could be made available.

By the close of 1994 agitation about the Long Island breast cancer epidemic forced the National Cancer Institute to mount a five-year study to determine the epidemic's causes, although no provisions were made to test the radioactivity of the local drinking water. The results will not appear until the turn of the century, which will presumably give Brookhaven sufficient time to deal with the pressing problem of hazardous waste disposal.

RADIOACTIVE WASTE ENDANGERS FISH

In August 1995 BNL took one step in this direction and was granted permission by the New York State Department of Environmental Conservation to upgrade the BNL sewage system by a "dewatering" process to begin early in November that would involve discharging "to the Peconic River of up to 1 million gallons per day of excess water." This water was admitted to contain nearly half a century's build-up of radioactive and heavy metal wastes, but with unspecified radioactivity levels described by BNL as "below federal and state drinking water standards."

By mid-October of 1995, two weeks before this dangerous process was to begin, William N. Smith, the director of a nonprofit recreational fishing association called Fish Unlimited, asked us for help in challenging the legality of the permit. There were no studies on how the proposed dewatering process would impact recreational and commercial fishing in the Peconic River, estuaries, and surrounding bodies of water, which are of key importance to the economy of the east end of Long Island. Dr. Sternglass and I quickly prepared affidavits on the health effects of radioactive discharges from BNL for submission to the Suffolk County Supreme Court hearing scheduled for the following week.

Within a few days, Smith was able to secure sufficient support from major business interests and local politicians in the east end to force Brookhaven to announce they would "reconsider" the proposal and promised to secure local consent before making any additional large-scale discharges into the Peconic River. BNL admitted that in the past millions of gallons of waste water with high tritium levels had been discharged into the river, but insisted that they were within safe state and federal regulations. In 1985, for example, a year in which a "brown tide" infestation of unknown etiology wiped out the prized east end bay scallops, the level of tritium in the Peconic River near BNL was reported by the New York State Health Department to be 100 times higher than the yardstick level observed in Albany.[60]

Smith was especially struck by our citation of an AEC study showing that young fish exposed to accepted levels of tritium quickly developed immune system deficiencies.[61]

I found it somewhat ironic that potential harm to fish appeared
to outranked harm to humans in arousing public opposition to radioactive pollution. We were immediately asked by another group of recreational and commercial fishermen for affidavits to oppose the disposal
of radioactive sludge from the submarine base at Groton into the Long
Island Sound near Fishers Island.

An environmental group called the Fishers Island Conservancy,
including the town of Southold, the Long Island Sound Lobstermen's
Association, the North Shore Baymen's Association, and Concerned
Citizens of Montauk were suing the U.S. Navy to stop them from
dumping sludge into the Long Island Sound at a site just off Fishers
Island—long one of the most productive fishing areas on the Atlantic
coast.

Like Brookhaven, the Groton submarine base near New London
on the Connecticut shore, was an EPA Superfund site with nearly four
decades of build-up of radioactive waste resulting from nuclear submarine refueling and waste disposal. The Fishers Island Conservancy
suit had secured the support of New York State Senators D'Amato and
Moynihan along with Governor Pataki and most Long Island elected
officials of both parties. The Navy, supported by Connecticut Senators
Dodd and Lieberman, denied there was any dangerous radioactivity
in the sludge but proposed to cover the waste by a problematic cap-
ping procedure.

In a Federal District Court in Long Island in November 1995, I was
permitted, along with other witnesses, to testify to the health effects
of radioactive wastes on both humans and fish, but after three weeks,
the court ruled in favor of the U.S. Navy, by which time the dumping
had been completed.

BROOKHAVEN'S DEFENSE ON PUBLIC-ACCESS TV

The arrogance displayed by officials operating DOE nuclear facilities
in ignoring public apprehension of their activities is illustrated by the
following account of local reaction to the ill-advised BNL proposal.
Richard Rosenthal, a producer at the local public-access television

station, invited Smith and me and BNL scientists to discuss the issue on October 16, 1995. Mona Rowe, the BNL publicist, said that BNL scientists were "too busy to participate." After the broadcast, she told Rosenthal that she would bring a BNL expert to the studio on October 30 to refute my statement, but was unwilling to do so face to face.

It is easy to see why the BNL expert—Dr. S.V. Musolino—was so intimidated of me. He exposed his ignorance of a basic precept of epidemiology—namely that a difference between any two mortality rates cannot be deemed to be truly significant unless the probability that the difference could be due to chance can be shown to be infinitesimal.

For example, Musolino charged that I "selected" evidence by displaying to viewers our figure 8–3, which traces the movement of breast cancer mortality rates in New York City and Westchester since 1960, as reported by the New York State Department of Health. It shows that in 1960, both rates began at about 21 deaths per 100,000 persons and moved up somewhat in the 1960s after the start-up of Indian Point in 1962. After the 1970s the rates for the affluent county of Westchester rose sharply to a peak of about 28 deaths in the 1980s, while the rate for less affluent city residents declined to 20 deaths. We have explained this epidemiological anomaly, which could not possibly be due to chance, as reflecting the fact that after the 1970s city residents shifted their water supply to the Catskill water shed, far from the Croton reservoirs, which are vulnerable to possible contamination from the nearby Indian Point reactors.

Unbelievably, Musolino then showed that if the same data were plotted on a scale that started at zero deaths, the visual perception of the statistically significant difference between the Westchester and city rates in the 1980s would appear diminished based on the same principle that the distance between two objects would appear to contract with the observer's distance from the objects. The statistical significance of the divergent movements of course remains unchanged.

Musolino then turned to our demonstration that the combined breast cancer incidence rate for 220,000 women living in 24 towns within 15 miles of the laboratory was significantly higher than the Suffolk County average. Musolino again ignored this fact in claiming he could find no pattern among the rates for the 24 towns in terms of the directions of known groundwater flows or prevailing wind patterns. We have been claiming that the only credible explanation for local variations in breast cancer rates might be found if we had independent local surveys of the radioactivity of the drinking water resulting from a 45-year build-up of radioactive waste at BNL. Such surveys, which could include evaluations of strontium–90 in baby teeth and cesium–137 in local firewood ash, could be performed for a tiny fraction of the half billion dollars of taxpayer money allotted to BNL by the Department of Energy each year.

A flood of letters published subsequently in the *East Hampton Star* indicated that efforts were now under way to organize public town meetings to force BNL officials to explain the absence of radioactivity measures of local drinking water and perhaps raise sufficient funds to undertake independent surveys. It seemed clear that BNL could not forestall public hearings about their waste disposal practices, despite the promised long-term NCI study.

BLOWING THE WHISTLE ON BROOKHAVEN ON COMMERCIAL TELEVISION

As this book was going to press in January of 1996, a series of events occurred that began with a Brookhaven concession that there was sufficient concern about the quality of drinking water south of the laboratory to warrant their offer of "free public water hookups to every house that currently uses well water in the area of northern Shirley." The town of Shirley is close to the towns of Brookhaven, Bellport, and Medford, which we had identified among those with the highest breast cancer incidence rates in Suffolk County, according to the New York State Tumor Registry. This offer, which was initially extended to about 800 families, was immediately followed by a series of evening news reports on New York City-based WPIX TV by investigative reporter Frank Ucciardo, who learned of mishandling of radioactivity at Brookhaven from two DOE whistle-blowers.

Each night from January 10 to January 17, WPIX ran a story on Brookhaven, beginning with the testimony of Joseph Carson, an Oak Ridge radiation specialist. Carson performed an official DOE review of the cover-up of safety violations that led to the March 1994 fire at the BNL High Flux Beam reactor. Next, Ucciardo interviewed Kenneth Dobreuenaski, a BNL radiation specialist who, prior to emerging as a whistle-blower, video taped the continuous discharge of radioactive waste and other chemicals into the groundwater, which ultimately flowed into nearby private wells. The tape also showed malfunctioning pumps spilling radioactive waste throughout the laboratory grounds, which endangered the lives of BNL employees. New York Senator D'Amato was so shaken by Dobreuenaski's video that he demanded a Senate investigation, saying that "a videotape I viewed recorded what appear incredible lapses in safety procedures . . . that has the potential to impact upon the health and safety of thousands of people."

Ucciardo also televised a public meeting at BNL on the evening of January 16. About 600 angry and bewildered residents of the town of Shirley attended. The town residents could not understand why the Brookhaven National Lab had just offered them free water hookups to public Suffolk County water along with simultaneous assurances that their private wells were perfectly safe. Apparently BNL had just discovered that contaminated ground water at a level 200 feet underneath BNL was moving in a southward direction. It proved to be too difficult a question for the panel of two dozen BNL and state and county environmental and public health experts to answer.

This was the most emotionally charged public meeting I have ever attended, reminiscent of my meeting in Oak Ridge before an audience torn between concern for their health and concern about continued employment. Here there was no such division of opinion among the 100 or more residents who quickly lined up to question the panelists after their fruitless attempt to explain what was clearly inexplicable. The panelists initially displayed an unbelievable insensitivity to the mood of the hostile audience. For example, when challenged, the county director of health services—Dr. Mahfouz Zakhi—offered a long and labored explanation that a given level of contamination in water that could kill mice need not be necessarily regarded as harmful to humans. He was continually interrupted by shouts of "Liar!" and "You are killing our children!" When one distraught resident accused the panel of murdering his wife, who had just died of breast cancer, he was politely thanked for his comments by Bill Gunther, the chief BNL apologist. For the next three hours, the town residents heatedly voiced their fear that BNL was responsible for both the loss of lives and the value of their homes. All of this was captured on videotape by the WPIX television crew and finally fairly described by the *New York Times* reporter John Rather in the January 28, 1996, Long Island Sunday supplement.

When my turn came, I said I was here as both a resident of Suffolk County and as an epidemiologist who had found the highest breast cancer rates in the county in towns just south of the laboratory, which were now being offered the free water hookups. I was glad to see that while these extraordinary rates could be explained by the southerly direction of the groundwater's flow, the fact remains that the county as a whole had registered the highest breast cancer mortality rates in the nation, with an increase since 1950, when BNL began operating, that was 40 times greater than the corresponding increase in the national rate. Did this not suggest, I asked, the need for performing independent radioactivity assays in all parts of the county?

Apparently anticipating my appearance, Robert Casey, BNL division head of environmental safety, rose from the audience to display the same enlarged maps and charts used by Dr. Musolino in his attempt to refute our findings on an earlier public-access television program, from which I had been barred. Casey went on to make the following statement:

> We frankly disagree with Dr. Gould and Dr. Sternglass, but we are also aware that the level of trust expressed here tonight is low. We do not want to conduct these proposed radioactivity tests ourselves and would in the future welcome input from Dr. Gould and Dr. Sternglass in their preparation.

This was an amazing shift. I wondered if it was the first step toward a policy of co-option; it is well known that some leaders of the women's breast cancer survivor groups were offered official positions in an effort to dampen their militant stand.

DEMAND FOR CLASS ACTION SUITS AGAINST BROOKHAVEN

The next day I received a dozen calls, three from upstate New York, New Jersey, and Connecticut and the rest from Long Island. All were from persons who had lived near Brookhaven and whose family members had sustained some form of cancer that, after viewing the WPIX newscast, they suspected was due to exposure to Brookhaven discharges. The callers had two questions: 1) Could they sue Brookhaven? 2) Could I be engaged as an expert witness for such a suit? One call was from a law firm that represented about 100 residents of Shirley and wanted to meet with me as soon as possible.

I tried to give them some idea of the difficulties involved. I told them that the class action mounted by 2,500 plaintiffs against the operator of the stricken Three Mile Island reactor had still not come to trial after 14 years. Despite the fact that 300 cases had been settled on the condition that the plaintiffs not reveal the amounts involved, the *New York Times* had not regarded the suit as newsworthy. On the other hand, the *New York Times* published the fact that some 27,000 plaintiffs were preparing a class action suit against the companies operating the Hanford Nuclear Weapons facility in Washington State. This followed the admission by the Department of Energy in 1992 that there were many cases of thyroid cancer following large releases of radioactive iodine from Hanford in the 1940s. So it really was a question of numbers: a sufficient number of persons enlisting in a class action suit could not be ignored.

I felt certain that eventually both the *Times* and the Long Island *Newsday* would have to take note of Ucciardo's remarkable revelations, and with the resulting widespread publicity one could hope to overcome a legal strategy designed to wait until all plaintiffs died. I agreed to help. I believe it is possible to enlist many thousands of plaintiffs in a class action suit and to raise sufficient funds for independent studies supporting radioactivity measures.

BROOKHAVEN'S DUPLICITY

Ucciardo's newscast on the evening of January 18 offered another surprise, and one that threw additional light on the feasibility of a class action suit against BNL. It appeared that there was already a $50 million suit in progress against the top BNL officials and the 9 universities that apparently shared responsibility for the direction of the BNL research program, for withholding the development of a promising mode of removing radioactive metals from BNL waste.

Ucciardo interviewed the plaintiff—an industrialist named Sanford Rose, head of the Transtech Development Corporation, who appeared so knowledgeable about the inner workings of Brookhaven that I immediately arranged through Ucciardo to meet with him. From Rose I learned the following:

As John Rather reported, "With the end of the Cold War, the mission of Brookhaven and the eight other national laboratories came into question. . . . As the need for nuclear arsenals declined the labs switched their emphases to alliances with industries to create job-producing technologies." Congress passed a Technology Transfer Act under which the national laboratories have entered into about 1,000 Cooperative Research and Development Agreements (called CREDAS), in which laboratory scientists share their expertise with such companies as ATT, IBM, Dow Chemical, Goodyear, Proctor and Gamble, who can supply the entrepreneurial funds necessary for the commercial development and application of any new scientific discovery of promise. The national laboratories are unsuited for such commercial development and, in fact, are legally constrained from using tax dollars to compete with private enterprise in such activities.

Rose, a well-respected technology entrepreneur, was particularly interested in Brookhaven's basic research program, in which many billions of dollars had been invested since 1947, resulting in four Nobel prizes in physics, a claim that was prominently featured in BNL public relations brochures. In 1992 he was invited to review BNL basic research programs to see whether they would lend themselves to commercial development.

He was disappointed to find little of commercial value, but he did find that one BNL researcher, Dr. A. J. Francis, developed a strain of bacteria that appeared capable of facilitating the removal of certain heavy radioactive metals from contaminated water. After bringing in his own technical and financial experts, Rose estimated that it would require a venture capital investment of perhaps $20 million to scale the process up from the test tube level to that of a pilot plant to test its commercial applicability. There was no guarantee of its success, of course, but as Rose explained, it was the nature of such venture capital investments; high risks bring high returns to all concerned. He was also keenly aware that its commercial success rested on the pressing social need for such beneficial waste treatment technologies. If successful, there was literally no limit to its profitability for himself, the U.S. government, and many communities all over the world in need of it. He made it clear, however, that his primary motivation was that of an investor.

BNL apparently initially welcomed his interest. By the close of 1992 he had worked out satisfactory contractual arrangements, and he began to assemble personnel and plant facilities for the new enterprise. Then early in the following year, for reasons that are still not clear to him, the top BNL officials suddenly drew back, saying initially that the process was really worthless and that in any case they could not proceed with the contractual obligation laboriously worked out over the previous year. Instead, he was offered an alternative contract in which, after assuming all risks, he would be obliged to share profits with other undesignated private parties. After two frustrating years, Rose realized that BNL had no intention of permitting him to undertake the successful exploitation of this process, and he began his suit in 1995.

To his horror he found that BNL officials were using private detectives to approach all of his business associates over the past three decades to press them into declaring that Rose had perjured himself in depositions, using threats of IRS investigations. He was particularly incensed to find that BNL introduced into the hearings the last will and testaments of his long deceased parents in an effort to deprecate his financial worth.

Rose decided to fight back. He found evidence that BNL officials had in the past made illegal contributions to prominent local politicians and that they had funneled lucrative contracts to favored contractors. Rose wondered, based on this evidence, whether the process that he agreed to invest in was being reserved for others who would be more likely to make private "special arrangements" with top BNL officials. Rose described an immoral culture of illegal "sweetheart" deals at BNL, along with other problems that were systematically being concealed from the public. Rose brought the two DOE whistle-blowers to the attention of Frank Ucciardo of WPIX as a first step in his one-man attempt to close Brookhaven down. He had assembled detailed documentation on past BNL corruption, which when shown to Senator D'Amato and Congressman Forbes apparently persuaded them to immediately abandon any hope of salvaging BNL from congressional investigation.

I interrupted his recital to ask whether he had received any physical threats. With some amusement, he replied that several of his friends and associates had reacted to their interrogations by sending him copies of the Karen Silkwood film, but that he had decided that nothing would deter him from proceeding with his suit.

I then asked whether the demise of Brookhaven would not jeopardize the radioactive waste treatment process that he prized so highly. Not in the least, he replied. Brookhaven itself was the obstacle to the few good scientists at the laboratory who hoped to realize the full beneficial potential of their discoveries. They were trapped in a high paying but corrupt bureaucratic culture devoted solely to the maintenance of nuclear technology; everything else, such as the medical application of radionuclides, was window dressing that could best be pursued elsewhere. For example, the few dollars allotted by BNL to explore benign solar technologies had been used in an attempt to show that photovoltaic cells and geothermal energy were bad for one's health.

He went on to explain the mind-set of top BNL officials in the following way. The success of the Manhattan Project, achieved under the direction of Dr. Robert Oppenheimer and a unique collection of the world's greatest physicists, conferred on their successors at the various national nuclear laboratories devoted to refining nuclear weapons an undeserved aura of prestige. (I reflected that Stuart Udall, a former secretary of the interior, had recently accused Dr. Norris Bradbury, who replaced Oppenheimer as director of the Los Alamos Laboratory, as one who—after denying there was any fallout danger from the Nevada Test site—took pains to secretly remove his own family from the danger zone.)[64]

For nearly half a century top BNL officials found themselves with unlimited funds at their disposal and unlimited power to spend such funds on the development of nuclear technology without any outside control of such expenditures—all under the protective mantle of national security considerations. Rose suspected that their reluctance to permit him to develop a promising commercial use of a biotechnical process would expose BNL's research programs to an unwanted public review.

I had never met Rose before, but I found his words strangely familiar. In 1966 I wrote a book called *The Technical Elite*,[3] which made a similar argument that the successful American postwar application of science in business enterprise was greatly facilitated by the availability of venture capital. After writing the book, I took my own advice, formed my own company and raised a small venture capital grant, which secured my own financial independence.

I saw in Sanford Rose a kindred spirit. I wrote that the great American economist Thorstein Veblen was the first to realize that men like Samuel Morse, Alexander Bell, and Thomas Edison exemplified the peculiarly American phenomenon which he called the "captain of industry" who could combine the expertise of the scientist and engineer with the necessary entrepreneurial funds that could only come from what Veblen called "the pecuniary interest." There was tension in any such technological enterprise, which only the "captain of industry" could resolve, because the pecuniary interest was also prone to such socially unproductive activities as monopolization, financial speculation, bribery, and bureaucratization. All the latter characteristics, according to Rose, could now be found in Brookhaven.

I asked Rose why he included the nine universities in his suit. Surely, I said they could not have known the details of what he uncovered? He replied that he was aware that a suit against Brookhaven alone would run into legal delays that could quickly exhaust his own funds, but that the nine universities—Columbia, Cornell, Harvard, Johns Hopkins, MIT, Princeton, Rochester, University of Pennsylvania and Yale—had ample endowment funds to cover his claims. He was certain that they had no knowledge of what was really going on at Brookhaven and hoped that they would want to disassociate themselves from a protracted legal suit.

He explained that in 1946 an educational charter had been established in New York State to permit the nine Associated Universities Inc.(AUI) to operate the Brookhaven research program, originally funded by the Atomic Energy Commission and now by the Department of Energy. The universities really served as window dressing but they would benefit from the huge amounts of research-and-development money and use of the facilities. Professors from the nine universities were enlisted as trustees to satisfy the charter, although neither they nor their respective schools were permitted a real corporate voice in the choice of research programs.

Rose showed me a letter he had just written to the presidents of each of the universities and to the 24 professorial trustees who shared legal responsibility for "directing" Brookhaven's research program, although under the terms of the 1946 charter they were promised indemnification from the government for any losses incurred. He felt certain that they would be horrified to learn of the following allegations he included in his letter:

Decades later AUI/BNL, after taking billions of taxpayer dollars can claim only modest scientific achievements. However, their morally flawed policies have left a most deplorable legacy:

- Years of dumping thousands of tons of hazardous waste on their site, much of it buried and lost forever leaching into the environment.
- Lack of any record keeping for decades of storing this waste.
- Contaminating drinking water without warning residents of possible lethal consequences.
- Abusing the public trust by transporting radioactive waste through heavily populated areas. In an effort to protect the lives and property of its citizens, New York City, New York State, and Suffolk County sued AUI to halt the transporting of radioactive waste through their streets. In defiance of findings by independent experts A.D. Little & Co. that "AUI/BNL was causing a risk to society whose consequences could be catastrophic," AUI continues to this day to transport large quantities of radioactive material through densely populated areas in violation of health codes, with complete disregard for the public safety.
- Syphoning $500 million of taxpayer money to clean up its site, which will take until 2020.
- (AUI/BNL) has a management culture that supports employees' misrepresenting and falsifying federal documents and scientists colluding to derail development for personal gain.
- Authorizes its key personnel to give thousands of dollars to local politicians.
- Condones employees running their own companies out of the lab while using lab personnel and machinery for personal profit.

After reading his letter, I informed Rose that I could supplement his sensational charges by providing the epidemiological evidence in this book that not only showed Suffolk County registered the greatest increase in breast cancer mortality since 1950 in the nation, but that was also true of all 14 counties in which the 7 oldest national nuclear laboratories had been located.

As I write these words in late January of 1996, I am getting daily word of hundreds of potential plaintiffs and attorneys calling Bill Smith of Fish Unlimited, asking whether a class action similar to that mounted by the 27,000 Hanford plaintiffs could be prepared against the Brookhaven National Laboratory. At this early juncture I think it possible that a very large number of potential plaintiffs may emerge.

That is where the matter rests today; not only in Suffolk County, but potentially in every one of the counties close enough to reactor sites to warrant the concerns expressed in this book. What is unusual about Long Island is that public awareness of the danger has quite suddenly reached an extraordinary level, which I could not have hoped for when I began to write this book. Long Island politicians can no longer ignore the questions being raised not only by breast cancer survivors, but by business interests, lawyers, real estate interests, fishermen, etc. With both political parties looking for ways to cut bloated federal expenditures, Brookhaven and the national nuclear laboratories may find themselves exceedingly vulnerable. Ultimately, with the threat to property values from radioactive pollution, it will become increasingly difficult for public officials to deny the magnitude and significance of the evidence presented in this book.

BREAST CANCER AND REACTORS IN CONNECTICUT

Although the epidemic rise of breast cancer in Connecticut matches that of neighboring Long Island, public awareness in Connecticut lags behind. No household surveys have been undertaken by breast cancer survivors as in Long Island. I was therefore delighted to receive an invitation from the Connecticut League of Women Voters to present my views on the health effects of emissions from Connecticut reactors at a meeting held near the Haddam Neck reactor on April 30, 1995.

The League had been given some funds to promote public discussion on the disposal of used fuel assemblies that were (temporarily!) stored on site for nearly 30 years in pools of water. The water requires constant cooling until the highly radioactive short-lived fission products lose some of their potency. I pointed out that the disposal problem could not be addressed as long as the reactors continued to operate and spent fuel rods were being constantly added. But I was happy to agree with representatives for Northeast Utilities and the Nuclear Regulatory Commission, who participated in the panel discussion, that the problem was one of great urgency. I also stressed the urgent need to examine the adverse health effects of the Millstone and Haddam Neck reactors, with respect to both the breast cancer mortality and incidence data that was particularly available for Connecticut— home of the best and oldest Tumor Registry in the nation.

Questions from the audience centered around why the incidence of breast cancer was increasingly affecting younger women. They were astonished to learn that, according to the Connecticut Tumor Registry, the almost threefold increase in breast cancer incidence among older women had (as shown in figure 2–1) started in 1945, with the initial introduction of nuclear fallout into a pristine atmosphere. A second boost in the steady annual increase came in 1970s, after the start-up of the Haddam Neck and Millstone reactors.

I also displayed figure 2–2 to show that younger women under the age of 50, born after the Nuclear Age began, are increasingly diagnosed with breast cancer. Another exhibit that shocked the audience was figure 8–6. Here, using the National Cancer Institute breast cancer mortality database, I revealed how high the breast cancer mortality rates were in Middlesex and New London Counties, where the Haddam Neck and Millstone reactors are located. For both counties combined, the increase in age-adjusted breast cancer mortality rates from 1950–54 to the 1980s reflect mainly the impact of emissions after 1970s, which matched the extraordinary increases registered by the nation's oldest DOE reactor sites.

URBAN COUNTIES WITH THE HIGHEST BREAST CANCER MORTALITY RATES

The location of the Brookhaven National Laboratory and the Indian Point, Haddam Neck, and Millstone reactors in the heavily populated urban counties of Suffolk, Westchester, Middlesex, and New London must be seen as an unfortunate consequence of the lack of understanding of the biological effects of ingesting fission products. These four counties are not alone. There are four dozen large urban counties that are fairly close to reactor sites and have by far the nation's highest breast cancer mortality rates.

In table 8–3 we list four dozen counties with 1985–89 age-adjusted breast cancer mortality rates that exceed the corresponding U.S. rate by a margin equal to two or more standard deviations. They are almost all large urban counties, and they are all within 100 miles of a reactor site; most of them are located in the northeastern states in which reactor sites are most heavily concentrated.

It is clear from table 8–3 that these mainly urban counties have extraordinarily high breast cancer rates relative to the U.S. rate. In the aggregate, they have a combined current rate of 28.7 deaths per 100,000, which is much higher than the U.S. rate of 24.6. Based on 42,306 deaths, chance probability is less than one out of trillions of cases. Moreover 28 of these 48 counties reached their peak, not in the years when DDT was widely used or when fallout was heaviest from nuclear testing, but in 1985–89, after nuclear reactors had produced their largest releases, including those from TMI, Chernobyl, and other large releases from the Oyster Creek, Nine Mile Point, Indian Point, Millstone, and Pilgrim plants as listed in appendix C.

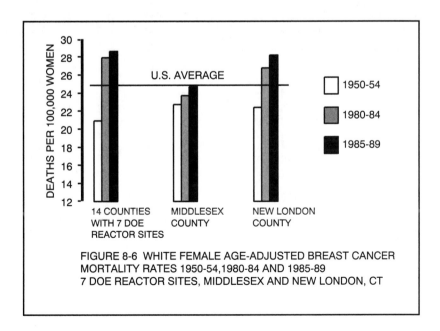

FIGURE 8-6 WHITE FEMALE AGE-ADJUSTED BREAST CANCER MORTALITY RATES 1950-54,1980-84 AND 1985-89
7 DOE REACTOR SITES, MIDDLESEX AND NEW LONDON, CT

**TABLE 8-3 WHITE FEMALE BREAST CANCER MORTALITY RATES
48 MAINLY URBAN COUNTIES WITH
SIGNIFICANTLY HIGH 1985-89 RATES**

County	ST	Age-Adjusted Mortality Rates			Percent Change		Number of Deaths		
		1950-54	80-84	85-89	80-84/ 1950-54	85-89/ 1950-54	1950-54	80-84	85-89
NEW ENGLAND									
MIDDLESEX	MA	29.2	28.9	29.8	0.99	1.02	1000	1393	1463
ESSEX	MA	29.3	27.9	27.7	0.96	0.95	532	690	721
BARNSTABLE	MA	42.1	28.8	31.4	0.68	0.75	72	215	271
ROCKINGHAM	NH	25.9	22.7	31.3	0.88	1.21	58	132	199
GRAFTON	NH	29.0	34.4	34.6	1.19	1.20	41	72	76
FAIRFIELD	CT	28.1	27.4	27.7	0.98	0.99	425	768	805
MIDDLE ATLANTIC									
ALBANY	NY	32.0	28.6	33.8	0.89	1.06	245	297	391
ERIE	NY	31.8	29.1	32.0	0.92	1.01	793	1020	1095
HUDSON	NJ	28.8	27.8	30.3	0.96	1.05	508	523	526
MONMOUTH	NJ	29.7	32.5	31.9	1.10	1.07	213	542	579
MORRIS	NJ	28.6	31.3	28.4	1.10	1.00	146	388	378
PHILADELPHIA	PA	29.4	30.4	30.0	1.03	1.02	1518	1331	1328
SCHENECTADY	NY	30.5	27.4	31.9	0.90	1.05	134	163	196
DELAWARE	PA	28.5	32.2	31.7	1.13	1.11	313	624	631
MONTGOMERY	PA	25.8	28.0	28.1	1.09	1.09	283	667	718
ALLEGHENY	PA	25.2	27.9	27.5	1.11	1.09	977	1476	1485
NEW YORK	NY	31.8	29.4	28.3	0.92	0.89	6817	6102	5755
GLOUCESTER	NJ	25.4	25.1	31.4	0.99	1.24	62	139	189
BERGEN	NJ	32.0	32.9	31.0	1.03	0.97	514	1035	1019
CAMDEN	NJ	27.6	28.3	28.8	1.03	1.05	224	399	422
ESSEX	NJ	31.8	31.2	32.3	0.98	1.02	792	693	696
EAST NORTH CENTRAL									
DU PAGE	IL	31.7	28.7	29.9	0.91	0.94	141	495	575
LAKE	IN	23.7	25.9	29.9	1.09	1.26	166	309	365
FRANKLIN	OH	26.5	28.1	28.2	1.06	1.06	352	621	665
HURON	OH	12.9	23.1	35.7	1.79	2.76	17	43	64
COOK	IL	29.3	28.4	28.5	0.97	0.97	3399	3963	3916
ALLEN	OH	25.4	22.2	32.3	0.87	1.27	63	77	113
CUYAHOGA	OH	28.4	29.4	30.2	1.03	1.06	1034	1385	1420
HAMILTON	OH	30.0	29.7	29.5	0.99	0.98	615	759	803
OAKLAND	MI	25.2	27.9	27.7	1.11	1.10	228	800	877
WAYNE	MI	28.6	28.0	27.8	0.98	0.97	1461	1406	1359
MILWAUKEE	WI	32.0	28.3	28.2	0.88	0.88	781	916	905
MACOMB	MI	23.1	26.6	28.9	1.15	1.25	85	520	647
WEST NORTH CENTRAL									
LANCASTER	NE	23.7	24.2	30.5	1.02	1.29	90	138	185
ST LOUIS CITY	MO	27.5	25.5	28.8	0.93	1.05	631	357	329
NICOLLET	MN	13.3	23.1	44.8	1.73	3.37	8	21	33

TABLE 8-3 CONTINUED
WHITE FEMALE BREAST CANCER MORTALITY RATES
48 MAINLY URBAN COUNTIES WITH
SIGNIFICANTLY HIGH 1985-89 RATES

County	ST	Age-Adjusted Mortality Rates			Percent Change		Number of Deaths		
					80-84/	85-89/			
		1950-54	80-84	85-89	1950-54	1950-54	1950-54	80-84	85-89
SOUTH ATLANTIC									
JAMES CITY	VA	22.1	26.3	29.8	1.19	1.35	53	174	222
OHIO	WV	30.2	27.2	33.7	0.90	1.12	65	70	82
FAIRFAX	VA	24.9	28.4	27.7	1.14	1.11	154	631	705
CLAYTON	GA	15.5	26.5	33.0	1.71	2.12	6	73	106
NEW CASTLE	DE	22.7	28.8	29.6	1.27	1.31	126	315	355
BALTIMORE CITY	MD	28.6	26.9	30.5	0.94	1.07	608	446	480
SOUTH EAST CENTRAL									
JEFFERSON	KY	24.8	26.9	27.8	1.09	1.12	295	565	576
PACIFIC									
SAN FRANCISCO	CA	28.2	30.5	27.9	1.08	0.99	658	566	529
SAN MATEO	CA	26.0	25.8	27.9	0.99	1.07	166	458	510
SAN DIEGO	CA	25.5	28.8	26.6	1.13	1.05	392	1501	1613
CONTRA COSTA	CA	27.2	27.5	28.2	1.01	1.04	141	515	580
LOS ANGELES	CA	27.4	27.1	27.0	0.99	0.99	3546	5264	5349
ALL 48		29.1	28.4	28.7	0.98	0.99	30948	41057	42306

HIGH BREAST CANCER RATES NEAR THE GREAT LAKES

We have seen that large urban counties like those in New York City were the first to suffer from the radioactive contamination of drinking water from the first wave of above-ground nuclear bomb tests. This was also true of the Great Lakes—the nation's largest expanse of surface waters. Since the turn of the century the Great Lakes have also served as the repository of chemical wastes from the American industrial heartland. Beginning in the 1970s, three dozen U.S. and Canadian civilian nuclear power reactors have poured their radioactive effluents into the Great Lakes.

Recognizing that the Great Lakes would therefore serve as an ideal laboratory to test Rachel Carson's characterization of strontium-90 and industrial chemicals as "sinister partners" in inducing carcinogenesis, Greenpeace asked us to calculate the combined current breast cancer mortality rate of 81 U.S. counties bordering the Great Lakes from Wisconsin to New York. The 81 border counties, listed in table 8–4, turned out to have a combined current rate that was extraordinarily high—27.8 deaths per 100,000, supported by 15,397 deaths in 1985–89. The probability that so great a difference from the corresponding U.S. rate of 24.6 deaths could be due to chance is infinitesimal.

As shown in table 8–4, mortality rates in the border counties were also extraordinarily high in 1950–54, so that just as in the case of New York the slight decline of 2 or 3 percent since 1950–54 cannot be regarded as a sign of improvement but rather the response of a highly contaminated area at the flat plateau stage of the logarithmic dose response relationship, which is now known as the Petkau Effect. As in the case of New York City, there are three reasons why in the years 1950–54 the Great Lakes border counties had already had above-average exposure to all the environmental causes of breast cancer—long-standing chemical pollution, immediate contamination from the first wave of bomb test radiation, and early overexposure to X rays.

There are a total of 15 reactor sites in the Great Lakes states, as can be seen from the maps in appendix B. In every one, there is evidence that rural counties closest to the reactors have registered significant upward divergences in breast cancer mortality since 1950–54; and in almost every case, all counties within a 100-mile radius have a combined current mortality rate significantly above that of the nation.

BREAST CANCER MORTALITY NEAR MINNESOTA REACTORS

In May 1994 we were asked by a concerned citizens group in Minnesota for preliminary figures from our analysis of breast cancer rates near the Prairie Island reactor. We found a significant breast cancer mortality increase in 12 rural counties close to the Monticello and Prairie Island reactors in Minnesota, and these findings were introduced in legislative hearings on dry-cask storage of high-level nuclear waste at the Prairie Island reactor. In May 1995, the Minnesota Department of Health published an attack on our findings. By including annual county figures on age-adjusted breast cancer mortality rates since 1950, the attack confirmed our findings in every respect.

TABLE 8-4 WHITE FEMALE BREAST CANCER MORTALITY RATES 1950-89: 81 US COUNTIES BORDERING ON THE GREAT LAKES
Deaths per 100,000 Women

FIPS Code	County	ST	Age-Adjusted Mortality Rates			Percent Change 80-84/ 85-89/		Number of Deaths		
			1950-54	80-84	85-89	50-54	50-54	50-54	80-84	85-89
17031	COOK	IL	29.3	28.4	28.5	-3%	-3%	3399	3963	3916
17097	LAKE	IL	37.4	26.0	27.6	-30%	-26%	162	274	339
18089	LAKE	IN	23.7	25.9	29.9	9%	26%	166	309	365
18091	LA PORTE	IN	28.9	26.9	24.2	-7%	-16%	57	90	89
18127	PORTER	IN	25.5	22.9	22.7	-10%	-11%	25	67	82
26001	ALCONA	MI	38.1	26.4	17.7	-31%	-54%	6	13	9
26003	ALGER	MI	0.0	25.7	24.0			0	9	6
26005	ALLEGAN	MI	22.4	27.6	22.2	23%	-1%	30	65	53
26007	ALPENA	MI	30.2	26.3	12.2	-13%	-60%	16	26	16
26009	ANTRIM	MI	19.4	20.8	20.4	7%	5%	6	12	14
26011	ARENAC	MI	26.7	27.1	14.1	2%	-47%	7	16	9
26013	BARAGA	MI	10.8	23.5	12.7	118%	18%	2	8	5
26017	BAY	MI	27.2	25.7	26.0	-5%	-4%	61	91	104
26019	BENZIE	MI	43.5	25.6	13.5	-41%	-69%	10	12	9
26021	BERRIEN	MI	24.1	22.9	24.3	-5%	1%	72	110	125
26029	CHARLEVOIX	MI	22.8	28.8	19.8	27%	-13%	11	20	15
26031	CHEBOYGAN	MI	15.3	21.5	17.5	41%	15%	6	18	18
26033	CHIPPEWA	MI	18.5	18.3	24.5	-1%	32%	12	17	21
26041	DELTA	MI	20.9	30.8	32.8	48%	57%	18	39	43
26047	EMMET	MI	26.9	13.1	17.7	-51%	-34%	14	14	16
26053	GOGEBIC	MI	16.6	23.5	14.4	42%	-13%	12	24	16
26055	GRAND TRAVERSE	MI	23.1	24.2	17.2	4%	-26%	22	46	41
26061	HOUGHTON	MI	29.3	14.7	17.8	-50%	-39%	33	20	31
26063	HURON	MI	25.6	21.5	21.4	-16%	-16%	21	28	33
26069	IOSCO	MI	28.2	33.2	28.9	18%	2%	8	32	30
26083	KEWEENAW	MI	41.7	56.5	4.1	35%	-90%	4	5	1
26089	LEELANAU	MI	18.8	26.0	17.9	39%	-5%	4	12	10
26095	LUCE	MI	4.9	21.6	14.1	342%	189%	1	4	2
26097	MACKINAC	MI	24.4	30.4	25.5	25%	5%	5	10	13
26099	MACOMB	MI	23.1	26.6	28.9	15%	25%	85	520	647
26101	MANISTEE	MI	31.0	28.2	16.9	-9%	-46%	17	24	19
26103	MARQUETTE	MI	25.9	26.7	16.7	3%	-36%	32	53	38
26105	MASON	MI	22.0	21.7	23.0	-1%	5%	12	24	29
26109	MENOMINEE	MI	30.2	25.6	30.5	-15%	1%	20	24	32
26115	MONROE	MI	23.0	23.0	30.6	-0%	33%	41	86	120
26121	MUSKEGON	MI	22.5	27.5	25.7	22%	15%	61	134	120
26127	OCEANA	MI	15.9	22.4	14.5	41%	-9%	8	16	12
26131	ONTONAGON	MI	22.8	15.3	20.9	-33%	-8%	5	6	8
26139	OTTAWA	MI	30.9	23.8	23.4	-23%	-24%	58	104	123
26141	PRESQUE ISLE	MI	24.0	13.8	22.9	-42%	-5%	7	9	13
26147	ST CLAIR	MI	29.0	27.0	23.2	-7%	-20%	71	110	107
26151	SANILAC	MI	30.9	16.6	27.7	-46%	-11%	27	26	40

TABLE 8-4 CONTINUED

WHITE FEMALE BREAST CANCER MORTALITY RATES 1950-89:
81 US COUNTIES BORDERING ON THE GREAT LAKES
Deaths per 100,000 Women

FIPS Code	County	ST	Age-Adjusted Mortality Rates			Percent Change 80-84/ 85-89/		Number of Deaths		
			1950-54	80-84	85-89	50-54	50-54	50-54	80-84	85-89
26153	SCHOOLCRAFT	MI	8.0	16.2	17.2	103%	115%	2	7	7
26157	TUSCOLA	MI	15.0	26.7	21.1	78%	40%	14	44	38
26159	VAN BUREN	MI	22.8	22.3	23.7	-2%	4%	28	47	51
26163	WAYNE	MI	28.6	28.0	27.8	-2%	-3%	1461	1406	1359
27031	COOK	MN	17.3	18.2	26.6	5%	54%	1	3	3
27075	LAKE	MN	18.9	16.4	12.1	-13%	-36%	4	8	8
27137	ST LOUIS	MN	21.5	26.7	28.8	24%	34%	125	216	230
36011	CAYUGA	NY	25.0	17.8	26.0	-29%	4%	58	49	76
36013	CHAUTAUQUA	NY	23.8	31.3	30.1	31%	26%	108	171	169
36029	ERIE	NY	31.8	29.1	32.0	-8%	0%	793	1020	1095
36045	JEFFERSON	NY	24.1	27.4	23.3	13%	-3%	69	80	74
36055	MONROE	NY	30.4	30.1	30.6	-1%	1%	481	680	687
36063	NIAGARA	NY	25.1	30.6	26.6	22%	6%	124	227	211
36073	ORLEANS	NY	26.8	22.0	24.5	-18%	-9%	25	30	35
36075	OSWEGO	NY	25.6	23.9	28.9	-7%	13%	59	79	95
36117	WAYNE	NY	27.4	24.2	29.7	-11%	8%	53	67	81
39007	ASHTABULA	OH	22.8	25.3	27.1	11%	19%	52	85	107
39035	CUYAHOGA	OH	28.4	29.4	30.2	3%	6%	1034	1385	1420
39043	ERIE	OH	27.9	25.8	24.9	-8%	-11%	42	59	67
39085	LAKE	OH	27.4	27.6	25.5	0%	-7%	55	172	176
39093	LORAIN	OH	24.1	26.4	27.0	9%	12%	88	199	214
39095	LUCAS	OH	27.0	29.0	27.9	7%	3%	297	395	412
39123	OTTAWA	OH	25.5	18.7	19.6	-27%	-23%	21	31	32
39143	SANDUSKY	OH	23.1	18.0	24.5	-22%	6%	33	33	51
42049	ERIE	PA	25.6	31.1	26.2	21%	2%	148	270	251
55003	ASHLAND	WI	26.5	36.0	28.6	36%	8%	14	23	17
55007	BAYFIELD	WI	22.5	32.2	23.6	43%	5%	8	20	11
55009	BROWN	WI	24.3	23.3	25.9	-4%	7%	60	118	146
55029	DOOR	WI	28.6	14.7	14.4	-49%	-50%	16	20	19
55031	DOUGLAS	WI	17.7	22.3	32.0	26%	81%	23	38	55
55051	IRON	WI	17.6	35.7	27.9	103%	58%	4	10	6
55059	KENOSHA	WI	27.1	26.6	29.2	-2%	8%	56	103	116
55061	KEWAUNEE	WI	26.2	23.3	27.1	-11%	3%	12	19	19
55071	MANITOWOC	WI	28.4	33.0	28.4	16%	-0%	51	94	83
55075	MARINETTE	WI	23.5	16.9	23.8	-28%	1%	23	30	49
55079	MILWAUKEE	WI	32.0	28.3	28.2	-12%	-12%	781	916	905
55089	OZAUKEE	WI	26.1	25.4	31.3	-3%	20%	17	49	70
55101	RACINE	WI	29.2	24.1	18.9	-17%	-35%	89	121	106
55117	SHEBOYGAN	WI	25.3	26.7	26.4	5%	4%	62	103	107
TOTAL	ABOVE 81 COUNTIES		28.3	27.6	27.8	-3%	-2%	11025	14917	15397
TOTAL	UNITED STATES		24.4	24.9	24.6	2%	1%	91392	167803	178868

The Nuclear Regulatory Commission reported that the Monticello reactor released more than 11 curies of radioactive iodine and strontium in the years 1972 to 1975. As for the Prairie Island reactors, a pipe rupture on October 2, 1979, caused a record high release into the secondary steam-generating loop, which lead to a large environmental release via the generator building vents. This was followed by 5 serious steam-generator tube leakages reported as late as September 1992.

Our analysis of the data obtained from the NCI (table 5–1) showed that Minnesota registered a white female breast cancer mortality rate in 1985–89 that represented an 8 percent decline since 1950–54. Data from the Minnesota Health Department, using 1970 rather than 1950 as the standard population year, shows a 5 percent decline, from 28.8 deaths per 100,000 in the first period to 27.5 in the final period, not a significant difference from the decline reflected in the NCI data.

The Monticello and Prairie Island reactors can be seen from the map on page 208 to be close to 12 contiguous rural counties in both Minnesota and Wisconsin. These 12 rural counties, in contrast to the declining state trend, had registered a combined breast cancer mortality rate that had increased significantly by 12 percent, from 24.2 deaths per 100,000 in 1950–54 to 27.1 in 1985–89.

The Minnesota Health Department examined 10 rural counties in Minnesota within 50 miles of the 2 reactors. These 10 counties registered a 7 percent increase, from 26.5 deaths per 100,000 in 1950–54 to 28.5 in 1985–89. Both the Health Department data and that of the NCI show a significant difference between the decline for the state, as opposed to the increase for the rural counties that received the most direct impact of the reactor emissions that began in 1970s.

The Monticello and Prairie Island reactors, like most other reactors, are located in and near rural counties, which have so few deaths that any increase in the age-adjusted breast cancer mortality rates between 1950–54 and 1985–89 over the corresponding moderate 1 percent gain registered by the United States can only be shown to be statistically significant by combining a few adjoining counties. The 12 counties closest to the 2 reactors that we suggested were most likely to be adversely affected by reactor emissions include Wright, Sherburn, Benton, Meeker, Mcloud, Goodhue, Wabasha, and Dakota in Minnesota and Pierce, St.Croix, Dunn, and Pepin in Wisconsin.

By combining the counties we increase the number of deaths involved, thereby increasing the significance of the indicated 12 percent gain in breast cancer mortality when compared to the 8 percent decline in Minnesota as a whole. This difference is equivalent to four standard deviations and could not be due to chance.

The Minnesota Health Department data show a similarly significant rise in breast cancer mortality in the period after start-up of the plants. In figure 8–7, we have charted five-year moving averages of the annual rates—in order to smooth out the year-to-year fluctuations—together with the trend lines fitted to the 1950–70 period before start-up, rather than the entire 1950–92 period used by the Health Department.

In figure 8–7 we highlight the sharp upward movement observed in 1985–89 for both Minnesota and the ten rural "nuclear" counties close to the reactors after releases began. One can see that there was indeed a nearly parallel decline in breast cancer mortality for both the state and the ten "nuclear" counties before reactor start-up and that the rate for the rural counties was indeed lower than that of the state, with the exception of a period some five to ten years after the largest Nevada above-ground tests in the 1950s.

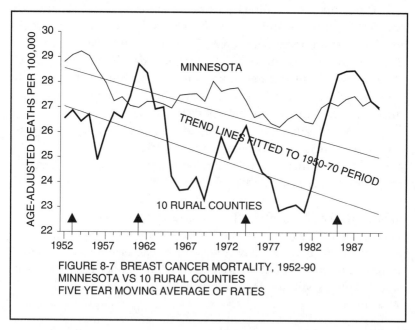

FIGURE 8-7 BREAST CANCER MORTALITY, 1952-90
MINNESOTA VS 10 RURAL COUNTIES
FIVE YEAR MOVING AVERAGE OF RATES

Some five to ten years after the Monticello plant began operations in the early 1970s, the previous long-term decline ended and was replaced by a rising trend in the 1980s. This trend was much steeper for the "nuclear" counties. The arrows indicate three earlier rises and declines, for which the Department of Health offers no explanation.

The first rise in the 1950–55 period represents the five-to-ten year delayed impact of the start of nuclear testing in 1945, in which year we have shown breast cancer incidence in Connecticut began a long-term two and one-half-fold rise after a previous declining trend. A second peak in 1960–65 reflects the delayed effect of the large atmospheric H-tests in the mid-1950s that ended in 1963. A third peak between 1970 and 1975 follows the large near-surface peaceful Plowshare tests in Nevada in the mid-60s, which ended in the early 1970s.

The last rise began about 1982, 5 to 10 years after the large releases of 11 curies from Monticello reported by the NRC from 1972 to 1975. These releases are almost equal to the figure reported for the stricken TMI reactor in 1979. The mortality rate is seen to have peaked in the years 1985–89, again some five to ten years after the steam generator tube ruptured at Prairie Island.

In fact, the Health Department's report shows a rise of 20 percent in the breast cancer mortality rate from 1965–69—just before start-up—to 1985–89 for the 10 "nuclear" counties. This while the rate remained unchanged for the state as a whole.

Although the methodology used in the report was specifically designed to refute our findings and hide the truth from the public, far from contradicting the results we had obtained with NCI data, the Minnesota Health Department's data fully supported the conclusion that currently permitted releases of fission products are a major neglected factor in the recent rise of breast cancer mortality in areas close to nuclear facilities.

"NUCLEAR" COUNTIES WITHIN 100 MILES OF REACTORS

We are now in a position to consider the results of adopting the more extensive definition of proximity to a reactor site—the one first used by Mangano in his classic study of cancer rates within 100 miles of Oak Ridge. In maps shown in appendix B we have drawn a circle with a radius of 100 miles around each reactor, taken all the counties within that 100-mile radius and calculated the combined age-adjusted breast cancer mortality rates for each of our 3 time periods. After eliminating the many duplicated counties, arising from overlapping radii, we were left with a total of 1,319 counties, which accounted for 69 percent of all breast cancer deaths in 1985–89.

We have summarized the results of this endeavor, first in table 8–5, in which we have calculated the combined breast cancer mortality rates for all counties within 100 miles of each of the 60 reactors in our study. Since there are about 400 duplicated counties, mainly in the regions east of the Mississippi, in table 8–6 we have eliminated the duplicated counties and arranged the remaining 1,319 "nuclear" counties by census region, to illuminate the varying environmental characteristics of each region.

By far the most important fact revealed by table 8–6 is that it effectively divides the nation into 2 parts: the first part is composed of the 1,319 "nuclear" counties that fall within 100 miles of each of the 60 reactors studied here and have a current combined age-adjusted breast cancer mortality rate of 25.8 deaths per 100,000 women. In the second part, at the other extreme, are the remaining 1,734 nonnuclear counties located mainly between the Rockies and the Mississippi River, furthest away from exposure to reactor emissions, with an

TABLE 8-5 BREAST CANCER MORTALITY RATES WITHIN 100 MILES OF 60 REACTOR SITES
Deaths per 100,000 Women

Facility	Number of Counties	Mortality Rate 1950-54	Mortality Rate 85-89	Ratio	Deaths 50-54	Deaths 85-89	Deaths per 100 Sq Miles 50-54	Deaths per 100 Sq Miles 85-89
GREAT LAKES STATES								
1 MONTICELLO/PRAIRIE ISLAND	46	26.9	23.9	0.89	1626	2503	2.59	3.98
2 KEWAUNEE/PT. BEACH	26	29.9	26.5	0.89	1403	2014	2.23	3.21
3 LACROSSE	33	24.5	22.8	0.93	619	922	0.99	1.47
4 BIG ROCK PT.	22	23.3	18.6	0.80	168	304	0.27	0.48
5 PALISADES/COOK	46	27.7	27.1	0.98	5443	8065	8.66	12.84
6 ZION	33	28.5	27.5	0.96	6149	8966	9.79	14.27
7 DRESDEN	44	28.4	27.2	0.96	6320	7684	10.06	12.23
8 FERMI/DAVIS BESSE	45	26.7	27.2	1.02	4679	7249	7.45	11.54
9 BEAVER VALLEY	53	24	26.7	1.11	4666	8074	7.43	12.85
10 WEST VALLEY	26	28.6	28.8	1.01	2315	3324	3.68	5.29
11 GINNA/FITZPATRICK/9 MILE PT.	25	28.5	28.8	1.01	2690	3870	4.28	6.16

TABLE 8-5 CONTINUED
BREAST CANCER MORTALITY RATES
WITHIN 100 MILES OF 60 REACTOR SITES

Facility	Number of Counties	Mortality Rate			Deaths		Deaths per 100 Sq Miles	
		1950-54	85-89	Ratio	50-54	85-89	50-54	85-89
NORTHEAST STATES								
12 MAINE YANKEE	14	24.5	24.7	1.01	589	954	0.94	1.52
13 VT.YANKEE/YANKEE-ROWE	45	28	28.2	1.01	7020	10753	11.17	17.11
14 PILGRIM	21	27.8	28.7	1.03	3253	7530	5.18	11.98
15 IND.PT./MILLSTONE/HADDAM/BRKHAVEN	49	30.1	28.8	0.96	15064	22124	23.98	35.21
16 OYSTER CREEK/SALEM	54	29.6	28.8	0.97	15938	24323	25.37	38.71
17 TMI/PEACH BOTTOM	56	23.9	27.2	1.14	1333	11010	2.12	17.52
SOUTHERN STATES								
18 CALVERT CLIFFS	53	25.1	26.3	1.05	2007	3036	3.19	4.83
19 NORTH ANNA	60	24.3	25.2	1.04	1409	3235	2.24	5.15
20 SURRY	46	21.6	25.6	1.19	733	2229	1.17	3.55
21 MCGUIRE	62	17.8	23.7	1.33	1033	3548	1.64	5.65
22 BRUNSWICK	19	17.2	21.6	1.26	173	610	0.28	0.97
23 OAK RIDGE	71	15.8	20.4	1.29	578	1652	0.92	2.63
24 SEQUOYAH	66	18	21.3	1.18	699	2101	1.11	3.34
25 SAVANNAH RIVER	53	18.2	21.3	1.17	329	912	0.52	1.45
26 ROBINSON	44	17.3	24	1.39	535	2086	0.85	3.32
27 OCONEE	66	17.5	22.5	1.29	591	2060	0.94	3.28
28 HATCH	58	16.3	19.7	1.21	207	564	0.33	0.90
29 BROWNS FERRY	49	18.4	21.1	1.15	658	1656	1.05	2.64
30 FARLEY	55	17.3	20.3	1.17	349	978	0.56	1.56
31 CRYSTAL RIVER	27	18.9	22.5	1.19	560	3833	0.89	6.10
32 ST. LUCIE/TURKEY PT.	18	18.3	23.3	1.27	531	5135	0.85	8.17
33 ARKANSAS ONE	42	15.9	20.5	1.29	336	1034	0.53	1.65
STATES WEST OF THE MISSISSIPPI								
34 HUMBOLDT BAY	7	20.9	24.8	1.19	97	299	0.15	0.48
35 RANCHO SECO	26	24.2	25.8	1.07	1717	5097	2.73	8.11
36 SAN ONOFRE	5	26.6	26.4	0.99	4418	9930	7.03	15.80
37 TROJAN	18	23.7	23.9	1.01	964	1953	1.53	3.11
38 HANFORD	17	19.6	23.1	1.18	169	417	0.27	0.66
39 IDAHO NATL. ENG. LAB (INEL)	16	14.2	19.8	1.39	50	162	0.08	0.26
40 SANDIA/LOS ALAMOS NATL. LAB	15	17.8	23.8	1.34	111	578	0.18	0.92
41 DUANE ARNOLD	43	24.9	22.8	0.92	970	1303	1.54	2.07
42 COOPER	56	23.4	22.8	0.97	1118	1591	1.78	2.53
43 FORT CALHOUN	50	25.3	22.8	0.90	881	1172	1.40	1.87
44 QUAD CITIES	41	24.4	24	0.98	1294	1865	2.06	2.97
45 PATHFINDER	46	23.3	23.1	0.99	484	709	0.77	1.13
46 FORT ST. VRAIN	24	25.2	22.7	0.90	643	671	1.02	1.07

TABLE 8-6 WHITE FEMALE BREAST CANCER MORTALITY RATES 1950-89: NUCLEAR AND NON-NUCLEAR COUNTIES
Deaths per 100,000 Women

Regions (# of Counties)	Age-Adjusted Mortality Rates			Percent Change		Number of Deaths		
	1950-54	80-84	85-89	80-84/ 50-54	85-89/ 50-54	50-54	80-84	85-89
Nuclear counties								
E. North Central (227)	26.6	26.7	26.3	0%	-1%	14790	22199	22876
New Eng./Mid Atlantic (188)	28.4	28.2	28.2	-1%	-1%	31041	45273	47071
S.Atlantic/E.S. Central (530)	19.9	23.1	23.2	16%	16%	7597	23023	26163
Pacific (70)	25.4	26.1	25.9	3%	2%	7296	16330	17532
Other (MT, WNC & WSC) (306)	23.9	23.2	23.0	-3%	-4%	5543	9156	9867
Total Nuclear counties (1319)	**26.0**	**26.0**	**25.8**	**0%**	**-1%**	**66267**	**115981**	**123509**
Total Non-nuclear Counties (1734)	**21.0**	**22.7**	**22.1**	**8%**	**6%**	**25125**	**51822**	**55359**
Total, All counties(3053)	24.4	24.9	24.6	2%	1%	91392	167803	178868

overall mortality rate of only 22.1 deaths per 100,000. This means that in the "nuclear" counties for every 100,000 women, there are nearly 4 more deaths today than in nonnuclear counties. Because of the large number of deaths in each sector, this is an extraordinarily significant difference.

This one fact destroys the credibility of the National Cancer Institute's insistence in its 1990 study that it could find no evidence that proximity to a nuclear facility had a significant effect on cancer mortality rates. The chance probability of so great a difference between the 1,319 "nuclear" counties and the remaining 1,734 nonnuclear rural counties is infinitesimal, or equivalent to 1,290 standard deviations!

The other surprising fact is that the 1,734 nonnuclear rural counties registered increases in their combined age-adjusted breast cancer mortality rate since 1950–54 of between 6 or 8 percent—significantly greater than the national increase of 1 or 2 percent and equivalent to nearly 10 standard deviations. What this means is that even the 100-mile definition of proximity to nuclear reactors is relative. Even those rural counties located furthest away from reactor sites were adversely affected by small amounts of ionizing radiation from both bomb tests and reactors, as we have found from our analysis of the logarithmic response of cancer mortality rates in pristine rural counties since 1950–54. Thus, there is no area in the nation today that can be considered to be free from the effects of continued releases of ionizing radiation from nuclear reactors.

Finally, it should be noted that the 1,734 nonnuclear counties roughly correspond to the Mountain and West South Central regions, shown (figures 3–7 and 3–8) to have had the least exposure to civilian reactor emissions and to have the nation's lowest current breast cancer and AIDS mortality rates. These nonnuclear counties account for only 31 percent of all breast cancer deaths. The "nuclear" counties—with nearly two-thirds of all deaths—dominate the national mortality trends. The nonnuclear areas offer us a mere glimpse of the benefits of living in a pollution-free nation.

If we analyze each county in terms of its proximity to one or more reactors we can see again how the concentration of reactors east of the Mississippi contribute to the increased breast cancer mortality in the "nuclear" counties. In table 8–7 we have divided the nation's counties into 9 groups, according to the number of reactors that fall within 100 miles of each county. There are 1,734 mainly rural counties that have no reactors within 100 miles, and these counties registered a breast can-

TABLE 8-7 BREAST CANCER MORTALITY RATES 1950-54, 1980-84 AND 1985-89 CORRELATED WITH NUMBER OF REACTORS WITHIN 100 MILES

Number of Reactors	Number of Counties	Deaths per 100,000		
		1950-54	80-84	85-89
0	1734	21.0	22.7	22.1
1	690	23.1	24.6	24.3
2	420	24.2	24.5	24.6
3	109	27.2	26.9	27.3
4	54	28.5	28.1	28.3
5	9	24.5	27.4	26.5
6	32	30.5	29.5	29.0
7	2	21.1	26.9	26.9
8	3	22.9	25.0	26.5
Total	3053	24.4	24.9	24.6
Correlation coefficient		0.43	0.69	0.78
Significance		not significant	0.05	0.01

cer mortality rate since 1950 that remained at a level below 23 deaths per 100,000 women. In the 1980s, it is clear that there was a significant positive correlation between breast cancer mortality and the number of reactors within 100 miles.

For example, there are 690 counties that are located within 100 miles of 1 reactor. They have aggregated breast cancer rates in the 1980s somewhat over 24 deaths per 100,000. There are 420 counties located within 100 miles of 2 reactors with rates of about 25 deaths per 100,000. Current rates greater than 26 deaths per 100,000 characterize those counties located within 100 miles of 4 or more reactors. There are even 5 counties that are located within roughly 100 miles of 8 of the nation's most troublesome reactors. These counties are New London and Tolland in Connecticut, Genessee in New York, and Bucks and Northampton in Pennsylvania. They are within roughly 100 miles of the following reactors: Three Mile Island, Peach Bottom, Oyster Creek, Millstone, Haddam Neck, Brookhaven, Indian Point, and Pilgrim.

What is interesting about table 8–7 is that it yields another example of the logarithmic dose-response relationship between breast cancer and reactor emissions. We can regard the number of reactors within 100 miles of a group of counties as a measure of the amount or intensity of exposure to reactor emissions. In table 8–7 we have correlated the breast cancer mortality rates of the nine groups of counties with the log values of the number of reactors. (Because there is no log value for zero, we have substituted the low value of .001. There can be no group of counties in the United States completely untouched by reactor emissions.)

We have recorded the three resulting correlation coefficients in table 8–7. It is noteworthy that in all three periods there is evidence of a positive correlation between breast cancer mortality and the log values of the number of nearby reactors. That correlation is only statistically significant in the 1980s, not in 1950–54 when only the seven DOE reactors were operating.

Figure 8–8 depicts the now familiar concave downward dose relationship of the 1985–89 breast cancer mortality rates to reactor emissions for the nine groups of counties shown in table 8–7.

As we move from those counties with very little exposure to reactor emissions to those with more exposure, the dose response rises quickly. When we reach those counties that are literally saturated with

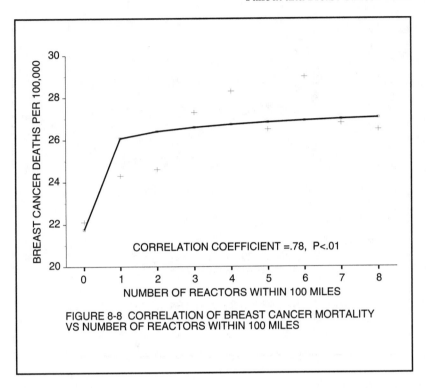

FIGURE 8-8 CORRELATION OF BREAST CANCER MORTALITY VS NUMBER OF REACTORS WITHIN 100 MILES

exposure from many reactors, the dose response flattens out. Note how similar this figure is to figure 3–9, which depicts the logarithmic dose response of current breast cancer mortality rates among nine census regions to cumulative *per capita* emissions of radioactive iodine and strontium.

The logarithmic dose response to ionizing radiation is probably the most difficult single issue for the National Cancer Institute to accept. It can be illustrated by figure 8–9, which demonstrates the highly significant negative correlation between the percentage gain in rates and the degree to which each of the areas in table 8–5 had rates in 1950–54 that were below the national average of 24.4 deaths per 100,000 (r=-.85, P<.001).

For example, note how in figure 8–9 the areas in the upper left quadrant that registered the greatest increases are those highly rural counties surrounding reactors either located in the South, such as Robinson (#26), Oconee (#27), Hatch (#28), Browns Ferry (#29), and

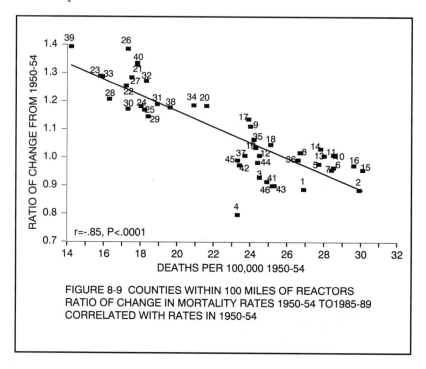

FIGURE 8-9 COUNTIES WITHIN 100 MILES OF REACTORS
RATIO OF CHANGE IN MORTALITY RATES 1950-54 TO1985-89
CORRELATED WITH RATES IN 1950-54

Farley (#30) along with the rural counties surrounding the old DOE reactors like Hanford (#38), INEL (#39), and Sandia/Los Alamos (#40). At the other extreme, with high initial and current mortality rates but moderate increases, are the more urban counties surrounding such Great Lakes reactors as Monticello/Prairie Island (#1), Kewaunee/Pt. Beach (#2), Lacrosse (#3), etc., and those in the Northeast, such as the Indian Point complex (#15), Oyster Creek/Salem (#16), and TMI/Peach Bottom (#17).

The impact of ionizing radiation in urban as opposed to rural counties is shown in figure 8–10, in which we note the significant positive correlation between population density and the current high mortality rates, with the same areas dominating the extremes in figures 8–9 and 8–10. If pesticides and herbicides were the principal factor in the breast cancer epidemic, one would not expect rural areas with low population density to have lower breast cancer rates than urban areas, since everyone by and large consumes the same contaminated fruits and vegetables and other foods.

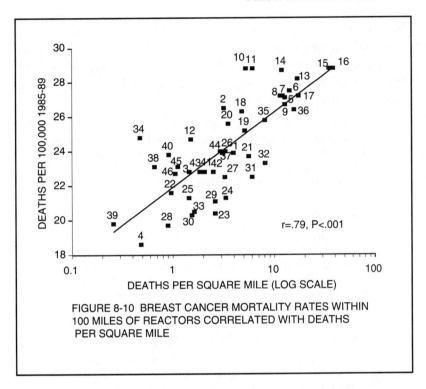

FIGURE 8-10 BREAST CANCER MORTALITY RATES WITHIN
100 MILES OF REACTORS CORRELATED WITH DEATHS
PER SQUARE MILE

MORTALITY RATES IN "NUCLEAR" VERSUS NONNUCLEAR COUNTIES

We have shown that counties within 100 miles of some 60 reactors registered about 4 more deaths per 100,000 women than was true for nonnuclear counties. How can we depict the enormous significance of this geographic difference?

For the roughly 100 million American women this difference comes to about 4,000 premature breast cancer deaths each year. There is at least an order of magnitude difference between breast cancer incidence and mortality. We can speculate that if all counties had the same low incidence rate, which can be presumed to characterize nonnuclear counties, there would be about 40,000 fewer cases of breast cancer reported each year. If we consider that other immune deficiency diseases such as AIDS and other kinds of cancer are also on the rise in counties most directly exposed to ionizing radiation from nuclear reactors, we begin to get a glimpse of the true magnitude of the current American health crisis. We must ask why this evidence has been so long ignored?

A partial answer can be found in a front-page story in the *New York Times* of August 2, 1995, entitled "Plunging Life Expectancy Puzzles Russia," which begins as follows:

> Life expectancy in Russia, already lower than in any other developed country, has plummeted again this year, and scientists and public health officials say they cannot explain the continuing steep decline. . . . Russia has become the first country in history to experience such sustained reversals in its health statistics.

And finally states:

> "What we have here is a disaster," said Dr. Aleksandr Chuchalin, a member of the Russian Academy of Science, who has been researching the health of children and the state of the environment. . . . Dr. Chuchalin and colleagues are beginning to examine the hypothesis that radiation produced by decades of nuclear irresponsibility—places like the Chernobyl power station but also at waste dumps and test sites across the country—is a major factor in the surge of illnesses and birth defects, but such links are never easy to demonstrate.

> "It was surprising that we could not seem to observe the genetic effects of what happened there," said Dr. David Hoel, chairman of the department of biometry and epidemiology at the Medical University of South Carolina, and an expert on the effects of radiation in populations. "Everyone assumes the connection. But it takes years of careful study to be sure."

Thus, ignoring the measures reported by the World Health Organization of mounting numbers of thyroid cancer cases in Belarus and the Ukraine since Chernobyl, Russian and American epidemiologists were prepared to wait for several generations for the genetic effects to show up before acknowledging concern. The National Cancer Institute displays the same unwillingness to acknowledge a truth that is becoming increasingly obvious.

The disingenuous use of the official cancer mortality data by the NCI to conceal the huge difference between mortality rates of "nuclear" versus nonnuclear counties is heightened by the fact, revealed in appendix D, that a confidential NCI memorandum circulated early in 1995 to discredit our preliminary findings performed an exercise similar to that summarized in tables 8–5 and table 8–6. In this memo the NCI, in effect, divided the nation into a "nuclear" sector, consisting of all counties within a radius of 50 miles of a reactor with an overall breast cancer mortality rate close to 27 deaths per 100,000, as compared to all other counties with a rate of 23.3 deaths. This reveals a difference of 4 deaths per 100,000 women between "nuclear" and nonnuclear counties, which translates to a chance probability equal to 200 standard deviations—a result hardly at variance with our own findings.

The highly urban "nuclear" counties defined as either those within a radius of 50 or 100 miles of a reactor accounted for the bulk of all deaths throughout the years from 1950 to 1989. The percent change in age-adjusted cancer mortality for the United States as a whole was dominated by these mainly urban counties, which probably always had significantly higher mortality rates than rural counties. The NCI memorandum argued that because these urban counties had a slight 1 or 2 percent decline from 1950–54 to 1985–89, breast cancer mortality improved over time.

Urban areas already had extremely high mortality rates by 1950–54 primarily due to early nuclear tests and high air and chemical pollution from the 1940s. The small and insignificant decline in mortality reflects the fact that they were already on the plateau of the logarithmic dose-response curve. Further contamination increased the cancer rates relatively little. By contrast, for the relatively pristine rural counties, the dose response to fission products in their drinking water was a much larger rise in cancer mortality.

Therefore it cannot be said that either urban or rural counties registered any significant improvement in breast cancer mortality from 1950–54 to 1985–89.

The good news is that while urban and rural cancer mortality rates are slowly converging, there is still a wide gap between the mortality rates of women living close to reactor sites and those living in rural counties far away from reactors. This is true when proximity to reactors is defined in any of the following ways:

1. As discussed in chapter 5, when the NCI limited the number of exposed counties to the 107 counties in which nuclear facilities were located, they found that after start-up the observed increase in breast cancer mortality in

these counties as an aggregate was equivalent to 9 standard deviations.

2. When the definition of exposed counties is extended to include 346 mainly rural counties within 50 miles of reactor sites, the observed increase in breast cancer mortality is equivalent to about 12 standard deviations.

3. Finally when the definition of exposed counties is extended to include urban counties within 50 to 100 miles of each reactor site, we do not find a significant divergence in the trend of breast cancer mortality rates compared with that of the United States, but the difference between the mortality rates of "nuclear" versus nonnuclear counties remains significantly great. The low rural mortality rates rose most rapidly because of the logarithmic nature of the dose-response curve to ionizing radiation. The overall trend of age-adjusted mortality rates of the large urban counties did not diverge from the national trend, on which they had a dominating influence. If rural counties close to reactors were so adversely affected, we can infer that urban counties close to reactors were also adversely affected.

Only such environmental factors as air and chemical pollution, urban stress along with nuclear reactor emissions can explain the much higher rates in densely populated urban areas. Each area in table 8–5, with a radius of 100 miles, extends over roughly 63,000 square miles; we have included in that table calculations of the number of deaths per 100 square miles to illustrate the fact that urbanized counties—particularly in the three northeast regions—have long had, and still by far have, the highest mortality rates along with the highest ratios of deaths per 100 square miles.

Reactors in the Northeast are surrounded by the most densely populated counties, which have an average current age-adjusted breast cancer mortality rate of about 28 deaths per 100,000. The highest rates in the nation—over 32 deaths per 100,000 are found in the New York metropolitan counties. "Nuclear" counties in the Great Lakes are somewhat less densely populated and have a current breast cancer mortality rate of about 26 deaths per 100,000.

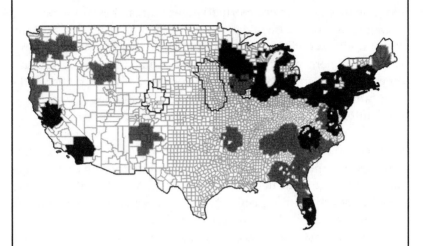

FIGURE 8-11 HIGH RISK COUNTIES
WITHIN 100 MILES OF NUCLEAR REACTORS

Nearly half of the nation's 3,000-odd counties can be defined as "nuclear" counties because they are located within 100 miles of reactor sites. They had more than two-thirds of all breast cancer deaths in 1985–89 and a combined age-adjusted breast cancer mortality rate (about 26 deaths per 100,000 women) that is significantly higher than that of all remaining counties (about 22 deaths per 100,000).

The "nuclear" counties at highest risk, depicted in this map with the darker shading, are mainly in the Northeast where the mortality rate of 28 deaths per 100,000 (with rates as high as 32 deaths per 100,000 in the New York Suburban counties) is associated with the greatest concentration of reactors. "Nuclear" counties in the Great Lakes and Pacific states also have combined mortality rates significantly higher than the U.S. rate of 24.6 deaths.

"Nuclear" counties in the southern states, along with those surrounding the DOE reactors at Hanford and the national laboratories in Idaho and New Mexico, are depicted with lighter shading and have had significantly greater increases since 1950 than the United States as a whole.

The nonnuclear counties—including those surrounding the five reactor sites that displayed no significant divergence from national norms—carry no shading and are seen to fall mainly between the Rocky Mountains and the Mississippi River.

"Nuclear" counties in the southern states are mainly rural and still have, on average, current mortality rates that fall below the national average. They have also registered significant increases in breast cancer mortality, about 20 percent, since 1950–54, which, when compared with the far more moderate increase for the United States, suggests that they may begin to catch up with the "nuclear" urban counties in the near future. This may also be true of the rural counties that surround the Hanford, INEL, and Sandia/Los Alamos reactor sites.

In figure 8–11 we generated a national county map that offers a visual summary of the data in tables 8–5, 8–6, and 8–7. The "nuclear" counties in the northeast regions—with significantly high current mortality rates—are indicated with a dark shading, while the southern rural "nuclear" counties, which have significantly increasing mortality rates, are indicated with a lighter shading.

While they still have mortality rates lower than the national rate, their combined rate has increased since 1950–54 by a significant 16 percent, as compared with 1 percent for the United States. For non-nuclear counties, the lowest rates (about 22 deaths) are found in the low-rainfall counties between the Rockies and the Mississippi River.

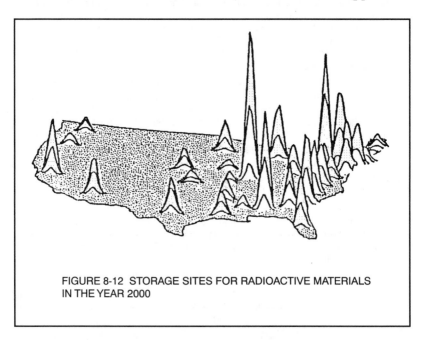

FIGURE 8-12 STORAGE SITES FOR RADIOACTIVE MATERIALS
IN THE YEAR 2000

These areas also have the lowest mortality rates from AIDS and other immune deficiency diseases. Of the 60 reactors, only 5—all in low-rainfall areas—display no increased risk of cancer for residents of neighboring counties and therefore are outlined above but carry no shading.

Three Department of Energy reactor sites (INEL, Sandia, and Los Alamos) in this low-rainfall area stand out as epidemiological anomalies, once again supporting the hypothesis that releases of nuclear fission products into the environment have contributed greatly to the rise in cancer since World War II.

Figure 8–11 effectively summarizes the findings of this book. It is strikingly similar to the map shown in figure 8–12 prepared by Ralph Nader's Public Citizen Group, which shows those parts of the nation that by the year 2,000 will be the storage sites for the largest amounts of radioactive materials. It should not come as a surprise that areas with large concentrations of radioactive waste should coincide with those areas whose residents' health would be most seriously affected.[62]

Chapter 9

IS IT TOO LATE?

One neglected contributor to the problem of radioactive pollution in "nuclear" counties is the incinerator, which recycles the long-lived fission products built up over time in wood and paper products into the surrounding atmosphere. Two Harvard scientists—Belton A. Burrows and Thomas C. Chalmers—have recently performed radioactive assays of firewood ashes from all over the world. They discovered that because most nuclear emissions have occurred in the Northern Hemisphere, the radioactivity of firewood ashes (judged by ratios of cesium-137 to potassium-40) in the Northern Hemisphere is 100,000 times higher than in the Southern Hemisphere.[63] They state that "whether or not these worldwide differences are the results of atomic bomb testing and fallout from prevailing winds, or of more local contamination by nuclear power plants, remains to be determined." This suggests that the radioactive pollution of any given area located near an incinerator is ongoing.

Loss of Biological Species

The discovery that levels of radioactivity are 100,000 times greater in the Northern Hemisphere than in the Southern Hemisphere may throw some light on the alarming rate at which biological species are now being lost, particularly in remote rain forest areas near the equator. Paleontologists have determined from fossil records that there have been five major extinctions of biota over the past half billion years. Over recent millennia we have been experiencing a man-made "sixth extinction."[64]

As a result of human population growth, consequent shifts in hunting and habitat patterns, and recent environmental abuses, it has been estimated that over the past few millennia biological species have been disappearing at a rate of 30,000 each year, a rate matching that of the Permian extinction 65 million years ago, when nearly 95 percent of all species were obliterated. One should consider, for example, that the current worldwide disappearance of frogs includes remote areas with inaccessible high altitudes, which cannot be attributed to industrial chemical pollution alone. European biologists have revealed the significant role of low-level radiation in accounting for the loss of large sections of the German Black Forest, as well as other plant life.[50]

In retrospect, it seems obvious that if low-level radiation can harm the human immune response, all other living beings would also be adversely affected. Certainly there has been considerable damage done in the past half century.

There Remain Some Pristine Areas

Despite the gradual convergence of rural and urban cancer mortality rates near reactors, it is good news that there remain nearly 2,000 rural counties that can still be regarded as relatively pristine with respect to environmental pollutants. This is a hopeful portent; it means that the breast cancer epidemic, as a man-made phenomenon, can be halted, as is happening in some rural areas far from nuclear reactors.

Probably most of the damage for women living in "nuclear" counties was done in the past, either because of above-average exposure to industrial chemicals, bomb-test radiation and over-exposure to X rays, which are now greatly reduced in dose per examination.

Reactor emissions, however, continue to exacerbate an already intolerable degree of environmental pollution. Unlike other environmental factors, this one can be stopped overnight with immediate observable improvements in public health. This was apparent during the brief period in 1987 when the notorious Peach Bottom reactors were closed by the NRC for several months. There was an almost immediate improvement in infant mortality in nearby Baltimore and Washington, D.C.

On August 2, 1995, the *New York Times* carried a story entitled "Move Abroad Can Change Breast Cancer Risk," based on a study published in the August 1995 issue of the *Journal of the National Cancer Institute,* which states:

> When a woman moves to a new country, her risk of dying will either rise or fall to match that of women native to her adopted land. . . . The work contradicts the notion that most of a woman's risk of breast cancer is set by puberty or early adulthood. It also suggests that by comparing migrant populations, scientists may get a handle on how women can modify their lives to avoid this hated malignancy.

Surely we would agree that it makes more sense to remove the environmental causes of breast cancer in a nation than to encourage migration to more pristine areas.

We have established that the location of the nation's nuclear reactors in effect divides the nation into two distinct geographic entities with respect to breast cancer mortality. We can speak of high-risk "nuclear" counties as opposed to the remaining nonnuclear counties, which are at lesser risk.

Our emphasis on the causal role of low-level radiation in the postwar epidemic rise of breast cancer does not mean that we believe it to be the only cause, merely one of the most overlooked causes—and one that exacerbates the role of toxic chemicals, bomb-test fallout, and past overexposure of women to X rays in affluent urban and suburban counties.

How to Deal with the Government

Stuart Udall, a former secretary of the Interior during the Kennedy and Johnson Administrations, is the highest ranking political figure with the courage and wisdom to denounce the secrecy with which postwar American nuclear policy has denied the lethal health effects of low-level radiation. In a recent book entitled *The Myths of August,* he describes how he learned that AEC officials lied about the cancers induced by the Nevada tests in the course of his unsuccessful legal representation of some of the downwinder victims. He regards the Nevada tests as "occupying a special niche in the annals of Nuremburg Code violations" and concludes that the AEC lied because they knew it would take several years "for the bomb-caused cancers to appear . . . and decided to adopt a pose that made the downwinders unsuspecting participants in a medical experiment."[65]

The Nevada downwinders' suits were unsuccessful. Despite winning their case in the lower courts, the Appellate Court ruled in favor of the AEC on the grounds that the U.S. government could not be held responsible. At one point, one of the lawyers for the plaintiffs sent a series of interrogatories to the AEC defense counsel with the following simple question: Who has the responsibility for the safety and welfare of persons and their property near areas of possible fallout?

The AEC answered as follows:

> It is the responsibility of the heads of families and owners of property to protect their families and their property from possible radioactive fallout.[29]

Thus the message to the rapidly rising number of women with breast cancer—and to all of us who are, in effect, downwinders—is that we must protect ourselves.

We must find a way to compel the federal government to accept the recent findings, which establish that our past knowledge of external exposures to the natural background radiation, medical X rays, and the direct radiation from atomic bombs misled us into underestimating the effect of low chronic exposures to fission products in the air and diet.

If we do not convince the government, the rising incidence of all cancers—along with increases in low-birthweight live births and other immune deficiency diseases—will destroy the financial stability of any modern society as medical and welfare costs rise uncontrollably. And this is precisely what is now happening, not only in the United States but also in the United Kingdom, the former Soviet Union, and France.

Since alternative means of protecting national security from the threat of nuclear weapons now exist and less toxic ways to meet our energy requirements are available, it is possible to end all releases of fission products into the environment and reverse the rising tide of illness and premature death that threatens our future.

I will close this chapter with a personal observation. I am a relative newcomer to that small band who have fought the good fight against ionizing radiation over the past three decades. I have been greatly influenced by the work of Ernest Sternglass, John Gofman, Rosalie Bertell, and Alice Stewart. Having come to this endeavor after retirement, I have not been exposed to the kind of scornful invective and dismissal by scientists employed by the nuclear establishment that moved the courageous John Gofman to denounce them as potential candidates "for Nuremburg-type trials for crimes against humanity for . . . gross negligence and irresponsibility. Now that we know the hazard of low-dose radiation, the crime is not experimentation—it's murder."[6]

I can therefore perhaps take a more balanced view of those scientists at the national nuclear laboratories who may have felt they were helping to realize the dream of the peaceful atom, but who today are resisting the fact that this dream has become a nightmare. Today even the electric utilities, facing deregulation pressures that may force them to jettison high cost reactors, are appealing for public support for ways to rid themselves of the dangerous used fuel assemblies on site that must be monitored for the next quarter of a million years.

My own interest in the nuclear power industry began back in 1984, when I published an article on "The Future of Nuclear Power,"[66] in which I pointed to the many indications that "the next fifteen years will witness an inexorable working out of a chain of dismal events embodied in three decades of massive commitments to a flawed technology."

I had discovered that free-market forces could not justify the economic viability of the nuclear power industry, which had come into being with massive federal governmental subsidies in the period 1950–79, in which the rated capacity of successive reactor designs rose fiftyfold without any operational experience to validate such rapid expansion.

That nuclear power can no longer be regarded as an economically viable alternative to other energy sources can still be inferred from the low ratings assigned by Wall Street to nuclear utility stocks and bonds. In 1984 I cited the case of Commonwealth Edison, which despite many years of high dividends had experienced no gain in its stock price over the past decade. By 1996 the Long Island Lighting Company, as a result of its $4 billion lost investment in the ill-fated Shoreham reactor, can be cited as possibly the worst single example of nuclear stupidity.

In 1984 I predicted that if the full costs of Shoreham were passed on to local rate payers, "the resulting doubling of the rate structure would turn Long Island into an economic wasteland." Today LILCO is facing the threat of public ownership at the hands of a Republican governor, despite his commitment to private enterprise.

Since 1984 my colleagues and I compiled the epidemiological evidence cited in this book, which shows that the economic waste of nuclear technology is dwarfed by its lethal health effects, with Long Island as a worst-case scenario illustrating both. If this fact were recognized in time and if the Brookhaven National Laboratory could be induced to promote solar rather than nuclear technologies, my prediction would be borne out that "Long Island could become the first area in the country to demonstrate the competitive viability of cogeneration units that convert natural gas into electricity, along with windmills and other solar technologies." I also predicted that "photovoltaic cells are expected to become competitive with high-cost centralized power systems within the next decade." The advent of the photovoltaic electric car may soon confirm the realism of this prediction.

The key qualification to the aforementioned rosy predictions is the factor of time. They were made before the Chernobyl disaster demonstrated that only an inexplicable factor of chance prevented the Three Mile Island meltdown of 1979 from inflicting comparable destruction on American society. A similar core meltdown accident is believed by many industry observers to have a 50 percent probability of occurring in any given decade.[67] Unless the EPA can be induced to resume monitoring the radioactivity of our milk and water, we may be forced to rely on international surveillance to even know what is happening.

A Race with Time

A crucial question can be posed by readers of both *Deadly Deceit* and *The Enemy Within*. Stated simply, we have argued that the struggle against low-level radiation is a race against time. After the cumulated build-up of man-made fission products can such a race be won in any meaningful sense? Along with the problem of the health effects of low-level radiation, there are the equally intractable environmental problems of chemical and fossil fuel pollution, global warming, the disappearance of the tropical rain forests, and the rapidly accelerating loss of countless precious biological species. Even though it may be possible to show that all environmental abuses are exacerbated by low-level radiation, how can one hope to convince the powers that rule the world to turn away from the nuclear option?

It is also true that the world today faces equally baffling social and economic problems in addition to those involving the degradation of the environment. It would not be unreasonable, however, to view low-level radiation as the principal evil, rather than merely one of many in a complex set of world problems.

I would like to offer one reason for believing that solving the problems of low-level radiation can ultimately lead to a rational reordering of a pollution-free global economy, one that will constitute a revolutionary break with an outmoded past. The process may begin at any moment, in the aftermath of the next inevitable nuclear accident of the magnitude of Chernobyl, which I don't believe any current political system will be able to survive.

My belief rests on the recognition that Chernobyl was the watershed event that will eventually be seen as the necessary counterpart to Hiroshima in changing the course of history. Despite the fact that Einstein said the nuclear bomb changed everything except the way people think, Chernobyl *has* begun to change the way people think. This is a fact still denied by the nuclear powers, who misread Chernobyl exactly as they failed in 1945 to see in Hiroshima its ultimate threat to human survival.

The Soviet rulers under Gorbachev fashioned the enlightened policies of glasnost and perestroika in 1986 only in the aftermath of the greatest accident in human history. It did not help; they were swept away by a consequent wave of civil disorder that effectively ended the Cold War but went on to engulf all of Eastern Europe and has even lead to the dismemberment of Yugoslavia. Western pundits prefer to see this period as merely a necessarily irrational prelude to the discovery of the virtues of a free-market economy. In this book, I have stated my grounds for believing instead that, in a single cataclysmic moment, Chernobyl revealed the Soviet rulers' massive deception of the Soviet population, which gave rise to the wave of civil disorder that continues today.

We have shown in this book that the Western powers that won World War II and saw in the nuclear bomb the promise of unlimited power are now also beset with an uncontrollable epidemic rise in radiation-induced illnesses and in the costs of medical care. All major nuclear powers today face the probability that the next nuclear accident of the magnitude of Windscale in 1957, Three Mile Island in 1979, and Chernobyl in 1986 will severely challenge their political legitimacy.

Indeed, the mindless zeal with which governments now permit the earth's fragile environment to be undermined can be likened to the political idiocy of the European heads of state on the eve of World War I. I believe that their inevitable failure to cope with problems beyond their understanding means that they will ultimately suffer the same fate as Gorbachev and the leaders of the former Soviet Union.

It is true that their removal from power was followed by a political vacuum, in which various elite groups are exercising criminal powers of the most brutish nature against the interests of the Soviet population. There is a current belief that Western economic and military power can in time enforce a stable civil and democratic order, not only in Russia but in all of Eastern Europe and indeed in the rest of the world. Such powers may soon be seen to be highly overrated in a world coming apart at the seams.

Even in the former Soviet Union, suffering from a ten-year drop in life expectancy attributable to past misrule, I do not think the present state of near anarchy can continue indefinitely. I cannot believe that the highly literate, gifted Russian population, whose aspirations were championed by the great Andrei Sakharov, now certainly shorn of any illusions about the mortal dangers of environmental abuse, will permit themselves to be forever exploited. Someday, perhaps sooner than elsewhere, the genius of the Russian people will create a rationally organized democratic economy, fueled by solar energy, simply because there is no other way for a modern society to survive. After all, even the great plagues of the Middle Ages that wiped out a third of the population of Europe (when life expectancy was half that of today) failed to halt the regeneration of civilized life.

So this, then, is the basis of my belief that the struggle against environmental pollution is one that cannot be lost—humankind will not permit its extinction at the hands of those few whose wealth and power can be swiftly eroded in the wake of the consequences of environmental folly.

HOW TO CALCULATE
BREAST CANCER MORTALITY RATES
NEAR NUCLEAR REACTORS

Our finding that there are clusters of counties near reactor sites with significant long-term increases in age-adjusted breast cancer mortality rates suggests that something coming out of those reactors is contributing to our national breast cancer epidemic. This appendix will describe how we have focused on those counties closest to each reactor site, and how readers with access to personal computers can use our data to replicate our estimates. Women living in these counties, already exposed in the past to bomb-test fallout, are most likely to be affected by additional radiation exposures. This appendix may encourage some who may want to do their own research.

Any reader wishing to find additional problem areas around a particular point source, such as a reactor or an incinerator, can write to the Radiation and Public Health Project (via the publisher). For the cost of duplication we can offer a floppy disk with the county age-adjusted breast cancer mortality rates for any particular state or region. A rough approximation of the combined age-adjusted rate for any group of selected counties can be obtained by weighting each county rate by the number of deaths in a given period. A more sophisticated way to secure a combined age-adjusted mortality rate for several counties is discussed below.

The National Cancer Institute studied cancer risk near reactors but chose far too limited a definition of exposed counties, as demonstrated by Joseph Mangano's groundbreaking Oak Ridge study discussed in chapter 4, in which he found significant increased cancer rates within 100 miles of Oak Ridge. We found that there are other factors to be considered, such as variations in prevailing wind and rainfall patterns.

We extended the NCI definition of an exposed area by choosing counties located downwind of each reactor site. Because counties closest to reactors are likely to be small rural counties, it is necessary to select a large enough population base so that the combined mortality rate can be supported by a sufficient number of deaths. Any divergent trend in breast cancer mortality from the U.S. performance can then be tested for statistical significance. First, we combined an average of about 7 contiguous rural counties within 50 miles of each reactor, in which we almost always found that the current age-adjusted breast cancer mortality rate for the combined counties had registered a statistically significant increase since 1950–54 when compared either to the generally more moderate change in the state or in the United States.

Next, we adopted a more inclusive definition of proximity. We calculated the combined mortality rates for all counties within a 100-mile radius of a reactor, which enabled us to include most of the nation's large urban counties, which were excluded by the two previous definitions of proximity. This helped us to arrive at our second key finding—namely that women living in counties within 100 miles of a reactor have mortality rates significantly higher than women living elsewhere.

For each of the 60 reactor sites studied here, we began by adding a few contiguous counties closest to the reactor and sought to add contiguous counties to the north and northeast, which is the general direction of the prevailing wind pattern, or other counties with known relevant topographical characteristics that would extend the geographic area that may be at special risk. We continued adding until we had a sufficient number of deaths so that any divergence from a national norm could achieve statistical significance.

We found that in 55 out of the 60 reactor sites studied here, this trial-and-error process succeeded in isolating 346 mainly rural counties within roughly 50 miles of reactor sites that registered an aggregated percentage increase since 1950–54 large enough to warrant the belief that reactor emissions are a contributing factor to the observed significant upward divergence in breast cancer mortality.

Obviously such a trial-and-error procedure had best be performed by someone well acquainted with the topography of the local area, including prevailing wind and rainfall patterns, upstream and downstream patterns, and a knowledge of the presence of all other nearby point sources of toxic pollutants. That is why we hope this appendix and appendix B will be used by readers to isolate other problem groupings of counties with significantly high breast cancer mortality rates.

For any such grouping that the reader may bring to our attention, we will calculate the true age-adjusted rates by using a much larger database, which we secured from the National Cancer Institute to produce the estimated mortality rates in this book.

In this database we have for each county and in each time period the number of white women breast cancer deaths in each of eighteen different five-year age-groups along with the number of women in each age-group. William McDonnell, of the RPHP staff, has written a personal computer program for this database, which enabled us to secure the true age-adjusted mortality rate for any desired combination of counties, including state, regional, and U.S. totals. This program will produce, within a matter of minutes, combined age-adjusted rates for any desired grouping for up to 50 counties or more. In each case, the program in effect removes county boundaries and yields a combined age-adjusted rate that is only approximated by the simple process of weighting each county age-adjusted rate by the total number of county deaths. (However, the simple weighted estimate rate generally falls within 2 or 3 percent of the true combined rate.)

All state departments of health have the facility to perform their own calculations of age-adjusted cancer mortality rates. Here, again, RPHP will cooperate with any citizen group wishing our help to make such estimates, secured at public expense, truly publicly available.

SIXTY REACTOR SITES AND COMPUTER GENERATED MAPS OF NEARBY COUNTIES

In this appendix, for each of the 60 reactor sites we display maps showing those counties within roughly 50 and 100 miles of a reactor site and the corresponding aggregated breast cancer mortality data to highlight those clusters of nearby counties that diverge significantly from national norms. We shall distinguish two different levels of statistical significance as follows: * P<.05 or P<.01; ** P<.001, although in many cases the latter designation could be considered conservative.

Clusters of mainly rural counties within 50 miles of a reactor site are shaded on the maps and are generally seen, with a few exceptions, to register significant long-term percent increases in breast cancer mortality since 1950–54. On occasion we also carry a column showing the percent change between the mortality rates from 1980–84 to 1985–89. In general, we found that for the combinations of contiguous rural counties close to civilian reactors, there were statistically significant increases in breast cancer mortality in this most recent period as well as the period from 1950–54 to 1980–84. This may suggest that reactor emissions are still exerting malign effects along with the delayed effects of bomb-test fallout. Rural counties near the oldest DOE reactor sites register improved mortality rates from 1980–84 to 1985–89, suggesting the beneficial effects of curtailed activity at these sites in the 1980s.

"NUCLEAR" AND NONNUCLEAR REGIONS

There are three regions of the nation that have been most exposed to what Rachel Carson characterized as the two "sinister" partners that induce carcinogenesis—radioactive strontium and industrial chemical pollutants—the Great Lakes, the Northeast, and the South. As is evident from figure 8–11, states west of the Mississippi and the Mountain states east of the Pacific coast states tend to have the lowest exposure and the lowest breast cancer rates. We have arranged the 60 maps, beginning with the most heavily contaminated regions and ending with the 5 reactor sites that fail to show a significant increase in breast cancer mortality.

Unfortunately, we cannot do justice to the wealth of information that is provided here for each reactor site and can offer just a few lines of commentary for each. We will begin with a detailed discussion of the first map and supporting data for the Monticello/Prairie Island reactors in Minnesota. A more detailed analysis is warranted because it has been subjected to a critical review by the Minnesota Department of Health. We will then follow the distribution of reactor sites east of the Mississippi in other Great Lakes states, followed by those from Maine to Florida, before turning to those west of the Mississippi.

THE GREAT LAKES STATES

There are more than a dozen civilian power reactor sites in the Great Lakes states of New York, Ohio, Illinois, Michigan, Minnesota, and Wisconsin. Along with a score of Canadian reactors, they have added considerable amounts of radioactive fission products to the Lakes, which interact with the long-present industrial chemical pollutants. According to table 8–4, there are 81 U.S. counties bordering the Great Lakes, with a combined current age-adjusted breast cancer mortality rate of 27.8 deaths per 100,000. This rate is so much higher than the national rate of 24.6 deaths per 100,000 that the probability that the difference could be due to chance is infinitesimal. The fact that the mortality rate was equally high in 1950–54 suggests that even in the early years of the Nuclear Age the combination of nuclear fallout, the use of contaminated surface water, high doses from early X-ray examinations, and chemical toxins released into the air has long been highly carcinogenic.

Epidemiologists consider a geographic difference in mortality rates to be significant if the probability that it could be due to chance is less than 5 in 100, and that this "chance probability" (P<.05) varies inversely with the number of deaths involved. For example, the breast cancer mortality rate for the 81 counties bordering the Great Lakes (27.8 deaths per 100,000) was based on 15,397 deaths in the 1985–89 period. This is so large a number that the chance probability turns out to be infinitesimal. It would be difficult to estimate precisely how much of the high mortality could be assigned to nuclear fallout versus chemical toxins. We can demonstrate that a significant fraction of the elevated cancer mortality can be attributed to man-made fission products by showing that the closer women live to a reactor, the greater is the risk of dying of breast cancer.

MONTICELLO/PRAIRIE ISLAND

Most of the reactor sites in the east north central states discharge their liquid effluents directly into the Great Lakes—as do their Canadian counterparts. The Monticello/Prairie Island reactor sites, however, are well inland. Like most other reactors, they are located in and near rural counties, which have so few deaths that any above-average increase in the age-adjusted breast cancer mortality rates in the 1980s as compared to 1950–54 can only be shown to be statistically significant by combining several adjoining counties. The adverse health effects of emissions from these reactors can be found by combining the 12 rural counties located close to these neighboring reactors.

In the map on page 208 we have lightly shaded those counties closest to the two reactors that are most likely to be adversely affected by reactor emissions and added a heavy border—in effect eliminating county boundaries in this cluster of contiguous counties. We will determine that their combined current mortality rate shows a significantly greater than average percentage gain since 1950.

Typically, if the combined counties are primarily rural counties near the reactor, then its increase since 1950 will generally significantly exceed that of the state, counties much farther away, or the nation. If the combined counties include mainly large urban counties then its current rate will generally significantly exceed the current U.S. rate.

Around each reactor in this and all other maps we have drawn circles with a radius of 50 miles and 100 miles. The rural counties most directly affected are those located downwind of the reactors—generally within the 50-mile radius. Within 100 miles we will frequently find the large urban counties that carry a darker shading. There are 48 such counties in the United States, all within 100 miles of 1 or more reactor sites, which have a current mortality rate that is significantly higher than the U.S. rate.

For example, in the map for Monticello/Prairie Island you will note that Nicollet County (FIPS Code 27103) is well within 100 miles of each reactor. This county has an extraordinarily high current age-adjusted breast cancer rate of 44 deaths per 100,000 women—about twice the corresponding Minnesota level. (This anomaly apparently has not yet attracted public attention, and we do not know the circumstances surrounding this particularly high current rate.)

Below each map we list the change in the age-adjusted breast cancer rates and the number of deaths individually and combined for the counties closest to the reactor. We also provide the corresponding combined data for all counties within 100 miles. Corresponding data for the state and the United States is shown to indicate the norms used to determine the statistical significance of the rates or of the degree of change.

The Monticello reactor was reported by the NRC to have released more than 11 curies of radioactive iodine and strontium between 1971 and 1975. (See appendix C.) The Prairie Island reactors reported a pipe rupture on October 2, 1979, which caused a record high release into the secondary steam-generating loop, leading to a large environmental release followed by five serious steam-generator tube leakages reported as late as September 1992.

Our analysis of the Minnesota data obtained from the NCI white female breast cancer mortality database (adjusted to the U.S. population mix of 1950) showed that the state registered a white female breast cancer mortality rate in 1985–89 that represented an 8 percent decline from 1950–54—the first period for which age-adjusted rates were available. We showed that for 12 contiguous rural counties close to the 2 reactor sites, the combined breast cancer mortality rate increased significantly by 12 percent—from 24.2 deaths per 100,000 in 1950–54 to 27.1 in 1985–89.

This information was first released by the Prairie Island Coalition Against Nuclear Storage in June of 1994 and greatly upset the Minnesota Department of Health, which then produced its own study, described by the *Minneapolis Star Tribune* as proving that "while nobody wants to live near a nuclear plant, nevertheless living near a nuclear plant engenders no greater risk than living elsewhere in Minnesota."

While the Department used the year 1970, rather than 1950, for age adjustment and chose ten Minnesota counties to represent the rural "nuclear" counties, their data showed the same overall significant difference between the state trend, which declined by 5 percent and the corresponding trend for the 10 rural counties, which rose by 7 percent, completely confirming our findings.

Additional evidence of the greater vulnerability of the 12 rural counties close to the Monticello/Prairie Island reactors comes from the fact that they continue to display a significant increase of 13 percent in breast cancer mortality rates from 1980–84 to 1985–89, when compared with no change for Minnesota as a whole.

In the maps to follow, the reader's attention should be drawn to those cases in which neighboring rural counties display significant mortality increases from 1980–84 to 1985–89. They point to possible continued mortality deterioration traceable to ongoing reactor emissions. For example, sharp rises in breast cancer mortality can be seen from 1980–84 to 1985–89 for rural counties close to civilian reactors in the South, such as North Anna (10 percent), McGuire (21 percent), Oconee (12 percent), Farley (29 percent), Hatch (12 percent), and Arkansas (12 percent). On the other hand, it is encouraging to note the recent improvement in rural counties near reactor sites that stopped operating some time ago: as in the case of INEL (-11 percent), and Los Alamos/Sandia (-2 percent).

As mentioned above, the following maps and tables are arranged by region, beginning with the most heavily contaminated and ending with the sites that fail to show a significant increase in breast cancer mortality. To find a particular reactor site, look in the index under the heading "Reactor sites and maps of nearby counties."

Monticello
Initial criticality 12/10/70
Located 23 miles southeast of St. Cloud, MN

Prairie Island Unit 1 & 2
Initial criticality 12/21/74 and 12/17/74
Located 26 miles southeast of Minneapolis, MN

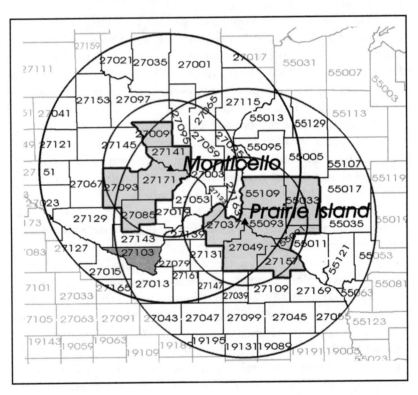

The 12 rural counties closest to the reactors are seen to have registered increases in combined age-adjusted breast cancer mortality rates since 1950–54, which are significantly greater than the corresponding changes for other Minnesota or Wisconsin counties. Note that the most significant increase occurred in the 1985–89 period.

Monticello and Prairie Island Unit 1 & 2

WHITE FEMALE BREAST CANCER MORTALITY RATES 1950-89
COUNTIES WITHIN 50 MILES OF
MONTICELLO AND PRAIRIE ISLAND
Deaths per 100,000 Women

FIPS Code	County	ST	Age-Adjusted Mortality Rates			Percent Change 80-84/ 85-89/		Number of Deaths		
			1950-54	80-84	85-89	50-54	50-54	50-54	80-84	85-89
MONTICELLO										
27171	WRIGHT	MN	34.3	22.7	22.7	-34%	-34%	26	33	36
27141	SHERBURNE	MN	22.1	36.2	22.2	64%	0%	6	27	22
27009	BENTON	MN	17.6	19.2	22.3	9%	26%	6	13	17
27093	MEEKER	MN	22.7	20.3	33.6	-11%	48%	12	16	20
27085	MC LEOD	MN	17.7	19.8	30.4	12%	72%	12	20	37
TOTAL	**ABOVE 5 COUNTIES**		**24.3**	**22.9**	**25.4**	**-6%**	**5%**	**62**	**109**	**132**
PRAIRIE ISLAND										
27049	GOODHUE	MN	22.8	23.4	30.2	3%	33%	24	36	52
27157	WABASHA	MN	30.4	12.2	32.1	-60%	5%	15	12	17
27037	DAKOTA	MN	23.2	26.5	30.0	14%	29%	27	115	159
55093	PIERCE	WI	30.7	31.0	25.8	1%	-16%	17	27	25
55109	ST. CROIX	WI	20.1	25.8	30.3	28%	51%	15	31	38
55033	DUNN	WI	24.5	22.2	13.0	-9%	-47%	18	21	16
55091	PEPIN	WI	17.7	19.1	24.9	8%	41%	3	5	7
TOTAL	**ABOVE 7 COUNTIES**		**24.1**	**24.5**	**27.9***	**2%**	**16%***	**119**	**247**	**314**
TOTAL	**ABOVE 12 COUNTIES**		**24.2**	**23.9**	**27.1***	**-1%**	**12%***	**181**	**356**	**446**
REMAINING 46 COUNTIES WITHIN 100 MILES OF THE REACTORS										
TOTAL	**46 COUNTIES**		**26.9**	**23.8**	**23.9**	**-12%**	**-11%**	**1626**	**2338**	**2503**
TOTAL	MINNESOTA		26.3	24.1	24.1	-8%	-8%	2165	3236	3431
TOTAL	WISCONSIN		26.9	25.7	24.3	-8%	-8%	2554	36991	4055
TOTAL	UNITED STATES		24.4	24.9	24.6	2%	1%	91392	167803	178868

*P<.01

Kewaunee
Initial criticality 3/7/74
Located 27 miles east-southeast of Green Bay, WI

Point Beach 1 & 2
Initial criticality 11/2/70 and 5/30/72
Located 15 miles north of Manitowoc, WI

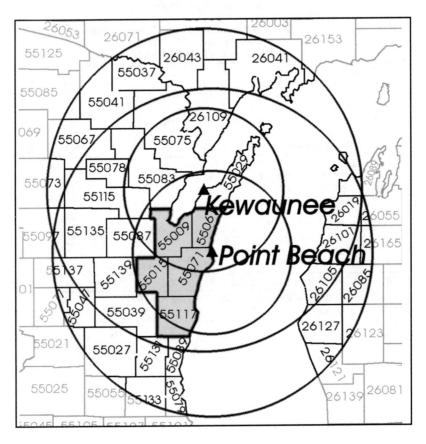

The 5 rural counties closest to the reactors have registered a combined increase in breast cancer mortality since 1950–54 that represents a significantly worse performance when compared with the sharp decline in breast cancer mortality registered by counties further away or when compared with the 10 percent improvement registered by the state of Wisconsin.

Kewaunee and Point Beach 1 & 2

WHITE FEMALE BREAST CANCER MORTALITY RATES 1950-89
COUNTIES WITHIN 50 AND 100 MILES OF KEWAUNEE/PT. BEACH
Deaths per 100,000 Women

FIPS Code	County	ST	Age-Adjusted Mortality Rates			Percent Change		Number of Deaths		
			1950-54	80-84	85-89	80-84/ 50-54	85-89/ 50-54	50-54	80-84	85-89
55015	CALUMET	WI	22.2	36.1	19.7	63%	-11%	11	30	19
55061	KEWAUNEE	WI	26.2	23.3	27.1	-11%	3%	12	19	19
55071	MANITOWOC	WI	28.4	33.0	28.4	16%	-0%	51	94	83
55117	SHEBOYGAN	WI	25.3	26.7	26.4	5%	4%	62	103	107
55009	BROWN	WI	24.3	23.3	25.9	-4%	7%	60	118	146
TOTAL5 COUNTIES			**25.6**	**27.3**	**26.1**	**6%**	**2%***	**196**	**364**	**374**
TOTAL	**26 COUNTIES**		**28.9**	**27.8**	**26.5**	**-4%**	**-8%**	**1403**	**2034**	**2014**
TOTAL	WISCONSIN		26.9	25.7	24.3	-4%	-10%	2554	3991	4055
TOTAL	UNITED STATES		24.4	24.9	24.6	2%	1%	91392	167803	178868

* P<.05

La Crosse
Initial criticality 7/11/67
Located 19 miles south of La Crosse, WI

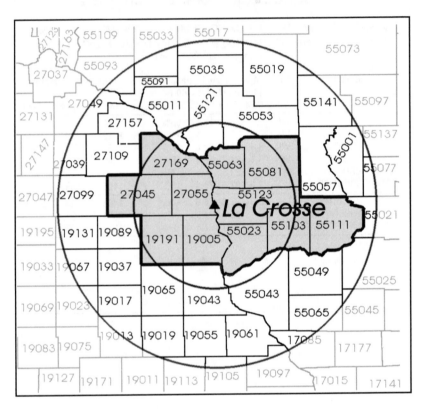

The counties closest to the reactor show no significant divergence from the national trend in age-adjusted breast cancer mortality since 1950–54. They do not do as well, however, as the surrounding counties within 100 miles. When the 2 percent increase registered by 1980–84 is compared with the 4 percent decline for Wisconsin as a whole, the chance probability is only .05, indicating some significant added risk near the reactor.

La Crosse

WHITE FEMALE BREAST CANCER MORTALITY RATES 1950-89
COUNTIES WITHIN 50 AND 100 MILES OF LA CROSSE
Deaths per 100,000 Women

FIPS Code	County	ST	Age-Adjusted Mortality Rates			Percent Change		Number of Deaths		
			1950-54	80-84	85-89	80-84/ 50-54	85-89/ 50-54	50-54	80-84	85-89
55123	VERNON	WI	16.9	17.5	15.2	4%	-10%	13	21	15
55063	LA CROSSE	WI	26.7	24.7	21.0	-7%	-21%	51	76	86
55081	MONROE	WI	21.4	18.8	16.9	-12%	-21%	19	30	25
55103	RICHLAND	WI	19.4	21.5	25.4	11%	31%	10	16	19
55111	SAUK	WI	14.7	13.3	25.3	-10%	72%	17	30	45
55023	CRAWFORD	WI	14.8	20.9	14.0	41%	-5%	6	13	12
19005	ALLAMAKEE	IA	23.9	17.5	26.9	-27%	13%	11	11	14
19191	WINNESHIEK	IA	22.3	22.3	26.3	-0%	18%	14	18	18
27055	HOUSTON	MN	17.6	21.5	17.7	23%	0%	8	13	11
27045	FILLMORE	MN	19.4	23.7	31.7	23%	64%	16	28	23
27169	WINONA	MN	27.1	32.7	18.3	21%	-32%	32	45	33
TOTAL	**11 COUNTIES**		**21.6**	**21.9**	**21.2**	**2%**	**-2%**	**197**	**301**	**301**
TOTAL	**33 COUNTIES**		**24.5**	**22.8**	**22.8**	**-7%**	**-7%**	**619**	**890**	**922**
TOTAL	WISCONSIN		26.9	25.7	24.3	-4%	-10%	2554	3991	4055
TOTAL	UNITED STATES		24.4	24.9	24.6	2%	1%	91392	167803	178868

Big Rock Point
Initial criticality 9/27/62
Located 4 miles northeast of Charlevoix, MI

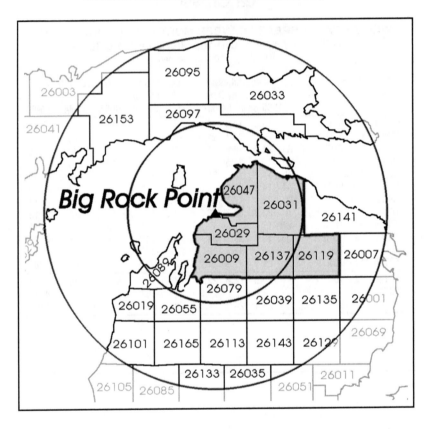

One of the nation's oldest civilian reactors, Big Rock Point is within 50 miles of 6 rural counties that in the aggregate have registered a significant 3 percent rise in breast cancer mortality since 1950–54, as compared to the 20 percent improvement in breast cancer mortality for all mainly rural counties within 100 miles.

Big Rock Point

WHITE FEMALE BREAST CANCER MORTALITY RATES 1950-89
COUNTIES WITHIN 50 AND 100 MILES OF BIG ROCK POINT
Deaths per 100,000 Women

FIPS Code	County	ST	Age-Adjusted Mortality Rates			Percent Change		Number of Deaths		
			1950-54	80-84	85-89	80-84/ 50-54	85-89/ 50-54	50-54	80-84	85-89
26029	CHARLEVOIX	MI	22.8	28.8	19.8	27%	-13%	11	20	15
26009	ANTRIM	MI	19.4	20.8	20.4	7%	5%	6	12	14
26031	CHEBOYGAN	MI	15.3	21.5	17.5	41%	15%	6	18	18
26047	EMMET	MI	26.9	13.1	17.7	-51%	-34%	14	14	16
26137	OTSEGO	MI	13.5	19.7	20.9	46%	56%	2	8	11
26119	MONTMORENCY	MI	0.0	20.8	31.7			0	6	14
TOTAL	6 COUNTIES		19.7	20.4	20.4	4%	3%*	39	78	88
TOTAL	22 COUNTIES		23.3	22.9	18.6	-2%	-20%	168	319	304
TOTAL	MICHIGAN		26.0	26.2	25.4	1%	-2%	3932	6492	6723
TOTAL	UNITED STATES		24.4	24.9	24.6	2%	1%	91392	167803	178868

* P<.05

Palisades
Initial criticality 5/24/71
Located 5 miles south of South Haven, MI

Donald C. Cook 1 & 2
Initial criticality 1/18/75 and 7/1/78
Located 11 miles south-southwest of St. Joseph, MI

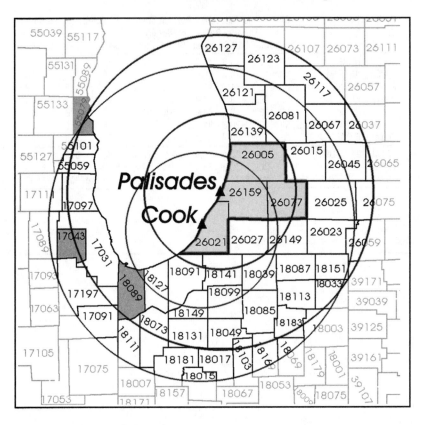

The 4 rural counties closest to the two reactor sites have registered a combined increase in age-adjusted breast cancer mortality of 12 percent since 1950–54, which is a significantly worse performance than the 2 percent decline registered in counties further away and in the state of Michigan. The 46 counties within 100 miles have a current rate of 27.1 deaths per 100,000, which is significantly above the national average of 24.6 deaths per 100,000.

Palisades and Donald C. Cook 1 & 2

WHITE FEMALE BREAST CANCER MORTALITY RATES 1950-89
COUNTIES WITHIN 50 AND 100 MILES OF PALISADES/COOK
Deaths per 100,000 Women

FIPS Code	County	ST	Age-Adjusted Mortality Rates			Percent Change 80-84/ 85-89/		Number of Deaths		
			1950-54	80-84	85-89	50-54	50-54	50-54	80-84	85-89
26159	VAN BUREN	MI	22.8	22.3	23.7	-2%	4%	28	47	51
26005	ALLEGAN	MI	22.4	27.6	22.2	23%	-1%	30	65	53
26077	KALAMAZOO	MI	19.8	27.0	26.0	37%	31%	69	164	165
26021	BERRIEN	MI	24.1	22.9	24.3	-5%	1%	72	110	125
TOTAL	**4 COUNTIES**		**21.9**	**25.1**	**24.5**	**15%**	**12%***	**199**	**386**	**394**
TOTAL	**46 COUNTIES**		**27.7**	**27.0**	**27.1****	**-3%**	**-2%**	**5443**	**7799**	**8065**
TOTAL	MICHIGAN		26.0	26.2	25.4	1%	-2%	3932	6492	6723
TOTAL	UNITED STATES		24.4	24.9	24.6	2%	1%	91392	167803	178868

* P<.01;** P<.001

Dresden 1, 2 & 3
Initial criticality 10/15/59, 1/7/70, and 1/31/71
Located 14 miles southwest of Joliet, IL

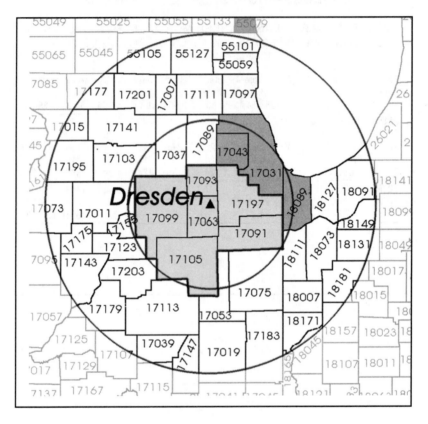

The Dresden reactors are among the nation's oldest civilian reactors, with the largest recorded volume of release since the 1970s of radioactive iodine and strontium—some 96 trillion picocuries. (See appendix C.) The six closest counties have registered an extraordinary increase in breast cancer mortality since 1950–54 when its combined rate was well below that of the state and the United States. The current combined rate for these 6 counties, along with that for the 44 large neighboring urban counties within the 100 mile radius, is among the highest in the nation and includes the nearby metropolitan Chicago counties.

Dresden 1, 2 & 3

**WHITE FEMALE BREAST CANCER MORTALITY RATES 1950-89
COUNTIES WITHIN 50 AND 100 MILES OF DRESDEN**
Deaths per 100,000 Women

FIPS Code	County	ST	Age-Adjusted Mortality Rates			Percent Change 80-84/ 85-89/		Number of Deaths		
			1950-54	80-84	85-89	50-54	50-54	50-54	80-84	85-89
17063	GRUNDY	IL	15.2	31.1	24.6	105%	62%	9	29	27
17093	KENDALL	IL	9.2	22.4	16.9	143%	83%	3	20	17
17091	KANKAKEE	IL	19.5	28.4	23.9	46%	23%	45	83	69
17099	LA SALLE	IL	27.6	29.3	28.6	6%	3%	85	132	125
17105	LIVINGSTON	IL	21.1	31.2	30.7	48%	46%	25	47	44
17197	WILL	IL	21.2	25.2	28.4	19%	34%	76	193	231
TOTAL	**6 COUNTIES**		**21.9**	**27.5**	**27.1****	**26%****	**24%****	**243**	**504**	**513**
TOTAL	**43 COUNTIES**		**28.4**	**27.5**	**27.2****	**-3%**	**-4%**	**5368**	**7505**	**7670**
TOTAL	ILLINOIS		26.6	26.8	26.2	1%	-2%	6320	8900	8981
TOTAL	UNITED STATES		24.4	24.9	24.6	2%	1%	91392	167803	178868

** P <.001

Zion 1 & 2
Initial criticality 6/19/73 and 12/24/73
Located 6 miles north of Waukegan, IL

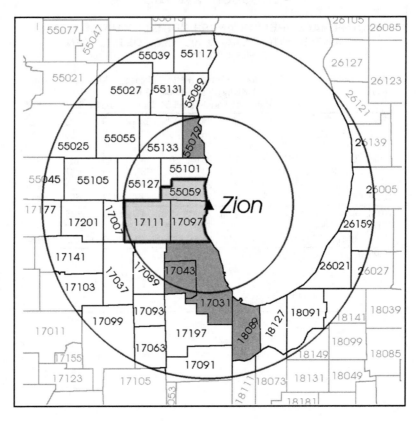

The 3 large urban counties closest to the Zion reactor as well as the counties within 100 miles and close to Lake Michigan have current age-adjusted breast cancer mortality rates significantly higher than the national average of 24.6 deaths per 100,000.

Zion 1 & 2

WHITE FEMALE BREAST CANCER MORTALITY RATES 1950-89
COUNTIES WITHIN 50 AND 100 MILES OF ZION
Deaths per 100,000 Women

FIPS Code	County	ST	Age-Adjusted Mortality Rates			Percent Change		Number of Deaths		
			1950-54	80-84	85-89	80-84/ 50-54	85-89/ 50-54	50-54	80-84	85-89
17097	LAKE	IL	37.4	26.0	27.6	-30%	-26%	162	274	339
17111	MC HENRY	IL	24.4	30.8	28.9	26%	19%	39	126	135
55059	KENOSHA	WI	27.1	26.6	29.2	-2%	8%	56	103	116
TOTAL	**3 COUNTIES**		**32.1**	**27.3**	**27.9****	**-15%**	**-13%**	**257**	**503**	**590**
TOTAL	**33 COUNTIES**		**28.9**	**27.6**	**27.5****	**-4%**	**-5%**	**6149**	**8661**	**8966**
TOTAL	ILLINOIS		26.6	26.8	26.2	1%	-2%	6320	8900	8981
TOTAL	WISCONSIN		26.9	25.7	24.3	-4%	-10%	2554	3991	4055
TOTAL	UNITED STATES		24.4	24.9	24.6	2%	1%	91392	167803	178868

** P<.001

Davis-Besse
Initial criticality 8/12/77
Located 21 miles east of Toledo, OH

Fermi
Initial criticality 6/21/85
Located at Laguna Beach, MI

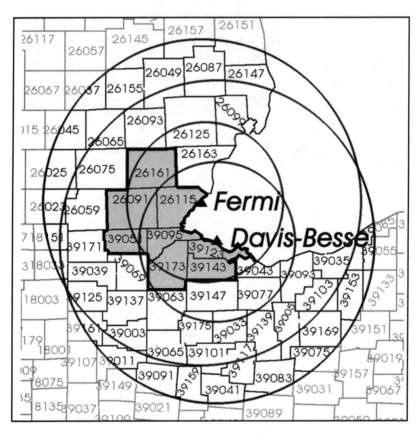

The 7 counties in Michigan and Ohio closest to these reactors have registered a combined age-adjusted increase in breast cancer mortality since 1950–54 that is significantly greater than the corresponding 1 percent national increase. The current rate, along with that of the 46 counties within 100 miles, is also significantly higher than the national average of 24.6 deaths per 100,000.

Davis-Besse and Fermi

WHITE FEMALE BREAST CANCER MORTALITY RATES 1950-89
COUNTIES WITHIN 50 AND 100 MILES OF DAVIS-BESSE/FERMI
Deaths per 100,000 Women

FIPS Code	County	ST	Age-Adjusted Mortality Rates			Percent Change 80-84/ 50-54	85-89/ 50-54	Number of Deaths		
			1950-54	80-84	85-89			50-54	80-84	85-89
39123	OTTAWA	OH	25.5	18.7	19.6	-27%	-23%	21	31	32
39095	LUCAS	OH	27.0	29.0	27.9	7%	3%	297	395	412
39051	FULTON	OH	24.2	19.9	27.0	-18%	11%	20	25	32
39173	WOOD	OH	21.2	24.8	22.8	17%	8%	35	70	73
39143	SANDUSKY	OH	23.1	18.0	24.5	-22%	6%	33	33	51
26115	MONROE	MI	23.0	23.0	30.6	-0%	33%	41	86	120
26091	LENAWEE	MI	23.0	28.1	25.7	22%	11%	41	74	75
26161	WASHTENAW	MI	22.4	25.8	26.2	15%	17%	70	132	153
TOTAL	**8 COUNTIES**		**25.1**	**25.8**	**26.6****	**3%**	**6%**	**558**	**846**	**948**
TOTAL	**45 COUNTIES**		**26.7**	**27.0**	**27.2****	**1%**	**2%**	**4769**	**6914**	**7249**
TOTAL	UNITED STATES		24.4	24.9	24.6	2%	1%	91392	167803	178868

** P<.001

Beaver Valley
Initial criticality 5/10/76
Located at Shippingport, PA

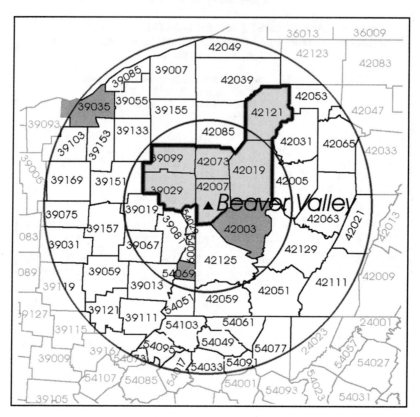

The 6 counties downwind of the reactor have registered a significant combined age-adjusted increase in breast cancer mortality
rates of 18 percent, compared with the corresponding national increase
of 1 percent. The 33 counties within 100 miles have a current combined
rate that is significantly higher than the national rate of 24.6 deaths per
100,000.

Beaver Valley

WHITE FEMALE BREAST CANCER MORTALITY RATES 1950-89
COUNTIES WITHIN 50 AND 100 MILES OF BEAVER VALLEY
Deaths per 100,000 Women

FIPS Code	County	ST	Age-Adjusted Mortality Rates			Percent Change		Number of Deaths		
						80-84/	85-89/			
			1950-54	80-84	85-89	50-54	50-54	50-54	80-84	85-89
42007	BEAVER	PA	23.2	23.1	25.5	-0%	10%	92	167	194
42019	BUTLER	PA	20.3	24.0	27.2	18%	34%	52	113	133
42073	LAWRENCE	PA	21.6	28.8	27.1	34%	26%	58	119	110
42121	VENANGO	PA	24.7	24.4	27.6	-2%	11%	46	50	64
39029	COLUMBIANA	OH	19.6	27.2	22.5	39%	15%	57	107	91
39099	MAHONING	OH	20.7	26.9	24.2	30%	17%	131	261	236
TOTAL	**6 COUNTIES**		**21.4**	**25.7**	**25.3**	**20%**	**18%****	**436**	**817**	**828**
TOTAL	**53 COUNTIES**		**24.0**	**26.8**	**26.7***	**12%**	**11%****	**4666**	**7804**	**8074**
TOTAL	PENNSYLVANIA		25.1	26.5	26.5	5%	5%	7005	10987	11522
TOTAL	UNITED STATES		24.4	24.9	24.6	2%	1%	91392	167803	178868

* P<.01   ** P<.001

West Valley

Radioactive landfill operation began in 1963.
Reprocessing of nuclear fuel began in April 1966
Located 30 miles southeast of Buffalo, NY

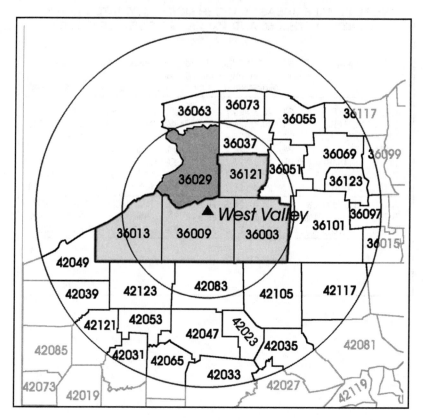

The four small counties closest to West Valley, operated by Nuclear Fuel Services, not only have registered a combined age-adjusted breast cancer mortality rate increase significantly above average, but that rate, along with that of all counties within a 100-mile radius, is significantly above the U.S. average.

West Valley

WHITE FEMALE BREAST CANCER MORTALITY RATES 1950-89
COUNTIES WITHIN 50 AND 100 MILES OF WEST VALLEY
Deaths per 100,000 Women

FIPS Code	County	ST	Age-Adjusted Mortality Rates			Percent Change 80-84/ 50-54	85-89/ 50-54	Number of Deaths		
			1950-54	80-84	85-89	50-54	50-54	50-54	80-84	85-89
36003	ALLEGANY	NY	23.4	27.6	30.2	18%	29%	33	45	49
36009	CATTARAUGUS	NY	29.3	32.4	25.8	10%	-12%	63	98	78
36013	CHAUTAUQUA	NY	23.8	31.3	30.1	31%	26%	108	171	169
36121	WYOMING	NY	24.8	27.0	29.4	9%	19%	24	36	35
TOTAL	**4 COUNTIES**		**25.3**	**30.6**	**28.8****	**21%***	**14%**	**228**	**350**	**331**
TOTAL	**26 COUNTIES**		**28.6**	**28.3**	**28.8****	**-1%**	**1%**	**2315**	**3214**	**3323**
TOTAL	UNITED STATES		24.4	2.9	24.6	2%	1%	91392	167803	178868

*P<.01,**P<.001

James A. Fitzpatrick
Initial criticality 11/17/74
Located 36 miles north of
Syracuse, NY

Ginna
Initial criticality 11/08/69
Located 16 miles northeast of
Rochester, NY

Nine Mile Point
Initial criticality 9/5/69
Located 8 miles northeast of Oswego, NY

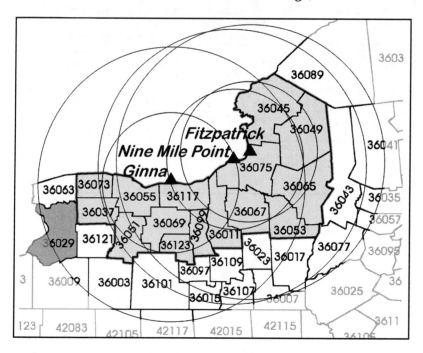

Emissions from these reactors affect the whole northwestern sector of New York State, perhaps even including Niagara County (36063), home of Love Canal. The 15 counties closest to the three reactors, as well as those within 100 miles, also affected by West Valley discharges in Cattaraugus County (36009), have a current combined age-adjusted breast cancer mortality rate that is just under 29 deaths per 100,000, which is significantly higher than the national average of 24.6 deaths and close to the highest levels in the nation. Note that the most significant increase occurred in 1985–89, as evidence of continued mortality deterioration.

James A. Fitzpatrick, Ginna, and Nine Mile Point

**WHITE FEMALE BREAST CANCER MORTALITY RATES 1950-89
COUNTIES WITHIN 50 AND 100 MILES OF FITZPATRICK,
GINNA, AND NINE MILE POINT**
Deaths per 100,000 Women

FIPS Code	County	ST	Age-Adjusted Mortality Rates 1950-54	80-84	85-89	Percent Change 80-84/ 50-54	85-89/ 50-54	Number of Deaths 50-54	80-84	85-89
36073	ORLEANS	NY	26.8	22.0	24.5	-18%	-9%	25	30	35
36037	GENESEE	NY	19.6	26.7	32.2	36%	64%	28	61	68
36051	LIVINGSTON	NY	27.7	30.3	25.5	10%	-8%	35	52	51
36055	MONROE	NY	30.4	30.1	30.6	-1%	1%	481	680	687
36117	WAYNE	NY	27.4	24.2	29.7	-11%	8%	53	67	81
36069	ONTARIO	NY	37.0	30.5	34.2	-18%	-8%	70	88	101
36123	YATES	NY	22.9	19.9	16.6	-13%	-28%	12	18	16
36099	SENECA	NY	20.8	20.9	27.1	0%	30%	22	26	34
36011	CAYUGA	NY	25.0	17.8	26.0	-29%	4%	58	49	76
36067	ONONDAGA	NY	28.7	28.2	29.2	-2%	2%	285	435	461
36075	OSWEGO	NY	25.6	23.9	28.9	-7%	13%	59	79	95
36045	JEFFERSON	NY	24.1	27.4	23.3	13%	-3%	69	80	74
36049	LEWIS	NY	19.3	16.4	16.1	-15%	-17%	12	13	16
36065	ONEIDA	NY	26.9	26.0	29.1	-3%	8%	184	264	291
36053	MADISON	NY	25.0	23.7	25.7	-5%	3%	37	54	55
TOTAL	**15 COUNTIES**		**28.2**	**27.3**	**28.6****	**-3%**	**1%**	**1426**	**1987**	**2108**
TOTAL	**25 COUNTIES**		**28.5**	**27.3**	**28.8****	**-4%**	**1%**	**2690**	**3660**	**3870**
TOTAL	UNITED STATES		24.4	24.9	24.6	2%	1%	91392	167803	178868

*P<.01,** P<.001

Maine Yankee
Initial criticality 10/23/72
Located 3.9 miles south of Wicassett, ME

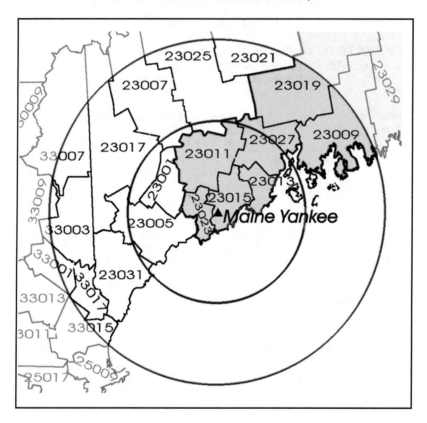

The 8 counties lying downwind of the reactor, when combined, registered a significant 14 percent increase in age-adjusted breast cancer mortality from 1950–54 to 1980–84, when compared with no observed change for Maine as a whole, which may be associated with a particularly large release reported by the NRC for the year 1973.

Maine Yankee

WHITE FEMALE BREAST CANCER MORTALITY RATES 1950-89
COUNTIES WITHIN 50 AND 100 MILES OF MAINE YANKEE
Deaths per 100,000 Women

FIPS Code	County	ST	Age-Adjusted Mortality Rates			Percent Change 80-84/ 85-89/		Number of Deaths		
			1950-54	80-84	85-89	50-54	50-54	50-54	80-84	85-89
23023	SAGADAHOC	ME	38.3	24.9	23.3	-35%	-39%	25	24	29
23015	LINCOLN	ME	18.6	41.3	21.0	123%	13%	13	42	27
23011	KENNEBEC	ME	23.3	23.8	23.3	2%	-0%	58	91	98
23013	KNOX	ME	28.0	22.3	27.1	-20%	-3%	31	34	42
23019	PENOBSCOT	ME	24.0	25.0	27.6	4%	15%	73	108	127
23027	WALDO	ME	12.4	28.2	15.7	127%	26%	10	29	19
23009	HANCOCK	ME	23.1	34.2	29.8	48%	29%	27	55	55
23029	WASHINGTON	ME	22.2	32.4	22.4	46%	1%	25	44	32
TOTAL	**8 COUNTIES**		**23.9**	**27.3**	**24.8**	**14%***	**4%**	**262**	**427**	**429**
TOTAL	**14 COUNTIES**		**24.5**	**24.6**	**24.7**	**0%**	**1%**	**589**	**889**	**954**
TOTAL	MAINE		24.5	24.6	24.1	0%	-2%	661	993	1040
TOTAL	UNITED STATES		24.4	24.9	24.6	2%	1%	91392	167803	178868

*P<.05

Vermont Yankee
Initial criticality 3/24/72
Located 5 miles south of Brattleboro, VT

Yankee Rowe
Initial criticality 8/19/60
Located 20 miles northwest of Greenfield, MA

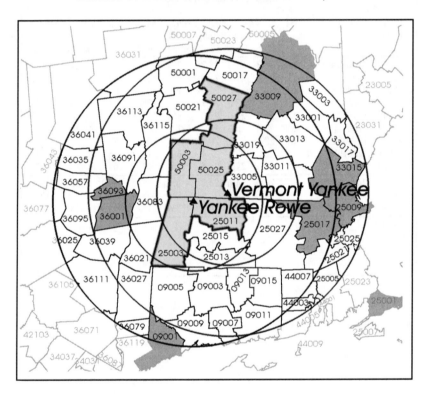

The 5 counties closest to these 2 reactors have registered a highly significant 12 percent increase in their combined age-adjusted breast cancer mortality rate since 1950–54, in sharp contrast to the more moderate increase in surrounding counties. Their 1985–89 rate of 28.6 deaths per 100,000 is even higher than that of the surrounding counties within a radius of 100 miles, which are affected by emissions from Pilgrim and Millstone. The Yankee Rowe reactor was finally closed in 1993, but unresolved decommissioning issues continue to pose public health problems.

Vermont Yankee and Yankee Rowe

WHITE FEMALE BREAST CANCER MORTALITY RATES 1950-89
COUNTIES WITHIN 50 AND 100 MILES OF
VERMONT YANKEE AND YANKEE ROWE
Deaths per 100,000 Women

FIPS Code	County	ST	Age-Adjusted Mortality Rates			Percent Change 80-84/ 50-54	85-89/ 50-54	Number of Deaths		
			1950-54	80-84	85-89	50-54	50-54	50-54	80-84	85-89
VERMONT YANKEE										
50025	WINDHAM	VT	28.4	22.1	24.9	-22%	-12%	30	31	35
50003	BENNINGTON	VT	22.8	30.7	29.7	35%	31%	16	42	40
50027	WINDSOR	VT	17.2	22.0	29.1	28%	69%	20	46	65
TOTAL	**3 COUNTIES**		**22.5**	**24.4**	**27.9**	**8%**	**24%**	**66**	**119**	**140**
YANKEE ROWE										
25011	FRANKLIN	MA	23.3	21.8	29.5	-7%	26%	43	52	76
25003	BERKSHIRE	MA	28.4	31.6	28.7	11%	1%	118	192	179
TOTAL	2 COUNTIES		27.0	28.7	28.8	6%	7%	161	244	255
TOTAL	**5 COUNTIES**		**25.5**	**27.2**	**28.6****	**7%**	**12%**	**227**	**363**	**395**
TOTAL	**45 COUNTIES**		**28.0**	**27.8**	**28.2****	**-1%**	**1%**	**7020**	**10117**	**10753**
TOTAL	MASSACHUSETTS		28.1	29.2	28.5	4%	1%	4238	6089	6164
TOTAL	VERMONT		24.2	25.8	26.2	7%	8%	270	441	480
TOTAL	UNITED STATES		24.4	24.9	24.6	2%	1%	91392	167803	178868

** P<.001

Pilgrim
Initial criticality 6/16/72
Located 25 miles southeast of Boston, MA

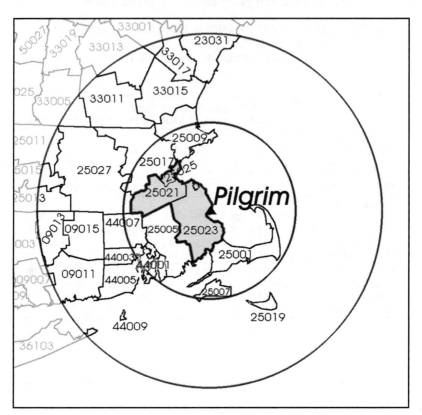

The three urban counties closest to the reactor are part of the Boston metropolitan area. Not only did they register a significant increase in breast cancer mortality since 1950–54, but its current rate of 30.6 deaths per 100,000 ranks with that of the New York metropolitan counties, exposed to emissions from Indian Point and Millstone, which have the highest breast cancer mortality rate in the nation.

Pilgrim

WHITE FEMALE BREAST CANCER MORTALITY RATES 1950-89
COUNTIES WITHIN 50 AND 100 MILES OF PILGRIM
Deaths per 100,000 Women

FIPS Code	County	ST	Age-Adjusted Mortality Rates			Percent Change		Number of Deaths		
			1950-54	80-84	85-89	80-84/ 50-54	85-89/ 50-54	50-54	80-84	85-89
25023	PLYMOUTH	MA	23.2	32.0	28.3	38%	22%	154	409	374
25025	SUFFOLK	MA	28.2	28.8	30.4	2%	8%	749	584	592
25021	NORFOLK	MA	30.3	31.6	31.8	4%	5%	412	723	755
TOTAL	**3 COUNTIES**		**28.1**	**30.6**	**30.6****	**9%**	**9%***	**1315**	**1716**	**1721**
TOTAL	**21 COUNTIES**		**27.8**	**28.3**	**28.7****	**2%**	**3%**	**4809**	**7131**	**7530**
TOTAL	MASSACHUSETTS		28.1	29.2	28.5	4%	1%	4238	6089	6164
TOTAL	UNITED STATES		24.4	24.9	24.6	2%	1%	91392	167803	178868

*P<.05,**P<.001

Millstone 1, 2 & 3
Initial criticalities 10/26/70, 1/17/75, and 1/23/86
Located 3.2 miles west-southwest of New London, CT

Haddam Neck
Initial criticality 7/24/67
Located 9.5 miles southeast of Middletown, CT

Brookhaven
Started in 1950
Located in central Suffolk County, NY

Indian Point 1, 2 & 3
Initial criticality 8/2/62, 5/22/73, and 4/6/76
Located 3 miles south of Peekskill, NY

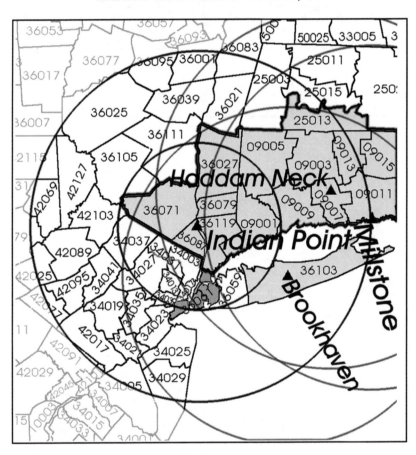

Millstone 1, 2 & 3, Haddam Neck, Brookhaven, and Indian Point 1, 2 & 3

Cumulated *per capita* emissions of radioactive iodine and strontium from these reactors since 1970s are five times the national average. There are eight counties closest to the four reactor sites. They have a current age-adjusted combined breast cancer mortality rate of 31 deaths per 100,000—the highest level in the nation—as well as significantly greater than average increases since 1950–54. Note, too, the high combined rate for the 29 counties within 100 miles of these reactors

Millstone 1, 2 & 3, Haddam Neck, Brookhaven, and Indian Point 1, 2 & 3

**WHITE FEMALE BREAST CANCER MORTALITY RATES 1950-89
COUNTIES WITHIN 50 AND 100 MILES OF MILLSTONE,
HADDAM NECK, BROOKHAVEN, AND INDIAN POINT**
Deaths per 100,000 Women

FIPS Code	County	ST	Age-Adjusted Mortality Rates 1950-54		80-84	85-89	Percent Change 80-84/ 50-54	85-89/ 50-54	Number of Deaths 50-54	80-84	85-89
INDIAN POINT											
36119	WESTCHESTER	NY	30.7		30.7	32.0	0%	4%	586	943	1011
36071	ORANGE	NY	26.4		29.6	28.3	12%	7%	133	219	238
36087	ROCKLAND	NY	24.3		29.9	33.1	23%	36%	69	220	265
36079	PUTNAM	NY	38.9		36.1	27.7	-7%	-29%	29	76	67
36027	DUTCHESS	NY	20.5		26.2	26.6	28%	30%	95	201	222
TOTAL ABOVE 5 COUNTIES			**28.3**		**30.1**	**30.7****	**6%**	**8%**	**912**	**1659**	**1803**
BROOKHAVEN											
36103	SUFFOLK	NY	23.2		31.3	32.4**	35%	40%**	232	1140	1285
HADDAM NECK/MILLSTONE											
09007	MIDDLESEX	CT	22.7		23.7	24.7	4%	9%	49	107	119
09011	NEW LONDON	CT	22.4		26.8	28.2	20%	26%	97	197	223
TOTAL 2 COUNTIES			**22.5**		**25.6**	**26.8****	**14%**	**19%****	**146**	**304**	**342**
TOTAL 48 COUNTIES			**30.1**		**29.3**	**28.8****	**-3%**	**-4%**	**15015**	**21466**	**21859**
TOTAL	NEW YORK CITY		31.8		29.4	28.3**	-8%	-11%**	6817	6102	5755
TOTAL	UNITED STATES		24.4		24.9	24.6	2%	1%	91392	167803	178868

** P<.001

Three Mile Island 1 & 2
Initial criticality 6/5/74 and 3/28/78
Major accident 3/28/79
Located 10 miles southeast of Harrisburg, PA

Peach Bottom 1, 2 & 3
Initial criticality 9/16/73 and 8/7/74
Unit 1 shut down in 1974
Located 17.9 miles south of Lancaster, PA

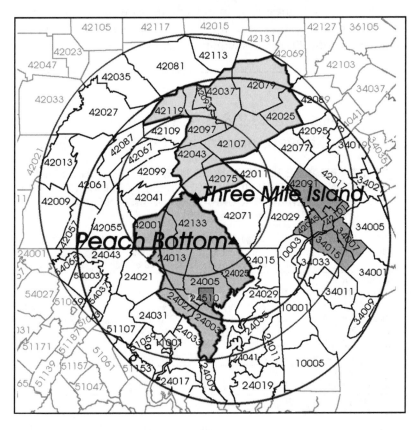

The 16 counties closest to these reactors have registered a significant 13 percent increase in breast cancer mortality since 1950–54. Their combined current rate of 27 deaths per 100,000 is close to the nation's highest. The same could be said for the even higher combined rate for all counties within a radius of 100 miles.

Three Mile Island 1 & 2 and Peach Bottom 1, 2 & 3

WHITE FEMALE BREAST CANCER MORTALITY RATES 1950-89
COUNTIES WITHIN 50 AND 100 MILES OF
THREE MILE ISLAND AND PEACH BOTTOM
Deaths per 100,000 Women

FIPS Code	County	ST	Age-Adjusted Mortality Rates			Percent Change 80-84/ 50-54	85-89/ 50-54	Number of Deaths		
			1950-54	80-84	85-89	50-54	50-54	50-54	80-84	85-89
THREE MILE ISLAND										
42043	DAUPHIN	PA	24.5	25.4	28.8	3%	17%	141	212	240
42075	LEBANON	PA	22.3	24.5	25.5	10%	14%	50	100	106
42097	NORTHUMBERLAND	PA	25.3	31.4	29.8	24%	18%	83	139	141
42107	SCHUYLKILL	PA	24.8	24.1	28.1	-3%	13%	134	184	199
42119	UNION	PA	18.5	14.4	25.5	-22%	38%	12	17	25
42093	MONTOUR	PA	22.5	35.5	25.5	58%	13%	15	26	20
42037	COLUMBIA	PA	19.6	29.7	33.1	51%	69%	31	70	73
42079	LUZERNE	PA .	22.6	25.2	25.5	11%	13%	243	383	387
42025	CARBON	PA	19.5	20.7	25.3	6%	29%	31	52	67
TOTAL	**9 COUNTIES**		**23.3**	**25.6**	**27.2***	**10%**	**17%**	**740**	**1183**	**1258**
PEACH BOTTOM										
42071	LANCASTER	PA	26.6	27.2	25.2	2%	-5%	182	351	356
42133	YORK	PA	24.5	27.9	26.1	14%	6%	143	294	309
24013	CARROLL	MD	20.7	21.0	25.8	2%	25%	28	58	86
24005	BALTIMORE	MD	27.5	24.9	28.4	-10%	3%	174	540	650
24025	HARFORD	MD	13.9	21.3	24.8	54%	79%	14	72	99
24027	HOWARD	MD	16.3	27.6	27.9	70%	72%	8	66	90
24003	ANNE ARUNDEL	MD	22.2	30.1	27.5	35%	24%	44	262	279
TOTAL	**7 COUNTIES**		**24.6**	**26.2**	**26.8****	**7%**	**9%***	**593**	**1643**	**1869**
TOTAL	**ABOVE 16 COUNTIES**		**23.9**	**26.0**	**27.0****	**9%**	**13%****	**1333**	**2826**	**3127**
TOTAL	56 COUNTIES		26.2	27.0	27.2**	3%	4%	6079	10226	11010
TOTAL	UNITED STATES		24.4	24.9	24.6	2%	1%	91392	167803	178868

* P<.01, ** P<.001

Calvert Cliffs
Initial criticality 10/7/74
45 miles southeast of Washington, D.C.

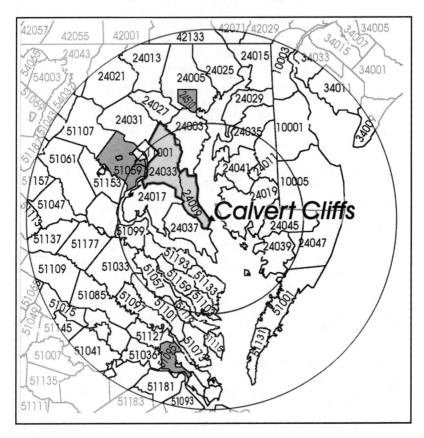

The 2 counties closest and downwind of the Calvert Cliffs reactor have registered a significant 12 percent increase in combined age-adjusted breast cancer mortality rates since 1950–54. Its current rate of 26.8 deaths per 100,000 is significantly higher than the U.S. rate of 24.6 deaths. The counties within 100 miles as well as the whole of Maryland are also impacted by emissions from the Peach Bottom reactor and have current mortality rates of the same high order.

Calvert Cliffs

WHITE FEMALE BREAST CANCER MORTALITY RATES 1950-89
COUNTIES WITHIN 50 AND 100 MILES OF CALVERT CLIFFS
Deaths per 100,000 Women

FIPS Code	County	ST	Age-Adjusted Mortality Rates			Percent Change 80-84/ 50-54	85-89/ 50-54	Number of Deaths		
			1950-54	80-84	85-89			50-54	80-84	85-89
24009	CALVERT	MD	38.8	15.8	18.8	-59%	-52%	7	13	20
24033	PRINCE GEORGES	MD	23.3	29.2	27.5	25%	18%	80	316	306
TOTAL	**2 COUNTIES**		**23.9**	**28.3**	**26.8**	**18%**	**12%**	**87**	**329**	**326**
TOTAL	**53 COUNTIES**		**25.1**	**26.8**	**26.2***	**7%**	**4%**	**2007**	**4365**	**4725**
TOTAL	MARYLAND		26.4	26.9	26.3	2%	-0%	1397	2893	3086
TOTAL	UNITED STATES		24.4	24.9	24.6	2%	1%	91392	167803	178868

* P<.001

Oyster Creek
Initial criticality 5/3/69
Located 9 miles south of Toms River, NJ

Salem
Initial criticality 6/30/77 and 12/11/76
Located 20 miles south of Wilmington, DE

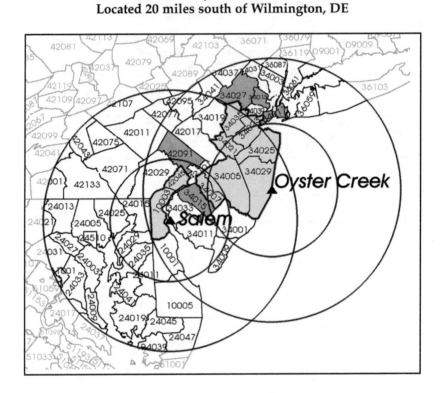

The 9 counties closest to these reactors have registered a combined age-adjusted breast cancer mortality increase since 1950–54 of 9 percent, which is significantly greater than the national increase of 1 percent. Possibly because the counties within 100 miles include some with the nation's highest concentrations of chemical wastes, their combined current rate of 28.8 deaths per 100,000 appears to be, along with that for New Jersey, among the highest in the nation.

Oyster Creek and Salem

WHITE FEMALE BREAST CANCER MORTALITY RATES 1950-89
COUNTIES WITHIN 50 AND 100 MILES OF
OYSTER CREEK AND SALEM
Deaths per 100,000 Women

FIPS Code	County	ST	Age-Adjusted Mortality Rates			Percent Change		Number of Deaths		
			1950-54	80-84	85-89	80-84/ 50-54	85-89/ 50-54	50-54	80-84	85-89
OYSTER CREEK										
34029	OCEAN	NJ	27.4	28.9	28.7	6%	5%	56	479	608
34005	BURLINGTON	NJ	27.3	26.6	28.6	-3%	5%	91	255	306
34025	MONMOUTH	NJ	29.7	32.5	31.9	9%	7%	213	542	579
34021	MERCER	NJ	26.7	27.4	28.7	2%	7%	165	248	286
34023	MIDDLESEX	NJ	27.6	30.3	30.5	10%	10%	184	534	601
34035	SOMERSET	NJ	27.6	30.4	27.7	10%	0%	72	196	197
TOTAL	**6 COUNTIES**		**28.0**	**29.6**	**29.7****	**6%**	**6%**	**781**	**2254**	**2577**
SALEM										
34007	CAMDEN	NJ	27.6	28.3	28.8	3%	5%	224	399	422
42045	DELAWARE	PA	28.5	32.2	31.7	13%	11%	313	624	631
10003	NEW CASTLE	DE	22.7	28.8	29.6	27%	31%	126	315	355
TOTAL	**3 COUNTIES**		**26.9**	**30.1**	**30.1****	**12%**	**12%***	**663**	**1338**	**1408**
TOTAL	**ABOVE 9 COUNTIES**		**27.5**	**29.8**	**29.9****	**8%**	**9%***	**1444**	**3592**	**3985**
TOTAL	53 COUNTIES		29.7	29.1	28.9**	-2%	-3%	16134	23683	28488
TOTAL	NEW JERSEY		29.4	29.3	29.3	-0%	-0%	3999	7007	7446
TOTAL	UNITED STATES		24.4	24.9	24.6	2%	1%	91392	167803	178868

*P<.01   ** P<.0001

North Anna 1 & 2
Initial criticality 4/5/78 and 6/12/80
Located 40 miles northwest of Richmond, VA

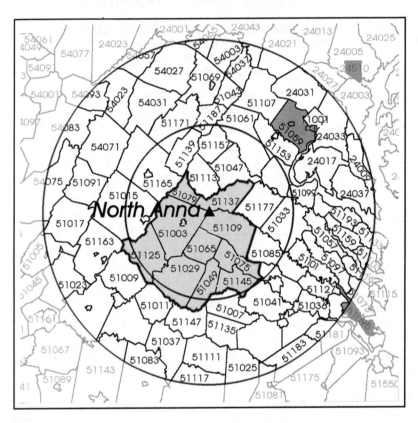

The 10 counties closest to the reactor registered an extraordinary 73 percent increase since 1950–54 in breast cancer mortality—significantly greater than the moderate 4 percent increase registered by the combined rate for all counties within 100 miles. The North Anna reactors have not been operating long. Much of this increase may be associated with the significant 24 percent increase since 1950–54 registered by Virginia, which may be affected by emissions from Oak Ridge.

North Anna 1 & 2

WHITE FEMALE BREAST CANCER MORTALITY RATES 1950-89
COUNTIES WITHIN 50 AND 100 MILES OF NORTH ANNA
Deaths per 100,000 Women

FIPS Code	County	ST	Age-Adjusted Mortality Rates			Percent Change 80-84/ 50-54	85-89/ 50-54	Number of Deaths		
			1950-54	80-84	85-89			50-54	80-84	85-89
51075	GOOCHLAND	VA	8.4	20.3	18.9	140%	124%	1	6	6
51065	FLUVANNA	VA	16.2	24.6	33.3	52%	106%	2	6	8
51003	ALBEMARLE	VA	14.8	20.8	21.9	40%	48%	16	53	60
51109	LOUISA	VA	15.3	17.2	26.2	12%	71%	4	7	12
51137	ORANGE	VA	10.5	19.4	20.4	85%	95%	3	12	14
51079	GREENE	VA	6.4	22.4	22.4	251%	250%	1	4	5
51049	CUMBERLAND	VA	25.4	30.5	9.2	20%	-64%	2	4	2
51029	BUCKINGHAM	VA	10.7	31.1	30.0	191%	181%	2	8	8
51145	POWHATAN	VA	0.0	11.4	25.1			0	3	7
51125	NELSON	VA	11.3	17.7	21.5	56%	90%	3	5	10
TOTAL	**10 COUNTIES**		**13.0**	**20.5**	**22.5**	**57%**	**73%****	**34**	**108**	**132**
TOTAL	**59 COUNTIES**		**24.4**	**27.1****	**25.2**	**11%**	**3%**	**1406**	**3104**	**3225**
TOTAL	VIRGINIA		19.7	24.0	24.5	22%	24%	1205	3226	3675
TOTAL	UNITED STATES		24.4	24.9	24.6	2%	1%	91392	167803	178868

** P<.001

Surry 1 & 2
Initial criticality 7/1/72 and 3/7/73
Located 19 miles northwest of Newport News, VA

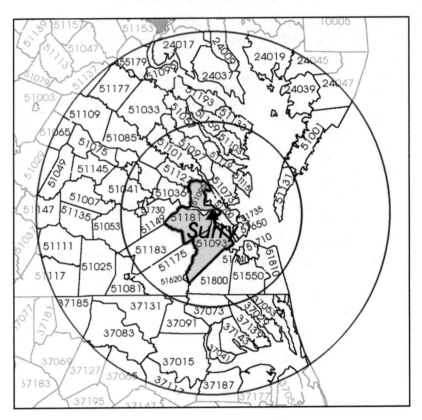

The three small rural counties closest to the Surry reactors have a combined current age-adjusted breast cancer mortality rate that is both significantly higher than that of the United States or Virginia as a whole and has risen significantly since 1950–54. The combined rate for counties within 100 miles has also registered a significant long-term increase.

Surry 1 & 2

WHITE FEMALE BREAST CANCER MORTALITY RATES 1950-89
COUNTIES WITHIN 50 AND 100 MILES OF SURRY
Deaths per 100,000 Women

FIPS Code	County	ST	Age-Adjusted Mortality Rates			Percent Change 80-84/ 85-89/		Number of Deaths		
			1950-54	80-84	85-89	50-54	50-54	50-54	80-84	85-89
51181	SURRY	VA	19.3	14.0	33.3	-27%	72%	2	2	4
51093	ISLE OF WIGHT	VA	37.1	23.7	22.3	-36%	-40%	7	9	12
51095	JAMES CITY	VA	22.1	26.3	29.8	19%	35%	53	174	222
TOTAL	**3 COUNTIES**		**23.2**	**25.9**	**29.4***	**12%**	**27%***	**62**	**185**	**238**
TOTAL	**46 COUNTIES**		**21.6**	**24.7**	**25.6**	**14%**	**18%****	**733**	**1930**	**2229**
TOTAL	VIRGINIA		19.7	24.0	24.5	22%	24%	1205	3226	3675
TOTAL	UNITED STATES		24.4	24.9	24.6	2%	1%	91392	167803	178868

* P<.01 **P<.001

McGuire 1 & 2
Initial criticality 8/8/81 and 8/5/83
Located 17 miles north of Charlotte, NC

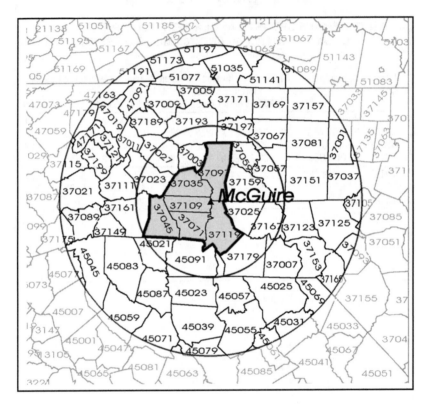

The McGuire reactors near Charlotte have not been operating long enough to be solely responsible for the highly significant 46 percent increase in the combined age-adjusted breast cancer mortality rates for the 6 counties closest to the reactors. Like most counties in North Carolina downwind of Oak Ridge, this increase may be largely associated with chronic exposure to Oak Ridge emissions sustained since 1943.

McGuire 1 & 2

WHITE FEMALE BREAST CANCER MORTALITY RATES 1950-89
COUNTIES WITHIN 50 AND 100 MILES OF MCGUIRE
Deaths per 100,000 Women

FIPS Code	County	ST	Age-Adjusted Mortality Rates			Percent Change 80-84/ 85-89/		Number of Deaths		
			1950-54	80-84	85-89	50-54	50-54	50-54	80-84	85-89
37071	GASTON	NC	12.2	18.8	19.3	54%	58%	22	89	101
37045	CLEVELAND	NC	22.9	18.8	27.9	-18%	21%	25	46	69
37119	MECKLENBURG	NC	20.2	25.2	30.7	25%	52%	69	233	325
37097	IREDELL	NC	19.5	21.1	28.9	8%	49%	21	47	77
37109	LINCOLN	NC	13.7	17.0	22.7	24%	65%	7	20	33
37035	CATAWBA	NC	18.3	20.0	23.1	10%	27%	20	66	88
TOTAL	**6 COUNTIES**		**18.0**	**21.7**	**26.3**	**21%**	**46%****	**164**	**501**	**693**
TOTAL	**62 COUNTIES**		**17.8**	**22.2**	**23.7**	**25%**	**33%****	**1033**	**2980**	**3548**
TOTAL	NORTH CAROLINA		17.7	22.1	23.3	25%	32%	1158	3330	3982
TOTAL	UNITED STATES		24.4	24.9	24.6	2%	1%	91392	167803	178868

** P<.001

Brunswick
Initial criticality 10/8/76
Located 20 miles south of Wilmington, NC

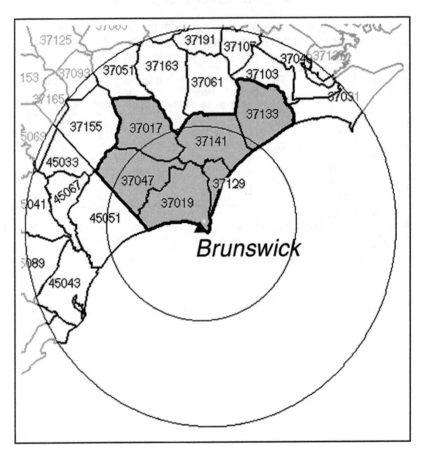

As in the case of McGuire the counties close to the Brunswick reactor have registered significant increases in age-adjusted breast cancer mortality rates, much of which could be associated with emissions from Oak Ridge, sustained since 1943. All the small counties within a radius of 100 miles have sufficient deaths to permit the observed 25 percent increase in age-adjusted breast cancer mortality since 1950–54 to be seen as statistically significant.

Brunswick

WHITE FEMALE BREAST CANCER MORTALITY RATES 1950-89
COUNTIES WITHIN 50 AND 100 MILES OF BRUNSWICK
Deaths per 100,000 Women

FIPS Code	County	ST	Age-Adjusted Mortality Rates			Percent Change 80-84/ 85-89/		Number of Deaths		
			1950-54	80-84	85-89	50-54	50-54	50-54	80-84	85-89
37017	BLADEN	NC	9.4	12.3	22.9	31%	144%	3	8	15
37019	BRUNSWICK	NC	16.3	24.8	13.9	52%	-15%	4	25	21
37047	COLUMBUS	NC	5.9	13.2	19.6	122%	231%	4	17	28
37129	NEW HANOVER	NC	28.5	20.7	22.6	-27%	-21%	32	54	73
37133	ONSLOW	NC	14.3	20.6	22.9	44%	60%	7	29	37
37141	PENDER	NC	19.2	24.6	22.5	28%	17%	4	12	15
TOTAL	**6 COUNTIES**		**18.0**	**19.5**	**21.1**	**8%**	**18%**	**54**	**145**	**189**
TOTAL	**19 COUNTIES**		**17.2**	**21.1**	**21.6**	**22%**	**25%***	**173**	**516**	**610**
TOTAL	NORTH CAROLINA		17.7	22.1	23.3	25%	32%	1158	3330	3982
TOTAL	UNITED STATES		24.4	24.9	24.6	2%	1%	91392	167803	178868

* P<.01

Oak Ridge National Laboratory
Selected on September 9, 1942, as a uranium enrichment site.
Code named Site X.
In full operation with 80,000 employees by late 1944.
Located 20 miles east of Knoxville, TN

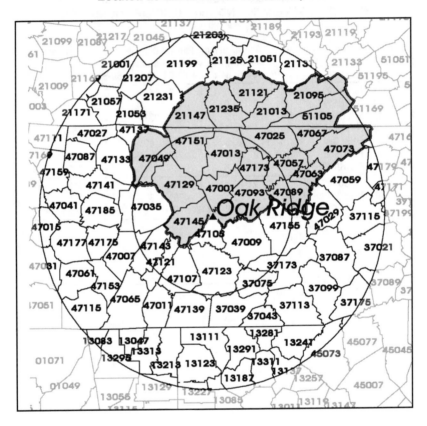

As one of the nation's oldest reactor sites (along with Hanford and Los Alamos), Oak Ridge has contributed to a 38 percent increase in the combined age-adjusted breast cancer rate of a group of 20 downwind counties. As in the case of all other DOE reactor sites located in rural areas with below-average initial mortality rates, the subsequent mortality increases are too large to be attributed to chance.

Oak Ridge National Laboratory

WHITE FEMALE BREAST CANCER MORTALITY RATES 1950-89
COUNTIES WITHIN 50 AND 100 MILES OF OAK RIDGE
Deaths per 100,000 Women

FIPS Code	County	ST	Age-Adjusted Mortality Rates			Percent Change 80-84/ 85-89/		Number of Deaths		
			1950-54	80-84	85-89	50-54	50-54	50-54	80-84	85-89
47001	ANDERSON	TN	18.7	21.6	23.9	16%	28%	17	50	58
47013	CAMPBELL	TN	14.6	28.8	20.4	97%	40%	9	35	29
47025	CLAIBORNE	TN	21.9	20.9	15.1	-5%	-31%	10	15	12
47049	FENTRESS	TN	4.1	23.2	6.4	458%	54%	1	10	4
47057	GRAINGER	TN	20.6	13.9	16.8	-33%	-18%	6	7	9
47063	HAMBLEN	TN	3.8	17.3	22.7	351%	492%	2	24	39
47067	HANCOCK	TN	22.3	7.3	44.4	-68%	99%	4	1	9
47073	HAWKINS	TN	20.6	22.0	21.7	7%	5%	13	30	30
47089	JEFFERSON	TN	15.7	21.5	25.3	36%	60%	7	23	28
47093	KNOX	TN	19.1	22.8	22.1	19%	16%	95	225	231
47129	MORGAN	TN	3.5	12.8	16.4	266%	368%	1	7	9
47145	ROANE	TN	21.6	16.9	16.5	-22%	-24%	14	27	30
47151	SCOTT	TN	10.7	15.1	12.2	40%	14%	3	7	7
47173	UNION	TN	10.7	13.1	28.2	22%	162%	2	5	11
21013	BELL	KY	5.1	23.1	21.5	350%	318%	4	24	22
21095	HARLAN	KY	11.0	15.8	22.1	43%	100%	11	21	28
21121	KNOX	KY	15.3	19.9	27.6	31%	81%	9	18	29
21147	MC CREARY	KY	3.5	17.7	23.3	405%	564%	1	7	10
21235	WHITLEY	KY	19.3	18.4	21.7	-5%	12%	13	21	25
51105	LEE	VA	6.3	24.2	18.5	284%	194%	4	20	18
TOTAL	**20 COUNTIES**			15.5	20.8	21.4	34%	38%**	226	577	638
TOTAL	**71 COUNTIES**			15.8	20.6	20.4	30%	29%**	578	1522	1652
TOTAL	UNITED STATES		24.4	24.9	24.6	2%	1%	91392	167803	178868

**P<.001

Oconee 1, 2 & 3
Initial criticality 4/19/73, 11/11/73, and 9/5/74
Located 30 miles west of Greenville, SC

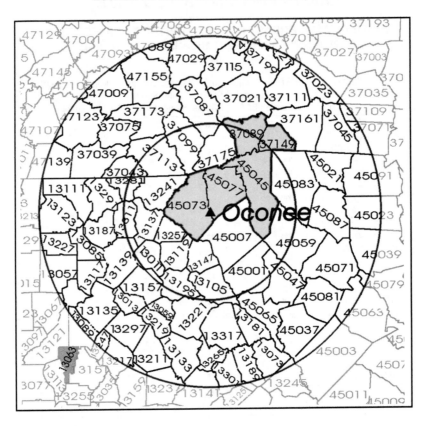

The 5 counties closest to the reactor have registered a 56 percent increase in their combined age-adjusted breast cancer rate since 1950–54, which is extraordinarily significant when compared with the corresponding 1 percent increase for the United States. The same is true for all 66 rural counties within 100 miles.

Oconee 1, 2 & 3

WHITE FEMALE BREAST CANCER MORTALITY RATES 1950-89
COUNTIES WITHIN 50 AND 100 MILES OF OCONEE
Deaths per 100,000 Women

FIPS Code	County	ST	Age-Adjusted Mortality Rates			Percent Change		Number of Deaths		
						80-84/ 50-54	85-89/ 50-54			
			1950-54	80-84	85-89			50-54	80-84	85-89
45073	OCONEE	SC	12.5	24.2	21.0	94%	68%	8	34	40
45045	GREENVILLE	SC	17.4	24.8	29.8	42%	71%	52	200	262
45077	PICKENS	SC	9.1	19.3	16.3	113%	80%	7	39	41
37089	HENDERSON	NC	23.8	19.8	26.7	-17%	12%	19	58	81
37149	POLK	NC	6.3	12.9	13.6	105%	116%	2	8	11
TOTAL	**5 COUNTIES**		**16.3**	**22.7**	**25.5**	**39%**	**56%****	**88**	**339**	**435**
TOTAL	**64 COUNTIES**		**17.8**	**21.9**	**22.7**	**23%**	**28%****	**576**	**1665**	**1979**
TOTAL	NORTH CAROLINA		17.7	22.1	23.3	25%	32%**	1158	3330	3982
TOTAL	SOUTH CAROLINA		18.4	22.7	22.2	23%	21%**	518	1577	1751
TOTAL	UNITED STATES		24.4	24.9	24.6	2%	1%	91392	167803	178868

** $P<.001$

H.B. Robinson
Initial criticality 9/20/70
Located 4.5 miles west-northwest of Hartsville, SC

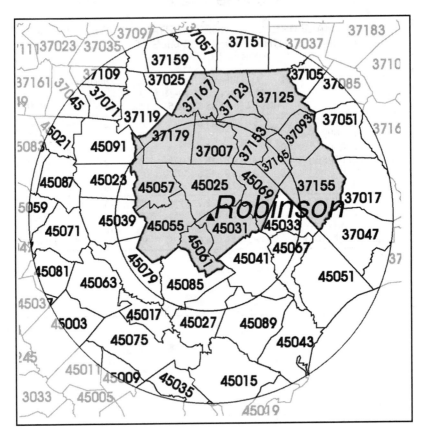

The 15 counties downwind of the Robinson reactor are all rural counties that registered a significant 27 percent increase in the combined age-adjusted breast cancer mortality rate since 1950–54, as compared to the 1 percent increase for the United States. The same is true for all 44 mainly rural counties within 100 miles.

H.B. Robinson

WHITE FEMALE BREAST CANCER MORTALITY RATES 1950-89
COUNTIES WITHIN 50 AND 100 MILES OF ROBINSON
Deaths per 100,000 Women

FIPS Code	County	ST	Age-Adjusted Mortality Rates			Percent Change 80-84/ 85-89/		Number of Deaths		
			1950-54	80-84	85-89	50-54	50-54	50-54	80-84	85-89
45025	CHESTERFIELD	SC	14.9	24.2	19.1	63%	29%	7	22	15
45031	DARLINGTON	SC	16.1	16.0	24.5	-1%	52%	9	22	35
45069	MARLBORO	SC	23.4	25.3	20.6	8%	-12%	8	15	11
45055	KERSHAW	SC	33.4	16.3	10.4	-51%	-69%	12	13	10
45061	LEE	SC	4.6	7.7	22.0	69%	379%	1	3	6
37007	ANSON	NC	12.0	16.4	15.7	36%	30%	4	12	9
37179	UNION	NC	12.7	20.2	30.3	60%	139%	9	34	62
37153	RICHMOND	NC	18.0	22.5	23.8	25%	32%	9	26	29
37155	ROBESON	NC	21.1	24.1	24.1	14%	14%	17	34	34
45057	LANCASTER	SC	17.1	18.0	19.1	5%	11%	9	23	29
37123	MONTGOMERY	NC	15.8	27.1	22.5	72%	42%	5	18	14
37093	HOKE	NC	7.0	23.7	17.6	241%	153%	1	5	5
37125	MOORE	NC	23.1	29.6	23.8	28%	3%	13	48	58
37165	SCOTLAND	NC	0.0	26.3	21.0			0	16	16
37167	STANLY	NC	20.7	22.4	20.1	8%	-3%	15	34	40
TOTAL	**15 COUNTIES**		**17.4**	**22.1**	**22.1**	**27%**	**27%***	**119**	**325**	**373**
TOTAL	**44 COUNTIES**		**17.3**	**21.8**	**24.0**	**26%**	**39%****	**535**	**1670**	**2086**
TOTAL	NORTH CAROLINA		17.7	22.1	23.3	25%	32%	1158	3330	3982
TOTAL	SOUTH CAROLINA		18.4	22.7	22.2	23%	21%	518	1577	1751
TOTAL	UNITED STATES		24.4	24.9	24.6	2%	1%	91392	167803	178868

* P<.01,** P<.001

Savannah River Plant
Established in 1950, began operations in 1952
Located 13 miles south of Aiken, GA and 20 miles
southeast of Augusta, GA

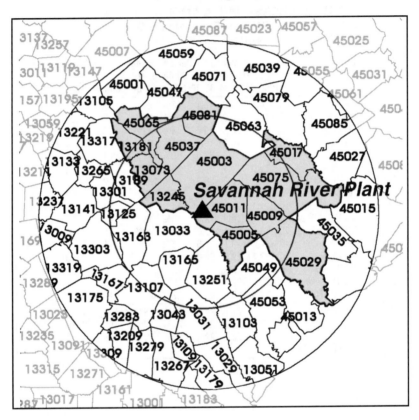

The 14 shaded counties closest to Savannah River have registered a significant increase of 20 percent in the combined age-adjusted breast cancer mortality rate from 1950–54 to 1980–84, when compared with the corresponding 2 percent increase for the United States, as is also true for the combined rate for all 53 counties within 100 miles.

Savannah River Plant

WHITE FEMALE BREAST CANCER MORTALITY RATES 1950-89
COUNTIES WITHIN 50 AND 100 MILES OF SAVANNAH RIVER PLANT
Deaths per 100,000 Women

FIPS Code	County	ST	Age-Adjusted Mortality Rates			Percent Change 80-84/ 85-89/		Number of Deaths		
			1950-54	80-84	85-89	50-54	50-54	50-54	80-84	85-89
13033	BURKE	GA	6.9	19.7	10.9	184%	57%	1	5	4
13073	COLUMBIA	GA	41.3	12.6	10.3	-69%	-75%	5	10	11
13181	LINCOLN	GA	22.7	12.5	24.4	-45%	7%	2	1	3
13245	RICHMOND	GA	16.0	23.1	23.2	44%	45%	26	79	78
45003	AIKEN	SC	18.9	20.0	21.8	6%	15%	16	50	64
45005	ALLENDALE	SC	23.1	25.3	4.2	9%	-82%	2	4	2
45009	BAMBERG	SC	12.1	24.4	23.1	102%	92%	2	7	6
45011	BARNWELL	SC	28.7	25.2	8.8	-12%	-69%	5	9	4
45017	CALHOUN	SC	7.5	22.5	14.1	202%	89%	1	5	3
45029	COLLETON	SC	6.3	24.9	23.0	297%	267%	2	19	15
45037	EDGEFIELD	SC	4.9	24.6	5.6	402%	15%	1	8	2
45065	MC CORMICK	SC	9.3	23.6	11.1	152%	19%	1	2	2
45081	SALUDA	SC	26.0	36.0	22.3	38%	-14%	6	15	12
45075	ORANGEBURG	SC	25.5	17.4	16.8	-32%	-34%	16	23	21
TOTAL	**14 COUNTIES**		**17.7**	**21.3**	**18.9**	**20%***	**6%**	**86**	**237**	**227**
TOTAL	**53 COUNTIES**		**18.2**	**22.2**	**21.3**	**22%****	**17%**	**329**	**860**	**912**
TOTAL	SOUTH CAROLINA		18.4	22.7	22.2	23%	21%	518	1577	1751
TOTAL	UNITED STATES		24.4	24.9	24.6	2%	1%	91392	167803	178868

*P<.05   ** P<.001

Sequoyah 1 & 2
Initial criticality 7/5/80 and 11/5/81
Located at Daisy, TN

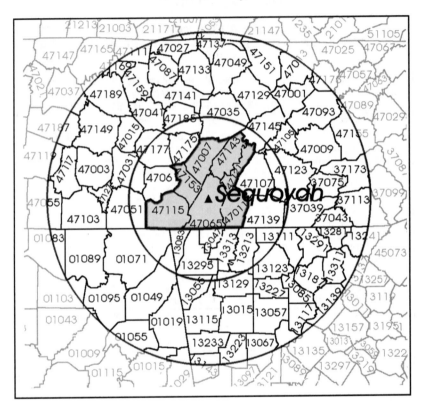

The 6 counties closest to the reactor have registered a combined age-adjusted breast cancer mortality rate increase of 24 percent since 1950–54—significantly higher than the 1 percent increase registered by the United States. The same is true for all counties within a 100-mile radius.

Sequoyah 1 & 2

WHITE FEMALE BREAST CANCER MORTALITY RATES 1950-89
COUNTIES WITHIN 50 AND 100 MILES OF SEQUOYAH
Deaths per 100,000 Women

FIPS Code	County	ST	Age-Adjusted Mortality Rates			Percent Change 80-84/ 85-89/		Number of Deaths		
			1950-54	80-84	85-89	50-54	50-54	50-54	80-84	85-89
47065	HAMILTON	TN	19.5	25.7	22.0	32%	13%	81	207	190
47011	BRADLEY	TN	13.4	16.4	22.6	23%	69%	9	33	49
47115	MARION	TN	17.8	14.8	16.6	-17%	-7%	7	11	12
47121	MEIGS	TN	18.6	17.9	13.4	-4%	-28%	2	4	3
47143	RHEA	TN	11.4	14.4	18.0	27%	58%	4	10	15
47153	SEQUATCHIE	TN	9.7	10.8	0.0	12%	-100%	1	3	0
TOTAL	**6 COUNTIES**		**18.0**	**22.3**	**20.9**	**24%***	**16%**	**104**	**268**	**269**
TOTAL	**66 COUNTIES**		**18.0**	**21.0**	**21.3**	**17%****	**18%**	**699**	**1883**	**2101**
TOTAL	TENNESSEE		18.1	20.8	21.1	15%	17%	1186	2706	2998
TOTAL	UNITED STATES		24.4	24.9	24.6	2%	1%	91392	167803	178858

* P<.01 ** P<.001

Browns Ferry 1, 2 & 3
Initial criticality 8/17/73, 7/20/74, and 8/8/76
Located 10 miles northwest of Decatur, AL

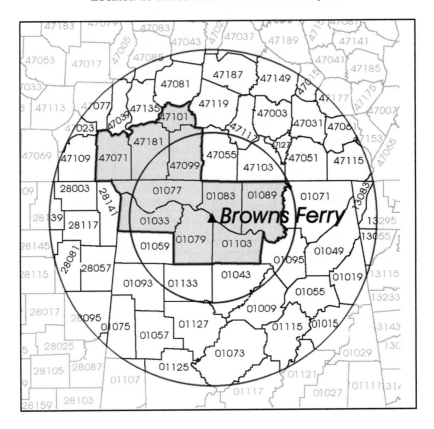

The 10 rural counties closest to the reactors, when combined, have registered a significant increase in breast cancer mortality since 1950–54, as have all 49 rural counties within 100 miles.

Browns Ferry 1, 2 & 3

WHITE FEMALE BREAST CANCER MORTALITY RATES 1950-89
COUNTIES WITHIN 50 AND 100 MILES OF BROWNS FERRY
Deaths per 100,000 Women

FIPS Code	County	ST	Age-Adjusted Mortality Rates			Percent Change 80-84/ 50-54	85-89/ 50-54	Number of Deaths		
			1950-54	80-84	85-89	50-54	50-54	50-54	80-84	85-89
01033	COLBERT	AL	21.7	23.7	19.2	9%	-12%	14	37	28
01083	LIMESTONE	AL	18.8	29.3	21.7	56%	15%	11	34	27
01077	LAUDERDALE	AL	19.5	20.2	22.0	4%	13%	19	48	54
01079	LAWRENCE	AL	20.4	26.1	12.9	28%	-37%	8	21	10
01103	MORGAN	AL	16.6	26.2	17.3	58%	4%	17	64	50
01089	MADISON	AL	15.9	23.8	27.6	50%	74%	20	106	149
47071	HARDIN	TN	13.5	19.1	20.6	41%	52%	5	14	17
47099	LAWRENCE	TN	15.6	23.7	22.2	52%	42%	10	29	28
47101	LEWIS	TN	14.7	24.8	21.9	69%	49%	2	8	7
47181	WAYNE	TN	10.4	15.6	12.8	50%	23%	3	7	6
TOTAL	**10 COUNTIES**			**17.5**	**23.8**	**21.9**	**36%****	**25%**	**109**	**368**	**376**
TOTAL	**48 COUNTIES**			**18.6**	**22.6**	**21.1**	**22%****	**13%**	**670**	**1665**	**1671**
TOTAL	ALABAMA		17.1	22.3	20.8	30%	22%	812	2167	2186
TOTAL	TENNESSEE		18.1	20.8	21.1	15%	17%	1186	2706	2998
TOTAL	UNITED STATES		24.4	24.9	24.6	2%	1%	91392	167803	178868

** P <.001

Joseph M. Farley 1 & 2
Initial criticality 8/9/77 and 5/5/81
Located in Dothan, AL

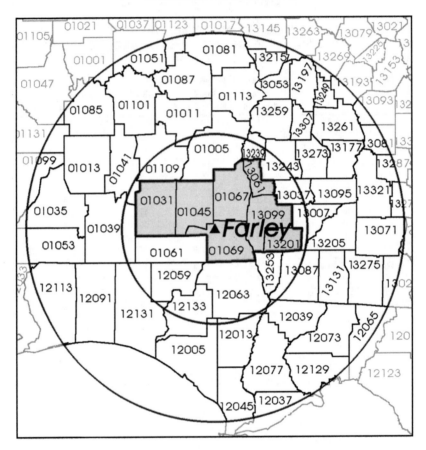

This is a fairly new reactor in southeast Alabama, surrounded by seven small rural counties. Their combined age-adjusted rate in 1985–89 is still well below the national average rate of 24.6 deaths per 100,000, and its 29 percent increase since 1950–54 is supported by too few deaths to be statistically significant. All 55 rural counties within 100 miles do have enough deaths to make the observed 18 percent increase since 1950–54 statistically significant. There may be some overlap with emissions from the three Browns Ferry reactors in northwest Alabama.

Joseph M. Farley 1 & 2

WHITE FEMALE BREAST CANCER MORTALITY RATES 1950-89
COUNTIES WITHIN 50 AND 100 MILES OF FARLEY
Deaths per 100,000 Women

FIPS Code	County	ST	Age-Adjusted Mortality Rates			Percent Change 80-84/ 50-54	85-89/ 50-54	Number of Deaths		
			1950-54	80-84	85-89			50-54	80-84	85-89
01069	HOUSTON	AL	18.4	13.2	17.6	-28%	-4%	14	27	35
01045	DALE	AL	12.4	25.5	20.5	105%	65%	5	22	20
01067	HENRY	AL	21.2	16.9	14.9	-20%	-30%	5	7	6
01031	COFFEE	AL	11.7	15.3	29.0	30%	147%	6	16	33
13099	EARLY	GA	16.2	16.0	15.3	-2%	-6%	3	5	5
13061	CLAY	GA	26.6	44.0	30.3	66%	14%	1	2	2
13201	MILLER	GA	21.4	23.1	24.7	8%	16%	3	5	4
TOTAL	**7 COUNTIES**		**16.1**	**17.4**	**20.8**	**8%**	**29%**	**37**	**84**	**105**
TOTAL	**55 COUNTIES**		**17.3**	**19.4**	**20.3**	**12%**	**18%***	**349**	**865**	**978**
TOTAL	ALABAMA		17.1	22.3	20.8	30%	22%	812	2167	2186
TOTAL	GEORGIA		18.3	20.6	21.8	13%	19%	1033	2599	3061
TOTAL	UNITED STATES		24.4	24.9	24.6	2%	1%	91392	167803	178868

* P<.05

Edwin I. Hatch 1 & 2
Initial criticality 9/12/74 and 7/4/78
Located 11 miles north of Baxley, GA

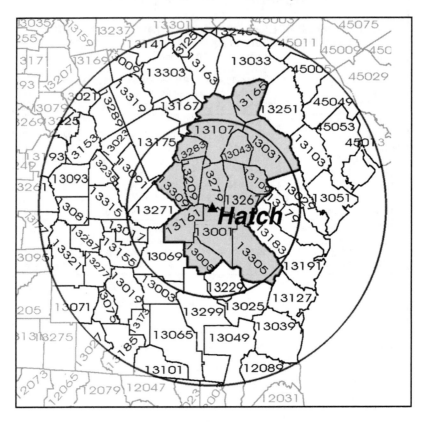

These reactors are surrounded by small rural counties; 14 of the closest contiguous counties have sufficient deaths to make the combined age-adjusted breast cancer mortality increase since 1950–54 statistically significant. The same is true for all counties within 100 miles.

Edwin I. Hatch 1 & 2

WHITE FEMALE BREAST CANCER MORTALITY RATES 1950-89
COUNTIES WITHIN 50 AND 100 MILES OF HATCH
Deaths per 100,000 Women

FIPS Code	County	ST	Age-Adjusted Mortality Rates			Percent Change 80-84/ 85-89/		Number of Deaths		
			1950-54	80-84	85-89	50-54	50-54	50-54	80-84	85-89
13001	APPLING	GA	4.7	6.9	11.0	47%	133%	1	3	4
13279	TOOMBS	GA	11.3	15.4	19.3	36%	71%	3	10	14
13043	CANDLER	GA	10.0	28.7	26.0	188%	160%	1	6	7
13107	EMANUEL	GA	9.8	13.2	29.1	35%	198%	3	7	14
13109	EVANS	GA	9.2	39.4	7.0	330%	-24%	1	7	1
13161	JEFF DAVIS	GA	7.7	16.0	10.9	108%	41%	1	4	5
13267	TATTNALL	GA	4.8	14.8	27.5	210%	477%	1	5	10
13005	BACON	GA	16.7	22.9	20.3	37%	21%	2	6	5
13165	JENKINS	GA	10.3	9.8	13.0	-6%	26%	1	2	3
13031	BULLOCH	GA	25.8	23.2	22.7	-10%	-12%	9	16	18
13309	WHEELER	GA	30.8	0.0	3.1	-100%	-90%	3	0	1
13305	WAYNE	GA	12.2	14.3	17.1	17%	40%	3	8	9
13209	MONTGOMERY	GA	0.0	10.5	0.0			0	3	0
13283	TREUTLEN	GA	0.0	6.5	8.3			0	1	2
TOTAL	**14 COUNTIES**		**12.0**	**16.2**	**18.2**	**35%**	**52%***	**29**	**78**	**93**
TOTAL	**57 COUNTIES**		**16.4**	**19.1**	**19.8**	**16%**	**21%***	**205**	**487**	**559**
TOTAL	GEORGIA		18.3	20.6	21.8	13%	19%	1033	2599	3061
TOTAL	UNITED STATES		24.4	24.9	24.6	2%	1%	91392	167803	178868

* P<.01

Crystal River
Initial criticality 1/14/77
Located 70 miles north of Tampa, FL

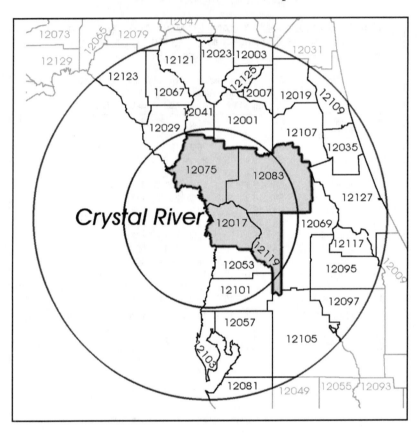

The 4 counties closest to the reactor have registered a significant 43 percent increase in combined age-adjusted breast cancer mortality increase since 1950–54, which is significantly greater than the corresponding increase for other counties within 100 miles, although many Florida counties may also be affected by emissions from the Turkey Point and St. Lucie reactors on the Atlantic coast.

Crystal River

WHITE FEMALE BREAST CANCER MORTALITY RATES 1950-89
COUNTIES WITHIN 50 AND 100 MILES OF CRYSTAL RIVER
Deaths per 100,000 Women

FIPS Code	County	ST	Age-Adjusted Mortality Rates			Percent Change 80-84/ 85-89/		Number of Deaths		
			1950-54	80-84	85-89	50-54	50-54	50-54	80-84	85-89
12017	CITRUS	FL	11.7	25.8	21.0	120%	79%	2	86	111
12075	LEVY	FL	12.0	22.8	29.0	90%	142%	2	16	26
12083	MARION	FL	18.0	23.5	23.2	30%	29%	13	111	161
12119	SUMTER	FL	19.6	12.9	32.0	-34%	63%	4	10	35
TOTAL	**4 COUNTIES**		**16.6**	**23.3**	**23.8**	**41%**	**43%****	**21**	**223**	**333**
TOTAL	**27 COUNTIES**		**18.9**	**22.6**	**22.5**	**20%**	**19%****	**560**	**3160**	**3833**
TOTAL	FLORIDA		18.4	22.8	22.8	24%	24%	1354	9070	10783
TOTAL	UNITED STATES		24.4	24.9	24.6	2%	1%	91392	167803	178868

** P<.001

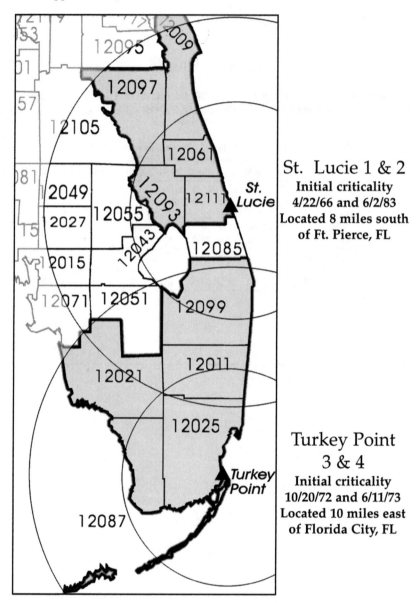

St. Lucie 1 & 2
Initial criticality
4/22/66 and 6/2/83
Located 8 miles south
of Ft. Pierce, FL

Turkey Point
3 & 4
Initial criticality
10/20/72 and 6/11/73
Located 10 miles east
of Florida City, FL

The ten counties closest to these reactors have clearly registered significant increases in age-adjusted breast cancer mortality rates since 1950–54 when compared with the corresponding national increases.

St. Lucie 1 & 2 and Turkey Point 3 & 4

WHITE FEMALE BREAST CANCER MORTALITY RATES 1950-89
COUNTIES WITHIN 50 AND 100 MILES OF
ST. LUCIE AND TURKEY POINT
Deaths per 100,000 Women

FIPS Code	County	ST	Age-Adjusted Mortality Rates			Percent Change 80-84/ 50-54	85-89/ 50-54	Number of Deaths		
			1950-54	80-84	85-89			50-54	80-84	85-89
ST. LUCIE										
12111	ST LUCIE	FL	6.5	20.7	23.5	221%	263%	3	74	112
12009	BREVARD	FL	18.8	24.4	26.9	30%	43%	16	262	361
12061	INDIAN RIVER	FL	17.2	19.3	24.5	12%	42%	6	67	97
12093	OKEECHOBEE	FL	30.1	22.3	13.3	-26%	-56%	2	14	9
12097	OSCEOLA	FL	14.4	27.1	24.0	89%	67%	10	62	70
TOTAL 5 COUNTIES			**16.0**	**23.3**	**24.8**	**46%**	**55%****	**37**	**479**	**649**
TURKEY POINT										
12025	DADE	FL	20.1	24.0	23.3	20%	16%	302	1447	1474
12087	MONROE	FL	14.3	21.0	21.2	47%	49%	7	51	52
12011	BROWARD	FL	15.0	22.8	24.1	52%	60%	52	1095	1293
12099	PALM BEACH	FL	16.6	24.0	23.9	44%	44%	58	696	913
12021	COLLIER	FL	22.8	23.5	21.5	3%	-6%	3	95	135
TOTAL 4 COUNTIES			**18.8**	**23.6**	**23.6**	**26%**	**26%****	**422**	**3384**	**3867**
TOTAL 18 COUNTIES			**18.3**	**23.4**	**23.3**	**28%**	**27%****	**531**	**4395**	**5135**
TOTAL	FLORIDA		18.4	22.8	22.8	24%	24%	1354	9070	10783
TOTAL	UNITED STATES		24.4	24.9	24.6	2%	1%	91392	167803	178868

** P<.001

Arkansas One 1 & 2
Arkansas One 1 initial criticality 8/6/74
Arkansas One 2 initial criticality 12/5/78
Located 6 miles west-northwest of Russellville, AR

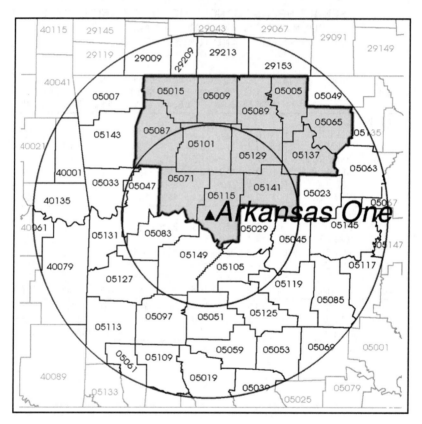

The 5 counties closest to the reactor have registered a 27 percent increase in combined age-adjusted breast cancer mortality rates since 1950–54, but without enough deaths to achieve statistical significance. If we included 12 contiguous counties to the north of the reactor, the resulting 39 percent overall increase, based on sufficient deaths (185) in 1985–89, would have a chance probability equivalent to three standard deviations (P< .001).

Arkansas One 1 & 2

WHITE FEMALE BREAST CANCER MORTALITY RATES 1950-89
COUNTIES WITHIN 50 AND 100 MILES OF ARKANSAS ONE
Deaths per 100,000 Women

FIPS Code	County	ST	Age-Adjusted Mortality Rates			Percent Change 80-84/ 50-54	85-89/ 50-54	Number of Deaths		
			1950-54	80-84	85-89			50-54	80-84	85-89
05115	POPE	AR	16.3	22.5	17.1	38%	5%	9	26	23
05071	JOHNSON	AR	20.4	21.6	20.6	6%	1%	8	13	15
05101	NEWTON	AR	6.5	12.9	18.9	100%	192%	1	3	5
05129	SEARCY	AR	3.9	13.9	13.2	260%	241%	1	5	5
05141	VAN BUREN	AR	12.4	14.9	16.4	20%	32%	3	8	13
05015	CARROLL	AR	18.1	21.5	25.2	19%	39%	7	16	18
05087	MADISON	AR	15.5	27.2	21.9	75%	41%	4	10	9
05009	BOONE	AR	9.2	21.6	22.6	136%	147%	4	18	26
05089	MARION	AR	9.4	6.9	11.7	-27%	23%	2	4	6
05005	BAXTER	AR	23.4	16.8	24.2	-28%	3%	6	30	47
05065	IZARD	AR	21.6	1.8	17.6	-92%	-19%	5	1	11
05137	STONE	AR	6.6	12.8	20.4	95%	209%	1	4	7
TOTAL	**12 COUNTIES**		**14.4**	**17.9**	**20.0**	**24%**	**39%***	**51**	**138**	**185**
TOTAL	**42 COUNTIES**		**15.9**	**19.5**	**20.5**	**23%**	**29%****	**336**	**878**	**1034**
TOTAL	ARKANSAS		15.4	19.1	19.5	24%	27%	545	1288	1466
TOTAL	UNITED STATES		24.4	24.9	24.6	2%	1%	91392	167803	178868

* P<.05,**P<.001

Hanford Reservation
Established in 1943
Located near Richland, Pasco, and Kennewick, Washington,
20 miles from the Yakima Reservation.

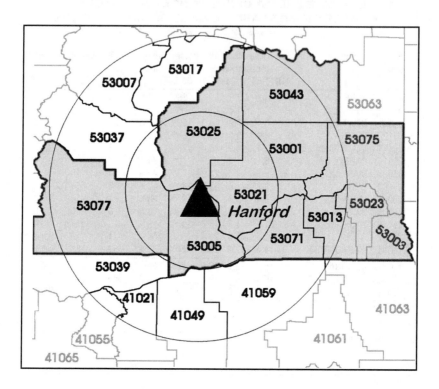

Eleven sparsely populated counties closest to Hanford, as well as all counties within 100 miles, have registered age-adjusted increases in breast cancer mortality since 1950–54 that are clearly significant when compared with the corresponding change for Washington State as a whole.

Hanford Reservation

WHITE FEMALE BREAST CANCER MORTALITY RATES 1950-89
COUNTIES WITHIN 50 AND 100 MILES OF HANFORD
Deaths per 100,000 Women

FIPS Code	County	ST	Age-Adjusted Mortality Rates			Percent Change 80-84/ 85-89/		Number of Deaths		
			1950-54	80-84	85-89	50-54	50-54	50-54	80-84	85-89
53001	ADAMS	WA	32.4	21.0	27.2	-35%	-16%	5	10	10
53003	ASOTIN	WA	15.9	17.2	23.0	9%	45%	5	13	12
53013	COLUMBIA	WA	23.6	13.6	15.9	-42%	-33%	4	1	3
53005	BENTON	WA	8.6	17.9	25.7	109%	200%	7	47	77
53021	FRANKLIN	WA	8.2	13.1	19.9	59%	142%	2	12	18
53023	GARFIELD	WA	5.5	21.2	11.2	281%	102%	1	2	2
53025	GRANT	WA	25.6	26.9	15.3	5%	-40%	10	37	23
53043	LINCOLN	WA	22.0	33.5	37.7	52%	71%	7	10	11
53071	WALLA WALLA	WA	21.5	26.1	20.5	21%	-4%	22	44	43
53075	WHITMAN	WA	28.1	21.3	40.5	-24%	44%	20	17	33
53077	YAKIMA	WA	19.9	22.6	23.8	14%	20%	61	123	137
TOTAL	**ABOVE 11**		**19.6**	**21.7**	**23.8**	**11%**	**21%***	**144**	**316**	**369**
TOTAL	**17 COUNTIES**		**19.6**	**21.7**	**23.1**	**10%**	**18%***	**169**	**365**	**417**
TOTAL	WASHINGTON		23.8	24.2	24.6	2%	3%	1489	2999	3411
TOTAL	UNITED STATES		24.4	24.9	24.6	2%	1%	91392	167803	178868

*P<.05

Trojan
Initial criticality 12/15/75
Located 35 miles northwest of Portland, OR

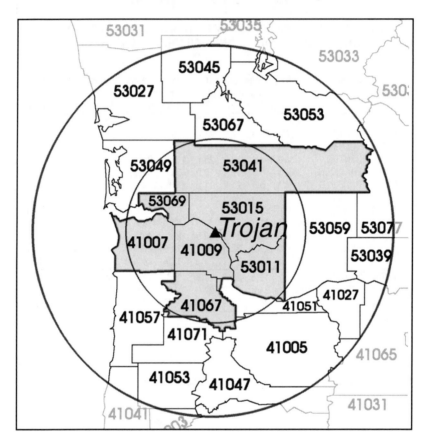

Counties close to the Trojan reactor, closed in 1992 in the wake of bitter local opposition, do not show a significant increase in age-adjusted breast cancer mortality since 1950–54, but NCI data do show a significant increase in cancer mortality in Columbia County in which the reactor began operations in 1975, in the period 1976–84 as compared with 1966–75.

Trojan

WHITE FEMALE BREAST CANCER MORTALITY RATES 1950-89
COUNTIES WITHIN 50 AND 100 MILES OF TROJAN
Deaths per 100,000 Women

FIPS Code	County	ST	Age-Adjusted Mortality Rates			Percent Change		Number of Deaths		
			1950-54	80-84	85-89	80-84/ 50-54	85-89/ 50-54	50-54	80-84	85-89
41009	COLUMBIA	OR	27.2	30.3	24.2	11%	-11%	15	34	24
41007	CLATSOP	OR	28.7	21.6	30.1	-24%	5%	23	28	38
41067	WASHINGTON	OR	20.1	24.8	26.2	23%	30%	35	163	206
53015	COWLITZ	WA	29.2	24.9	19.1	-15%	-35%	33	59	55
53069	WAHKIAKUM	WA	23.2	5.9	27.7	-75%	19%	2	1	3
53011	CLARK	WA	24.0	23.6	24.6	-2%	2%	50	129	148
53041	LEWIS	WA	18.2	21.0	26.0	15%	43%	25	42	58
TOTAL	**7 COUNTIES**		**23.8**	**24.0**	**25.1**	**1%**	**5%**	**183**	**456**	**532**
TOTAL	**19 COUNTIES**		**23.6**	**24.2**	**24.1**	**3%**	**2%**	**999**	**1983**	**2159**
TOTAL	OREGON		23.3	23.9	23.2	3%	-0%	956	2038	2151
TOTAL	UNITED STATES		24.4	24.9	24.6	2%	1%	91392	167803	178868

Humboldt Bay
Initial criticality 2/16/63
Located 3 miles southwest of Eureka, CA

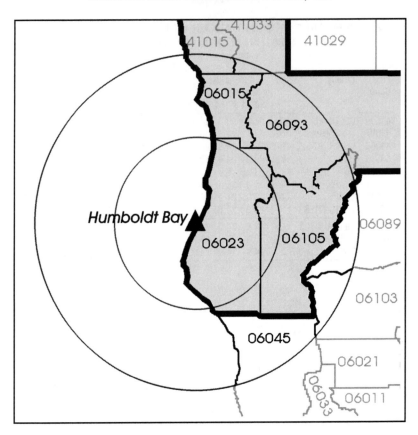

The 7 downwind counties closest to the reactor have sufficient deaths to indicate that the 22 percent combined increase in the age-adjusted breast cancer mortality rate since 1950–54 is statistically significant when compared with either the corresponding change for California or the United States.

Humboldt Bay

WHITE FEMALE BREAST CANCER MORTALITY RATES 1950-89
COUNTIES WITHIN 50 AND 100 MILES OF HUMBOLDT BAY
Deaths per 100,000 Women

FIPS Code	County	ST	Age-Adjusted Mortality Rates			Percent Change 80-84/ 85-89/		Number of Deaths		
			1950-54	80-84	85-89	50-54	50-54	50-54	80-84	85-89
06023	HUMBOLDT	CA	25.6	24.2	27.3	-6%	6%	42	72	96
06015	DEL NORTE	CA	19.4	27.1	17.4	40%	-10%	4	16	11
06093	SISKIYOU	CA	23.8	27.6	25.4	16%	7%	17	39	37
06105	TRINITY	CA	15.9	29.2	15.0	83%	-6%	2	11	7
41015	CURRY	OR	5.9	25.0	22.7	325%	287%	1	16	23
41033	JOSEPHINE	OR	15.5	25.2	25.6	63%	65%	11	58	61
TOTAL 6 COUNTIES			**21.5**	**25.4**	**24.7**	**18%**	**14%**	**77**	**212**	**235**
06045	MENDOCINO	CA	18.9	25.6	25.4	36%	35%	20	53	64
TOTAL	**7 COUNTIES**		**20.9**	**25.5**	**24.8**	**22%***	**18%**	**97**	**265**	**299**
TOTAL	CALIFORNIA		25.5	26.1	25.9	2%	1%	7653	17237	18541
TOTAL	UNITED STATES		24.4	24.9	24.6	2%	1%	91391	167803	178868

* P<.05

Idaho National Engineering Laboratory
Established in 1949 as the National Reactor Testing Station
Located 22 miles west of Idaho Falls, ID

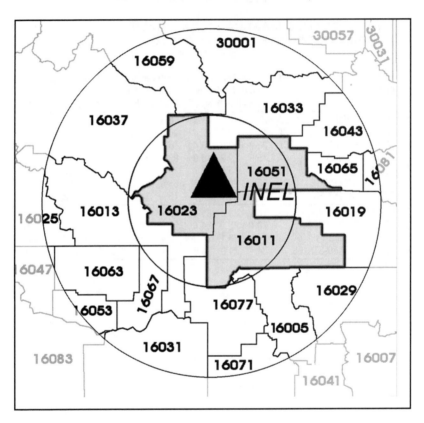

The three small rural counties closest to INEL, and indeed all counties within 100 miles, have registered significant increases in age-adjusted breast cancer mortality since 1950–54.

Idaho National Engineering Laboratory

**WHITE FEMALE BREAST CANCER MORTALITY RATES 1950-89
COUNTIES WITHIN 50 AND 100 MILES OF INEL**
Deaths per 100,000 Women

FIPS Code	County	ST	Age-Adjusted Mortality Rates			Percent Change		Number of Deaths		
			1950-54	80-84	85-89	80-84/ 50-54	85-89/ 50-54	50-54	80-84	85-89
16011	BINGHAM	ID	7.0	17.7	21.9	153%	213%	3	14	21
16023	BUTTE	ID	0.0	20.6	7.7			0	2	1
16051	JEFFERSON	ID	0.0	26.9	19.1			0	10	9
TOTAL	**3 COUNTIES**		**4.8**	**20.6**	**20.1**	**433%**	**322%****	**3**	**26**	**31**
TOTAL	**16 COUNTIES**		**14.2**	**22.3**	**19.8**	**57%**	**39%****	**50**	**161**	**162**
TOTAL	IDAHO		18.9	22.3	18.9	18%	0%	243	585	571
TOTAL	UNITED STATES		24.4	24.9	24.6	2%	2%	91392	167803	178868

** P<.001

Rancho Seco

Initial criticality 9/16/74
Located 25 miles southeast of Sacramento, CA

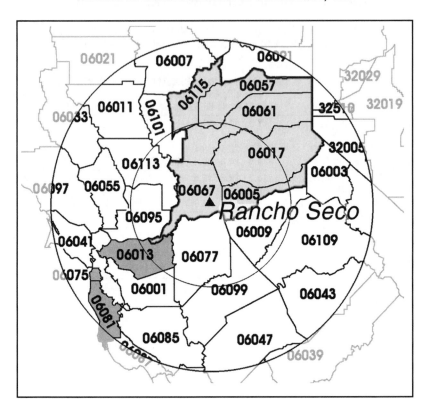

The 6 counties downwind of the reactor have registered a signifi-cant increase in the combined age-adjusted breast cancer mortal-ity rate since 1950–54 as have all counties within 100 miles, when com-pared with the corresponding change for either California or the United States.

Rancho Seco

WHITE FEMALE BREAST CANCER MORTALITY RATES 1950-89
COUNTIES WITHIN 50 AND 100 MILES OF RANCHO SECO
Deaths per 100,000 Women

FIPS Code	County	ST	Age-Adjusted Mortality Rates 1950-54	80-84	85-89	Percent Change 80-84/ 50-54	85-89/ 50-54	Number of Deaths 50-54	80-84	85-89
06067	SACRAMENTO	CA	21.8	25.8	27.3	18%	25%	153	565	675
06005	AMADOR	CA	32.4	30.6	26.4	-5%	-18%	8	25	24
06017	EL DORADO	CA	12.6	19.2	25.7	52%	104%	6	54	84
06057	NEVADA	CA	11.3	20.7	18.2	84%	62%	7	47	58
06061	PLACER	CA	17.5	28.7	26.8	64%	53%	21	110	131
06115	YUBA	CA	31.0	23.8	28.4	-23%	-8%	16	26	38
TOTAL	**6 COUNTIES**		**20.8**	**25.3**	**26.5****	**21%**	**27%****	**211**	**827**	**1010**
TOTAL	**26 COUNTIES**		**24.2**	**26.1**	**25.8****	**8%**	**7%****	**1717**	**4696**	**5097**
TOTAL	CALIFORNIA		25.5	26.1	25.9	2%	1%	7653	17237	18541
TOTAL	UNITED STATES		24.4	24.9	24.6	2%	1%	91392	167803	178868

** P<.0001

San Onofre 1, 2 & 3
Initial criticality 6/14/67, 7/26/82, and 8/29/83
Located 2.5 miles south of San Clemente

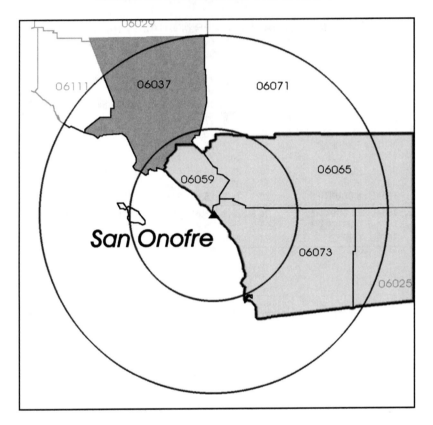

The 4 counties closest to the San Onofre reactors registered a highly significant 15 percent increase in combined age-adjusted breast cancer rates since 1950–54. Los Angeles County is included within a 100 mile radius, and for all 5 counties the current rate of 26.4 deaths per 100,000 is significantly above the U.S. rate of 24.6 deaths.

San Onofre 1, 2 & 3

WHITE FEMALE BREAST CANCER MORTALITY RATES 1950-89
COUNTIES WITHIN 50 AND 100 MILES OF SAN ONOFRE
Deaths per 100,000 Women

FIPS Code	County	ST	Age-Adjusted Mortality Rates			Percent Change 80-84/ 50-54	85-89/ 50-54	Number of Deaths		
			1950-54	80-84	85-89	50-54	50-54	50-54	80-84	85-89
06059	ORANGE	CA	20.3	25.7	25.9	27%	27%	163	1393	1554
06073	SAN DIEGO	CA	25.5	28.8	26.6	13%	5%	392	1501	1613
06065	RIVERSIDE	CA	20.9	24.2	23.3	16%	12%	111	589	685
06025	IMPERIAL	CA	15.0	21.2	13.7	42%	-9%	14	47	33
TOTAL	**4 COUNTIES**		**23.0**	**26.5**	**25.5**	**15%****	**11%**	**680**	**3530**	**3885**
06071	SAN BERNARDINO	CA	25.3	23.5	26.0	-7%	3%	206	591	729
06037	LOS ANGELES	CA	27.4	27.1	27.0**	-1%	-1%	3546	5264	5349
TOTAL	**6 COUNTIES**		**26.5**	**26.6**	**26.3****	**0%**	**-1%**	**4432**	**9385**	**9963**
TOTAL	CALIFORNIA		25.5	26.1	25.9	2%	1%	7653	17237	18541
TOTAL	UNITED STATES		24.4	24.9	24.6	2%	1%	91391	167803	178868

** P<.001

Los Alamos National Laboratory
Began operations in 1943
Located 25 miles northeast of Santa Fe,
60 miles north of Albuquerque, NM

Sandia National Laboratory
Began operations in 1945
Located immediately south of Albuquerque, NM

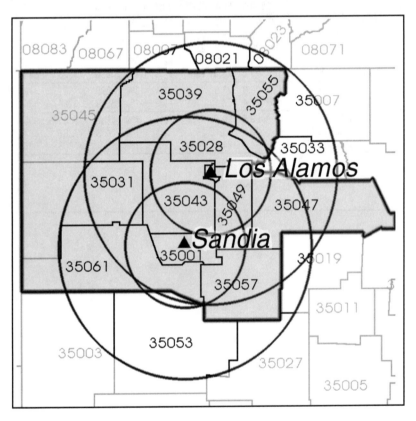

For the counties within 50 and 100 miles of the Los Alamos/Sandia DOE nuclear facility, the combined age-adjusted breast cancer rate has increased significantly since 1950–54. This is true for all counties close to the seven DOE reactor sites that began operations prior to 1950.

Los Alamos National Laboratory and Sandia National Laboratory

WHITE FEMALE BREAST CANCER MORTALITY RATES 1950-89
COUNTIES WITHIN 50 AND 100 MILES OF
LOS ALAMOS AND SANDIA LABS
Deaths per 100,000 Women

FIPS Code	County	ST	Age-Adjusted Mortality Rates 1950-54	80-84	85-89	Percent Change 80-84/ 50-54	85-89/ 50-54	Number of Deaths 50-54	80-84	85-89
35001	BERNALILLO	NM	22.3	25.6	26.7	15%	20%	62	285	342
35028	LOS ALAMOS	NM	63.1	49.9	18.9	-21%	-70%	2	21	10
35031	MC KINLEY	NM	4.5	30.3	12.3	575%	175%	1	12	6
35039	RIO ARRIBA	NM	7.3	17.3	21.9	136%	200%	3	11	16
35043	SANDOVAL	NM	0.0	24.7	24.2			0	20	30
35045	SAN JUAN	NM	10.3	18.1	23.0	76%	123%	3	24	36
35047	SAN MIGUEL	NM	12.3	20.7	23.4	68%	90%	6	12	18
35049	SANTA FE	NM	26.9	24.2	24.2	-10%	-10%	18	53	68
35055	TAOS	NM	7.4	9.8	11.7	32%	59%	2	5	8
35057	TORRANCE	NM	13.2	14.9	17.1	13%	29%	2	3	4
35061	VALENCIA	NM	4.6	25.4	16.4	457%	259%	2	30	25
TOTAL	**ABOVE 11**		**17.7**	**24.4**	**24.0**	**38%**	**36%****	**101**	**476**	**563**
TOTAL	**15 COUNTIES**		**17.8**	**23.9**	**23.8**	**35%**	**34%****	**111**	**486**	**578**
TOTAL	NEW MEXICO		16.3	22.7	21.3	39%	31%	192	766	845
TOTAL	UNITED STATES		24.4	24.9	24.6	2%	1%	91392	167803	178868

** p<.0001

Duane Arnold
Initial criticality 3/23/74
Located 8 miles northwest of Cedar Rapids, IA

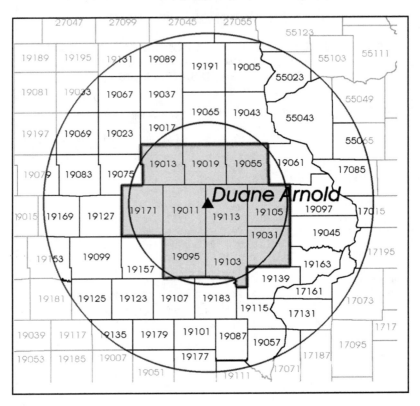

The 10 small rural counties within 50 miles of this reactor registered a combined age-adjusted breast cancer mortality increase of 11 percent since 1950–54, which is in significant contrast to the overall decline registered by counties farther away and by the state of Iowa.

Duane Arnold

WHITE FEMALE BREAST CANCER MORTALITY RATES 1950-89
COUNTIES WITHIN 50 AND 100 MILES OF DUANE ARNOLD
Deaths per 100,000 Women

FIPS Code	County	ST	Age-Adjusted Mortality Rates			Percent Change 80-84/ 85-89/		Number of Deaths		
			1950-54	80-84	85-89	50-54	50-54	50-54	80-84	85-89
19013	BLACK HAWK	IA	21.3	26.0	25.7	22%	20%	56	110	108
19019	BUCHANAN	IA	22.8	17.7	20.9	-22%	-8%	15	13	16
19055	DELAWARE	IA	17.3	22.8	20.4	32%	18%	9	19	14
19171	TAMA	IA	24.1	30.1	14.4	25%	-40%	15	29	16
19011	BENTON	IA	16.9	16.7	13.1	-1%	-22%	12	16	14
19113	LINN	IA	19.6	23.4	27.2	19%	39%	69	123	137
19105	JONES	IA	23.8	18.7	23.1	-21%	-3%	12	13	17
19031	CEDAR	IA	21.1	27.4	19.7	30%	-7%	11	20	15
19103	JOHNSON	IA	28.9	27.3	23.4	-6%	-19%	33	52	46
19095	IOWA	IA	26.6	22.2	22.7	-17%	-15%	14	17	14
TOTAL	**10 COUNTIES**		**21.7**	**24.2**	**24.1**	**12%**	**11%***	**246**	**412**	**397**
TOTAL	**43 COUNTIES**		**24.9**	**23.7**	**22.8**	**-5%**	**-8%**	**970**	**1293**	**1303**
TOTAL	IOWA		24.2	23.0	22.3	-5%	-8%	1877	2452	2443
TOTAL	UNITED STATES		24.4	24.9	24.6	2%	1%	91392	167803	178868

* P<.01

Cooper Station
Initial criticality 2/21/74
Located 70 miles south of Omaha, NE

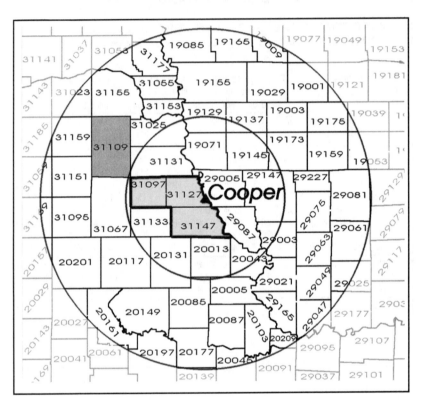

This reactor in the relatively dry state of Nebraska is 1 of only 5 of the 60 reactor sites in which we found no significant increase in breast cancer mortality rates near the reactor since 1950–54. This does not mean that no harm was done by reactor emissions, but that it was too small to be detected.

Cooper Station

WHITE FEMALE BREAST CANCER MORTALITY RATES 1950-89
COUNTIES WITHIN 50 AND 100 MILES OF COOPER STATION
Deaths per 100,000 Women

FIPS Code	County	ST	Age-Adjusted Mortality Rates			Percent Change 80-84/ 85-89/		Number of Deaths		
			1950-54	80-84	85-89	50-54	50-54	50-54	80-84	85-89
31127	NEMAHA	NE	29.2	27.5	14.8	-6%	-49%	10	11	4
31147	RICHARDSON	NE	24.3	26.6	27.1	9%	11%	13	11	12
31097	JOHNSON	NE	20.4	30.5	21.6	50%	6%	5	6	5
TOTAL	**3 COUNTIES**		**24.9**	**27.8**	**21.6**	**11%**	**-13%**	**28**	**28**	**21**
TOTAL	**12 COUNTIES**		**21.7**	**25.0**	**18.4**	**15%**	**-15%**	**127**	**142**	**116**
TOTAL	**43 COUNTIES**		**23.4**	**23.9**	**22.8**	**2%**	**-3%**	**1118**	**1539**	**1591**
TOTAL	NEBRASKA		23.7	24.4	23.3	3%	-2%	894	1276	1295
TOTAL	UNITED STATES		24.4	24.9	24.6	2%	1%	91392	167803	178868

Fort Calhoun
Initial criticality 8/6/73
Located 19 miles north of Omaha, NE

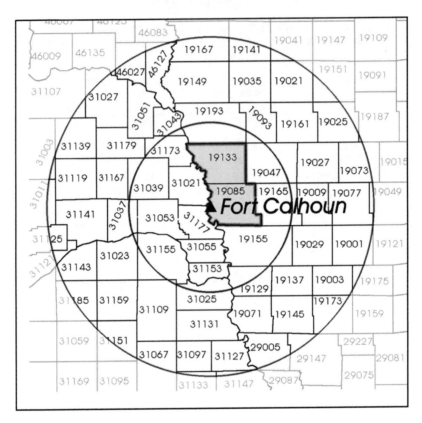

Two of the counties closest to this reactor nearly doubled their combined age-adjusted breast cancer mortality rate since 1950–54, but they are too small for this increase to be statistically significant.

Fort Calhoun

**WHITE FEMALE BREAST CANCER MORTALITY RATES 1950-89
COUNTIES WITHIN 50 AND 100 MILES OF FORT CALHOUN**
Deaths per 100,000 Women

FIPS Code	County	ST	Age-Adjusted Mortality Rates			Percent Change 80-84/ 85-89/		Number of Deaths		
			1950-54	80-84	85-89	50-54	50-54	50-54	80-84	85-89
19085	HARRISON	IA	16.6	28.9	11.8	74%	-29%	10	18	9
19133	MONONA	IA	20.7	37.3	24.8	80%	20%	9	17	15
TOTAL	**2 COUNTIES**		**18.2**	**32.9**	**17.3**	**80%***	**-5%**	**19**	**35**	**24**
TOTAL	**9 COUNTIES**		**27.0**	**26.0**	**24.3**	**-4%**	**-10%**	**338**	**469**	**464**
TOTAL	IOWA		24.2	23.0	22.3	-5%	-8%	1877	2452	2443
TOTAL	UNITED STATES		24.4	24.9	24.6	2%	1%	91392	167803	178868

* P<.05

Pathfinder
Initial criticality 1964
Located in Minnehaha County, SD

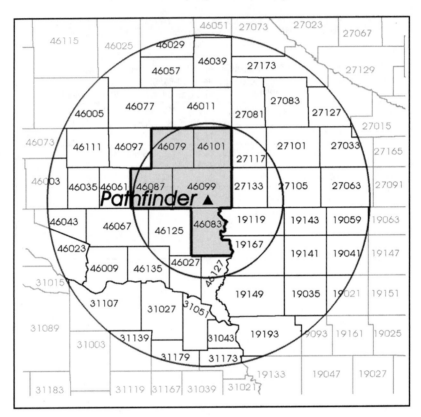

Like the Fort Calhoun reactor in Nebraska, the counties closest to the reactor show an increase in the combined age-adjusted breast cancer mortality rate since 1950–54 that is in sharp contrast to the decline registered by the rural counties farther away and in the state as a whole, but there are too few deaths to make that increase statistically significant.

Pathfinder

WHITE FEMALE BREAST CANCER MORTALITY RATES 1950-89
COUNTIES WITHIN 50 AND 100 MILES OF PATHFINDER
Deaths per 100,000 Women

FIPS Code	County	ST	Age-Adjusted Mortality Rates			Percent Change		Number of Deaths		
			1950-54	80-84	85-89	80-84/ 50-54	85-89/ 50-54	50-54	80-84	85-89
46083	LINCOLN	SD	14.0	23.1	15.0	66%	8%	5	17	12
46099	MINNEHAHA	SD	26.7	22.9	26.3	-14%	-1%	50	84	96
46087	MC COOK	SD	15.0	16.0	23.2	7%	55%	4	6	6
46079	LAKE	SD	30.9	23.3	27.7	-25%	-11%	10	12	15
46101	MOODY	SD	13.5	24.9	18.4	85%	37%	3	6	7
TOTAL	**5 COUNTIES**			**23.7**	**22.9**	**25.2**	**-3%**	**6%**	**72**	**125**	**136**
TOTAL	**11 COUNTIES**		**23.0**	**21.7**	**23.7**	**-6%**	**3%**	**122**	**194**	**203**
TOTAL	46 COUNTIES		23.3	22.9	23.1	-2%	-1%	464	678	709
TOTAL	SOUTH DAKOTA		22.6	23.6	22.8	4%	1%	358	542	547
TOTAL	UNITED STATES		24.4	24.9	24.6	2%	1%	91392	167803	178868

Fort St. Vrain
Initial criticality 1976
Located in Platteville, CO

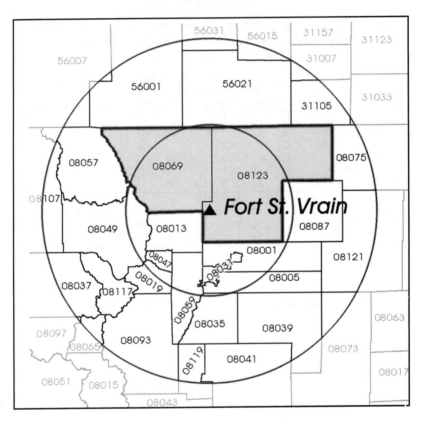

This reactor operated commercially only from 1979 to 1985. While the two counties closest to the reactor when combined have registered an above average percentage gain from 1950–54 to 1985–89, there are insufficient deaths to achieve statistical significance, and no such evidence within the 100-mile radius.

Fort St. Vrain

WHITE FEMALE BREAST CANCER MORTALITY RATES 1950-89
COUNTIES WITHIN 50 AND 100 MILES OF FORT ST. VRAIN
Deaths per 100,000 Women

FIPS Code	County	ST	Age-Adjusted Mortality Rates			Percent Change 80-84/ 50-54	85-89/ 50-54	Number of Deaths		
			1950-54	80-84	85-89			50-54	80-84	85-89
08123	WELD	CO	23.6	20.9	22.0	-11%	-7%	36	66	80
08069	LARIMER	CO	18.9	18.6	24.2	-1%	28%	25	74	117
TOTAL	**2 COUNTIES**		**21.7**	**19.7**	**23.2**	**-9%**	**7%**	**61**	**140**	**197**
TOTAL	**6 COUNTIES**		**26.7**	**22.7**	**23.2**	**-15%**	**-13%**	**475**	**756**	**826**
TOTAL	23 COUNTIES		25.2	22.8	22.5	-10%	-11%	615	1270	1409
TOTAL	COLORADO		23.9	21.8	21.5	-9%	-10%	849	1742	1929
TOTAL	UNITED STATES		24.4	24.9	24.6	2%	1%	91392	167803	178868

Quad Cities
Initial criticality 10/18/71
Located 20 miles northeast of Moline, IL

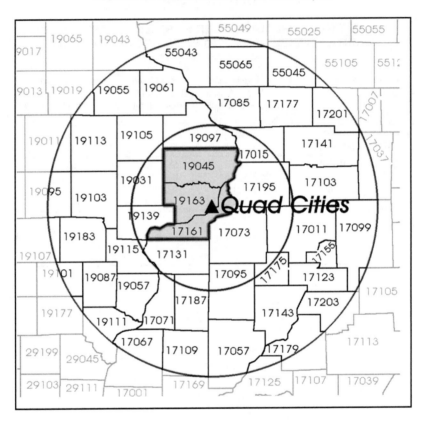

Rock Island, the largest county near the reactor, registered a 21 percent increase in age-adjusted breast cancer mortality since 1950–54, which was offset by a comparable decline in Scott County, which had an unusually above average rate in 1950–54. There is no evidence of a significant increase in counties within 50 or 100 miles.

Quad Cities

WHITE FEMALE BREAST CANCER MORTALITY RATES 1950-89
COUNTIES WITHIN 50 AND 100 MILES OF QUAD CITIES
Deaths per 100,000 Women

FIPS Code	County	ST	Age-Adjusted Mortality Rates			Percent Change 80-84/ 85-89/		Number of Deaths		
			1950-54	80-84	85-89	50-54	50-54	50-54	80-84	85-89
17161	ROCK ISLAND	IL	21.3	22.6	25.7	6%	21%	80	121	144
19163	SCOTT	IA	29.4	27.4	23.6	-7%	-20%	85	123	112
19045	CLINTON	IA	24.4	24.4	22.8	-0%	-6%	37	50	53
TOTAL	**3 COUNTIES**		**24.8**	**24.8**	**24.6**	**-0%**	**-1%**	**202**	**294**	**309**
TOTAL	**41 COUNTIES**		**24.6**	**24.9**	**23.9**	**1%**	**-3%**	**1324**	**1880**	**1883**
TOTAL	IOWA		24.2	23.0	22.3	-5%	-8%	1877	2452	2443
TOTAL	UNITED STATES		24.4	24.9	24.6	2%	1%	91392	167803	178868

RADIOACTIVE MATERIALS RELEASED FROM NUCLEAR POWER PLANTS

Each year the Nuclear Regulatory Commission releases a report prepared by the Brookhaven National Laboratory summarizing releases of radioactive materials from each civilian power reactor since the 1970s. Although there is evidence that these reports often greatly underestimate the releases, in the case of the Three Mile Island accident of 1979—they provide the public with tangible information, about which one can assess the degree of local danger from a particular radioactive release. We accordingly offer below tabular summaries (in curies) of the annual releases, from the 1970s to 1987, of three types of radioactive materials for each operating reactor, arranged by state and census region, as follows:

1. **Airborne Effluents of Iodine-131 and Particulates**
   This category includes all radionuclides with a half-life greater than 8 days and as such includes strontium- 90, with a half-life of about 30 years. As we have seen, radioactive iodine and strontium are associated with many immediate and delayed health effects. The cumulated total from the 1970s to 1987 is 370 curies— equivalent to 370 trillion picocuries in terms of the unit used to measure the radioactivity of a liter of milk or water.

2. Airborne Effluents, Total Fission, and Activation Gases
This category includes all radionuclides with half-lives less than eight days. The cumulated 1970–1987 total comes to 57,165 curies—or 57,165 trillion picocuries—a figure that was never published by the Nuclear Regulatory Commission. Such fission products never existed in nature prior to the Nuclear Age. Recent reports of corrosion problems in pressurized water reactors suggest that airborne short-lived fission products are not being monitored, constituting a serious new public health problem.

3. Liquid Effluents, Mixed Fission, and Activation Products
This category excludes short-lived noble gases, tritium, and alpha released in liquid effluents. For some reactors such as the #1 Millstone reactor on the Long Island Sound, such liquid releases in 1975 and 1976 were so large—about 400 curies (400 trillion picocuries)—that in conjunction with peak releases of I–131 and particulates in those years, they gave rise to the hypothesis that radiation mutated the spirochete responsible for Lyme disease,[11] which got its name from early reports of the disease in the nearby town of Old Lyme in the fall of 1975. The spirochete was harmless for previous generations, and today both Connecticut and downwind Rhode Island have by far the greatest *per capita* Lyme disease rates in the nation.

Unfortunately for the lay public, the Nuclear Regulatory Commission adopted a scientific mode of reporting radioactive releases, perhaps to avoid calling attention to the extraordinary magnitude of some of them. For example, the largest single annual release of I–131 and particulates is reported (in exponential format) for the #2 Three Mile Island reactor in 1979 as 1.42E+01 curies. In decimal format this is equal to 14.2 curies or 14.2 trillion picocuries. In the exponential format, it is not possible for the layman to add releases over time or by region—a great obstacle to any analysis of the health effects of such releases. Accordingly, we have converted the reported data on radioactive releases to decimal format. The reader should bear in mind that what appears to be a very small release of .01 curies is not so small when multiplied by 1 trillion, which yields the equivalent number of picocuries. A picocurie is the unit used to measure the radioactivity of milk and water.

The data here all come from the 1987 annual NRC report, covering the years 1970–87.[45] We chose not to use the succeeding reports for 1988 and 1989. In the latter two reports we have noted, for the first time since 1970, some drastic inexplicable downward revisions of back data that warrant suspicion. In 1985 and 1986, the reader will note that the Indian Point reactors reported releases of about 14 curies of radioactive iodine and strontium—equal to the 1979 TMI release. These huge releases were followed by sharp increases in the percentage of underweight live births in Westchester. In the 1988 annual NRC report, published in 1991, 6 years after the first large release, the 14 curie figure for the years 1985 and 1986 was revised downward to about 2 curies—still a large amount—equivalent to 2 trillion picocuries and capable of significantly raising the radioactivity of the water in the neighboring Hudson River and Croton reservoirs.

It should be pointed out that even the figure of 14 curies reported for TMI in 1979 is only an educated guess on the part of the NRC; since most of the monitoring devices did not function during the accident. Occasional reports now emerging from Department of Energy Dose Reconstruction Reports of releases of radioactive iodine and strontium from Hanford and Oak Ridge are several magnitudes larger than reported releases from civilian reactors.

HEALTH EFFECTS OF INDIAN POINT EMISSIONS ON NEARBY PEEKSKILL

In chapter 2, we showed that a significant rise in low-birthweight live births follows large-scale exposure to I–131 and particulates. Infant mortality is generally less sensitive because of the success with which modern medical technology can keep low-birthweight infants alive. The town of Peekskill, however, is so close to the Indian Point reactors (about four miles) that every large Indian Point release was followed by significant increases in Peekskill infant mortality rates.

For example, the Peekskill infant mortality rate rose 49 percent—from 10.7 deaths per 1,000 live births in 1984 to 15.9 in 1987, following the reported release of 14 curies from Indian Point in 1985 and

1986. Again, in 1976 the Peekskill IMR nearly quadrupled—from 5.3 in 1973 to 23.6 in 1976, after a reported release of 2.3 curies in 1974–76.

While no data on I–131 releases are available for the Indian Point start-up years 1962–65, the Peekskill IMR rose 138 percent—from 16.9 in 1962 to 40.3 in 1965. A *New York Times* story of November 5, 1965, entitled "Con Ed Accused of Harming Fish," reported that "Representative Richard Ottinger charged that hundreds of thousands to millions of fish had been killed in the Hudson River as a result of the building of an atomic power plant at Indian Point, south of Peekskill."

Thus we see that both in Westchester and Suffolk Counties the unfortunate decision to locate reactors near heavily populated areas resulted in increased mortality for both humans and fish. Readers wanting to ascertain the past health effects of reactor emissions in towns near their homes can press for past annual data on low birthweights and infant mortality from state and local health agencies and by reviewing past local news coverage. It may be difficult to obtain data from health agencies, but such data has been compiled and cannot be legally withheld from public view.

TABLE C-1 AIRBORNE EFFLUENTS OF IODINE-131 AND PARTICULATES (CURIES): BY STATE AND REGION 1970-87

HALF-LIFE EQUAL TO OR GREATER THAN 8 DAYS
BWR = Boiling Water Reactor; PWR = Pressurized Water Reactor

Reactor	St	Type	1970	1971	1972	1973	1974	1975	1976	1977	1978
MAINE YANKEE	ME	PWR			0.01	0.94	0.05	0.01	0.01	0.01	0.00
VERMONT YANKEE 1	VT	BWR			0.17	0.07	0.36	0.01	0.01	0.01	0.22
PILGRIM 1	MA	BWR			0.03	0.47	1.45	2.58	0.67	0.69	0.18
YANKEE ROWE 1	MA	PWR	0.01	0.01	0.01	0.19	0.53	0.01	0.01	0.00	0.00
HADDAM NECK	CT	PWR	0.01		0.02	0.05	0.01	0.01	0.01	0.00	0.01
MILLSTONE 1	CT	BWR		4.00	1.32	0.20	3.26	9.98	2.33	4.86	4.55
MILLSTONE 2	CT	PWR						0.01	0.01	0.00	0.00
MILLSTONE 3	CT	PWR									
NEW ENGLAND			**0.02**	**4.01**	**1.56**	**1.92**	**5.66**	**12.61**	**3.06**	**5.58**	**4.96**
INDIAN POINT 1 & 2	NY	PWR				0.01	0.43	1.62	0.24	0.06	0.21
INDIAN POINT 3	NY	PWR									0.01
JAMES A. FITZPATRICK	NY	BWR						0.04	0.68	0.17	0.28
NINE MILE POINT 1	NY	BWR	0.01	0.06	0.97	1.98	0.89	2.78	2.20	0.20	0.14
NINE MILE POINT 2	NY	BWR									
R. E. GINNA	NY	PWR	0.05	0.17	0.04	0.01	0.01	0.02	0.03	0.03	0.01
SHOREHAM 1	NY	BWR									
OYSTER CREEK 1	NJ	BWR	0.32	2.14	6.48	7.02	3.51	5.64	6.39	9.05	18.10
BEAVER VALLEY 1 & 2	PA	PWR							0.01	0.00	0.07
LIMERICK 1	PA	BWR									
PEACH BOTTOM 2 & 3	PA	BWR				0.01	0.01	0.04	0.98	0.27	0.10
SUSQUEHANNA 1 & 2	PA	BWR									
TMI 2/EPICOR	PA	PWR									
THREE MILE ISLAND 1	PA	PWR					0.01	0.01	0.01	0.03	0.14
THREE MILE ISLAND 2	PA	PWR									0.00
MIDDLE ATLANTIC			**0.38**	**2.37**	**7.49**	**9.03**	**4.86**	**10.15**	**10.54**	**9.81**	**19.05**
HOPE CREEK 1	DE	BWR									
SALEM 1	DE	PWR								0.00	0.04
SALEM 2	DE	PWR									
CALVERT CLIFFS 1 & 2	MD	PWR						0.07	0.14	0.31	0.14
NORTH ANNA 1 & 2	VA	PWR									0.03
SURRY 1 & 2	VA	PWR			0.01	0.04	0.14	0.05	0.35	0.12	0.06
BRUNSWICK 1 & 2	NC	BWR						0.01		0.93	0.41
HARRIS 1	NC	PWR									
MCGUIRE 1	NC	PWR									
MCGUIRE 2	NC	PWR									
CATAWBA 1	SC	PWR									
CATAWBA 2	SC	PWR									
H. B. ROBINSON 2	SC	PWR			0.03	0.30	0.05	0.02	0.10	0.00	0.00
OCONEE 1, 2 & 3	SC	PWR				0.01	0.03	0.01	0.27	0.54	0.22
SUMMER 1	SC	PWR									
EDWIN I. HATCH 1	GA	BWR									
EDWIN I. HATCH 2	GA	BWR									

TABLE C-1 CONTINUED
AIRBORNE EFFLUENTS OF IODINE-131 AND PARTICULATES (CURIES): BY STATE AND REGION 1970-87
HALF-LIFE EQUAL TO OR GREATER THAN 8 DAYS

Reactor	1979	1980	1981	1982	1983	1984	1985	1986	1987	Total
MAINE YANKEE	0.06	0.00	0.00	0.00	0.00	0.02	0.00	0.00	0.00	1.12
VERMONT YANKEE 1	0.44	0.02	0.00	0.00	0.00	0.01	0.01	0.01	0.01	1.36
PILGRIM 1	0.15	0.10	0.07	0.04	0.05	0.01	0.06	0.01	0.00	6.56
YANKEE ROWE 1	0.00	0.00	0.00	0.00	0.00	0.01	0.00	0.00	0.00	0.78
HADDAM NECK	0.05	0.01	0.01	0.00	0.01	0.06	0.00	0.01	0.00	0.27
MILLSTONE 1	0.59	0.33	0.15	0.21	0.06	0.06	0.05	0.05	0.03	32.03
MILLSTONE 2	0.01	0.02	0.11	0.32	0.06	0.04	0.01	0.01	0.01	0.60
MILLSTONE 3								0.00	0.01	0.01
NEW ENGLAND	**1.29**	**0.48**	**0.34**	**0.58**	**0.18**	**0.20**	**0.12**	**0.09**	**0.05**	**42.71**
INDIAN POINT 1& 2	0.45	0.06	0.04	0.04	0.02	0.15	5.67	8.36	0.02	17.38
INDIAN POINT 3	0.00	0.03	0.00	0.00	0.00	0.02	0.00	0.00	0.00	0.08
JAMES A. FITZPATRICK	0.01	0.13	0.28	0.77	0.38	0.21	0.17	0.09	0.14	3.34
NINE MILE POINT 1	0.05	0.03	0.01	0.03	0.01	0.02	0.03	0.02	0.02	9.44
NINE MILE POINT 2									5.17	5.17
R. E. GINNA	0.02	0.01	0.01	0.01	0.02	0.00	0.00	0.00	0.01	0.44
SHOREHAM 1										0.00
OYSTER CREEK 1	9.32	1.25	2.24	1.04	0.02	0.44	3.04	0.70	0.10	76.80
BEAVER VALLEY 1 & 2	0.00	0.00	0.01	0.00	0.05	0.01	0.00	0.01	0.01	0.18
LIMERICK 1								0.01	0.00	0.01
PEACH BOTTOM 2 & 3	0.26	0.03	0.04	0.04	0.05	0.10	0.07	0.05	0.02	2.06
SUSQUEHANNA 1 & 2			0.00	0.00	0.00	0.01	0.03	0.00	0.01	0.05
TMI 2/EPICOR		0.00	0.00	0.00	0.00	0.00				0.00
THREE MILE ISLAND 1	0.01	0.00	0.00	0.00	0.00	0.00	0.00	0.00	0.00	0.21
THREE MILE ISLAND 2	14.20	0.00	0.00	0.00	0.00	0.00	0.00	0.00	0.00	14.20
MIDDLE ATLANTIC	**24.32**	**1.53**	**2.64**	**1.94**	**0.55**	**0.96**	**9.01**	**9.24**	**5.49**	**129.36**
HOPE CREEK 1										
SALEM 1	0.01	0.22	0.48	0.01	0.06	0.00	0.04	0.00	0.00	0.87
SALEM 2		0.00	0.01	0.00	0.04	0.01	0.09	0.00	0.00	0.15
CALVERT CLIFFS 1 & 2	2.05	0.07	0.05	0.18	0.10	0.06	0.05	0.09	0.09	3.40
NORTH ANNA 1 & 2	0.06	0.01	0.48	0.03	0.33	0.09	0.09	0.02	0.02	1.16
SURRY 1 & 2	0.01	0.02	0.07	0.06	0.08	0.06	0.03	0.02	0.02	1.13
BRUNSWICK 1 & 2	0.95	2.12	0.89	1.99	6.25	0.35	0.06	0.05	0.18	14.19
HARRIS 1									0.00	0.00
MCGUIRE 1			0.00	0.00	0.00	0.01	0.01	0.03	0.06	0.12
MCGUIRE 2					0.00	0.01	0.01	0.03	0.06	0.12
CATAWBA 1							0.00	0.01	0.01	0.01
CATAWBA 2								0.01	0.01	0.01
H. B. ROBINSON 2	0.00	0.00	0.00	0.00	0.01	0.00	0.01	0.01	0.02	0.56
OCONEE 1, 2 & 3	0.23	0.13	0.32	0.26	0.11	0.11	0.00	0.04	0.15	2.43
SUMMER 1					0.00	0.00	0.00	0.00	0.00	0.00
EDWIN I. HATCH 1		0.43	0.21	0.18	0.07	0.07	0.04	0.02	0.25	1.27
EDWIN I. HATCH 2		0.01	0.01	0.07	0.02	0.01	0.03	0.02	0.12	0.29

TABLE C-1 CONTINUED
AIRBORNE EFFLUENTS OF IODINE-131 AND PARTICULATES (CURIES): BY STATE AND REGION 1970-87
HALF-LIFE EQUAL TO OR GREATER THAN 8 DAYS
BWR = Boiling Water Reactor; PWR = Pressurized Water Reactor

Reactor	St	Type	1970	1971	1972	1973	1974	1975	1976	1977	1978
VOGTLE 1	GA	PWR									
CRYSTAL RIVER 3	FL	PWR								0.00	0.00
ST. LUCIE 1	FL	PWR							0.01	0.15	0.52
ST. LUCIE 2	FL	PWR									
TURKEY POINT 3	FL	PWR									
TURKEY POINT 3 & 4	FL	PWR				0.06	3.63	0.43	0.42	1.04	0.46
TURKEY POINT 4	FL	PWR									
SOUTH ATLANTIC			**0.00**	**0.00**	**0.04**	**0.41**	**3.85**	**0.59**	**1.29**	**3.09**	**1.88**
DAVIS-BESSE 1	OH	PWR								0.00	0.00
PERRY 1	OH	BWR									
BRAIDWOOD 1	IL	PWR									
BYRON 1 & 2	IL	PWR									
CLINTON 1	IL	BWR									
DRESDEN 1	IL	BWR	3.30	0.67	2.75	0.04	0.68	0.96	0.84	4.93	2.28
DRESDEN 2 & 3	IL	BWR	1.60	8.68	5.89	6.70	6.50	4.31	5.49	6.86	3.13
LASALLE 1 & 2	IL	BWR									
QUAD CITIES 1 & 2	IL	BWR			0.75	5.50	8.88	1.31	1.33	1.69	2.15
ZION 1 & 2	IL	PWR				0.01	0.01	0.14	0.09	0.05	0.09
BIG ROCK POINT 1	MI	BWR	0.13	0.61	0.15	4.60	0.16	0.12	0.05	0.01	0.01
DONALD C. COOK 1 & 2	MI	PWR						0.01	0.01	0.07	0.11
FERMI 2	MI	BWR									
PALISADES	MI	PWR			0.01	0.31	0.01	0.38	0.04	0.02	0.02
KEWAUNEE	WI	PWR					0.02	0.66	0.01	0.02	0.01
LA CROSSE	WI	BWR	0.06	0.01	0.71	0.20	0.04	0.10	0.07	0.17	0.03
POINT BEACH 1 & 2	WI	PWR		0.01	0.03	0.55	0.16	0.07	0.02	0.01	0.03
EAST NORTH CENTRAL			**5.09**	**9.98**	**10.29**	**17.91**	**16.46**	**8.06**	**7.95**	**13.83**	**7.85**
SEQUOYAH 1 & 2	TN	PWR									
BROWNS FERRY 1, 2 & 3	AL	BWR					0.12	0.27	0.07	0.10	0.23
JOSEPH M. FARLEY 1	AL	PWR									0.04
JOSEPH M. FARLEY 2	AL	PWR									
GRAND GULF 1	MS	BWR									
EAST SOUTH CENTRAL			**0.00**	**0.00**	**0.00**	**0.00**	**0.12**	**0.27**	**0.07**	**0.10**	**0.27**
MONTICELLO	MN	BWR	0.04	0.58	1.20	5.70	3.71	0.17	0.09	0.05	0.03
PRAIRIE ISLAND 1 & 2	MN	PWR				0.01	0.01	0.02	0.01	0.01	0.00
DUANE ARNOLD	IA	BWR						0.00	0.08	0.02	0.04
CALLAWAY 1	MO	PWR									
COOPER	NE	BWR					0.24	0.05	0.04	0.02	0.01
FORT CALHOUN 1	NE	PWR				0.01	0.01	0.01	0.02	0.01	0.01
WOLF CREEK 1	KS	PWR									
WEST NORTH CENTRAL			**0.04**	**0.58**	**1.20**	**5.72**	**3.97**	**0.25**	**0.24**	**0.12**	**0.09**

TABLE C-1 CONTINUED
AIRBORNE EFFLUENTS OF IODINE-131 AND
PARTICULATES (CURIES): BY STATE AND REGION 1970-87
HALF-LIFE EQUAL TO OR GREATER THAN 8 DAYS

Reactor	1979	1980	1981	1982	1983	1984	1985	1986	1987	Total
VOGTLE 1									0.00	0.00
CRYSTAL RIVER 3	0.02	0.01	0.02	0.00	0.00	0.00	0.00	0.00	0.00	0.06
ST. LUCIE 1	0.20	0.06	0.08	0.42	0.21	0.26	0.79	0.27	0.04	3.00
ST. LUCIE 2					0.01	0.28	0.19	0.04	0.06	0.59
TURKEY POINT 3							0.01	0.02	0.01	0.04
TURKEY POINT 3 & 4	0.08	0.07	0.03	0.22	0.14	0.03				6.61
TURKEY POINT 4							0.01	0.00	0.01	0.02
SOUTH ATLANTIC	**3.60**	**3.16**	**2.64**	**3.43**	**7.45**	**1.34**	**1.48**	**0.68**	**1.11**	**36.04**
DAVIS-BESSE 1	0.01	0.00	0.06	0.01	0.01	0.00	0.00		0.00	0.08
PERRY 1								0.00	0.00	0.00
BRAIDWOOD 1								0.00	0.00	0.00
BYRON 1 & 2							0.00	0.05	0.01	0.07
CLINTON 1									0.00	0.00
DRESDEN 1	0.02	0.01	0.01	0.00	0.00	0.00	0.00			16.50
DRESDEN 2 & 3	6.97	11.00	9.87	0.95	0.63	0.13	0.16	0.07	0.15	79.08
LASALLE 1 & 2			0.00	0.02	0.01	0.02	0.07	0.05	0.18
QUAD CITIES 1 & 2	1.57	0.59	1.27	0.41	0.44	0.09	0.61	0.11	0.09	26.79
ZION 1 & 2	0.07	0.00	0.01	0.09	0.02	0.04	0.03	0.04	0.00	0.70
BIG ROCK POINT 1	0.00	0.03	0.01	0.00	0.00	0.13	0.08	0.08	0.03	6.20
DONALD C. COOK 1 & 2	0.07	0.07	0.36	0.13	0.06	0.02	0.18	0.02	0.06	1.17
FERMI 2								0.00	0.01	0.01
PALISADES	0.02	0.03	0.04	0.02	0.03	0.00	0.05	0.00	0.03	1.02
KEWAUNEE	0.00	0.00	0.00	0.00	0.00	0.00	0.00	0.01	0.01	0.74
LA CROSSE	0.03	0.01	0.02	0.01	0.01	0.01	0.01	0.01	0.00	1.48
POINT BEACH 1 & 2	0.01	0.00	0.20	0.01	0.02	0.00	0.01	0.00	0.00	1.13
EAST NORTH CENTRAL	**8.78**	**11.75**	**11.84**	**1.63**	**1.24**	**0.44**	**1.14**	**0.47**	**0.45**	**135.16**
SEQUOYAH 1 & 2		0.00	0.01	0.12	0.00	0.02	0.00	0.00	0.00	0.17
BROWNS FERRY 1, 2 & 3	0.05	0.11		0.19	0.28	0.17	0.02	0.00	0.00	1.62
JOSEPH M. FARLEY 1	0.02	0.00	0.62	0.09	0.05	0.01	0.01	0.00	0.00	0.84
JOSEPH M. FARLEY 2			0.00	0.00	0.00	0.00	0.00	0.00	0.00	0.01
GRAND GULF 1					0.00	0.00	0.00	0.00	0.00	0.01
EAST SOUTH CENTRAL	**0.07**	**0.11**	**0.64**	**0.40**	**0.33**	**0.20**	**0.03**	**0.01**	**0.01**	**2.64**
MONTICELLO	0.03	0.03	0.09	0.04	0.03	0.10	0.07	0.17		12.13
PRAIRIE ISLAND 1 & 2	0.00	0.00	0.00	0.00	0.01	0.00	0.01	0.00	0.00	0.10
DUANE ARNOLD	0.03	0.09	0.03	0.01	0.02	0.02	0.01	0.07	0.14	0.55
CALLAWAY 1						0.00	0.00	0.00	0.00	0.00
COOPER	0.18	0.15	0.01	0.16	0.02	0.01	0.02	0.01	0.03	0.95
FORT CALHOUN 1	0.00	0.00	0.00	0.00	0.00	0.01	0.01	0.00	0.01	0.11
WOLF CREEK 1							0.00	0.00	0.00	0.00
WEST NORTH CENTRAL	**0.25**	**0.28**	**0.14**	**0.21**	**0.08**	**0.14**	**0.12**	**0.26**	**0.17**	**13.84**

TABLE C-1 CONTINUED
AIRBORNE EFFLUENTS OF IODINE-131 AND PARTICULATES (CURIES): BY STATE AND REGION 1970-87
HALF-LIFE EQUAL TO OR GREATER THAN 8 DAYS
BWR = Boiling Water Reactor; PWR = Pressurized Water Reactor

Reactor	St	Type	1970	1971	1972	1973	1974	1975	1976	1977	1978
ARKANSAS ONE 1	AR	PWR					0.05	0.74	0.06	0.01	0.00
ARKANSAS ONE 2	AR	PWR									
RIVER BEND 1	LA	BWR									
WATERFORD 3	LA	PWR									
WEST SOUTH CENTRAL			**0.00**	**0.00**	**0.00**	**0.00**	**0.05**	**0.74**	**0.06**	**0.01**	**0.00**
FORT ST. VRAIN	CO	GAS									
PALO VERDE 1	AZ	PWR									
PALO VERDE 2	AZ	PWR									
PALO VERDE 3	AZ	PWR									
MOUNTAIN			**0.00**	**0.00**	**0.00**	**0.00**	**0.00**	**0.00**	**0.00**	**0.00**	**0.00**
WNP-2	WA	BWR									
TROJAN	OR	PWR							0.02	0.05	0.01
DIABLO CANYON 1 & 2	CA	PWR									
HUMBOLDT BAY 3	CA	BWR	0.35	0.30	0.48	0.29	0.84	1.06	0.08	0.00	0.00
RANCHO SECO 1	CA	PWR						0.01	0.01	0.01	0.03
SAN ONOFRE 1	CA	PWR	0.01	0.01	0.01	1.61	0.01	0.04	0.01	0.00	0.00
SAN ONOFRE 2 & 3	CA	PWR									
PACIFIC			**0.36**	**0.31**	**0.49**	**1.90**	**0.85**	**1.11**	**0.12**	**0.06**	**0.05**
U.S. TOTAL			**5.89**	**17.25**	**21.07**	**36.89**	**35.82**	**33.78**	**23.32**	**32.60**	**34.14**

Reactor	1979	1980	1981	1982	1983	1984	1985	1986	1987	Total
ARKANSAS ONE 1	0.00	0.17	0.01	0.00	0.00	0.00	0.00	0.00	0.00	1.05
ARKANSAS ONE 2	0.00	0.01	0.01	0.00	0.01	0.00	0.00	0.00	0.00	0.04
RIVER BEND 1								0.00	0.00	0.00
WATERFORD 3							0.00	0.01	0.00	0.01
WEST SOUTH CENTRAL	**0.01**	**0.17**	**0.02**	**0.01**	**0.01**	**0.00**	**0.01**	**0.01**	**0.00**	**1.10**
FORT ST. VRAIN	0.00	0.00	0.00	0.26	0.00	0.00	0.00			0.26
PALO VERDE 1							0.00	0.01	0.06	0.07
PALO VERDE 2								0.00	0.01	0.02
PALO VERDE 3										0.00
MOUNTAIN	**0.00**	**0.00**	**0.00**	**0.26**	**0.00**	**0.00**	**0.00**	**0.01**	**0.07**	**0.35**
WNP-2						0.38	0.24	0.07	0.08	0.77
TROJAN	0.03	0.03	0.08	0.01	0.01	0.01	0.01	0.01	0.00	0.26
DIABLO CANYON 1 & 2						0.00	0.00	0.00	0.00	0.00
HUMBOLDT BAY 3	0.00	0.00	0.00	0.00	0.00	0.00	0.00	0.00	0.00	3.41
RANCHO SECO 1	0.01	0.01	0.00	0.03	0.00	0.02	0.01	0.00	0.00	0.14
SAN ONOFRE 1	0.00	0.84	0.01	0.00	0.00	0.00	0.00	0.00	0.00	2.56
SAN ONOFRE 2 & 3				0.00	0.16	0.41	0.45	0.16	0.42	1.60
PACIFIC	**0.04**	**0.88**	**0.09**	**0.04**	**0.16**	**0.82**	**0.70**	**0.24**	**0.50**	**8.73**
U.S. TOTAL	**38.36**	**18.36**	**18.35**	**8.50**	**10.01**	**4.11**	**12.63**	**11.01**	**7.87**	**369.94**

TABLE C-2 AIRBORNE EFFLUENTS: TOTAL FISSION AND ACTIVATION GASES (TOTAL CURIES) BY STATE AND REGION 1970-87

Figures represented in 1,000 curie units
BWR = Boiling Water Reactor; PWR = Pressurized Water Reactor

Reactor Name	Type	ST	1970	1971	1972	1973	1974	1975	1976	1977	1978
MAINE YANKEE	PWR	ME			0	0	6	4	1	0	1
VERMONT YANKEE	BWR	VT			55	180	64	4	3	3	5
PILGRIM	BWR	MA			18	230	546	46	183	413	33
YANKEE ROWE	PWR	MA	0	0	0	0	0	0	0	0	1
HADDAM NECK	PWR	CT	0	0	0	0	0	0	0	3	2
MILLSTONE 1, 2 & 3	B&P	CT		276	726	79	912	2970	509	622	567
NEW ENGLAND			**0**	**276**	**799**	**489**	**1528**	**3025**	**696**	**1042**	**609**
INDIAN POINT 1, 2 & 3	PWR	NY				0	6	8	12	16	15
JAMES A. FITZPATRICK	BWR	NY						4	44	23	6
NINE MILE POINT 1 & 2	BWR	NY	10	253	517	872	558	1300	176	4	3
R.E. GINNA	PWR	NY	0	0	0	1	1	10	6	3	1
SHOREHAM 1	BWR	NY									
OYSTER CREEK 1	BWR	NJ	110	516	866	810	279	206	167	177	998
BEAVER VALLEY 1 & 2	PWR	PA							0	0	0
LIMERICK 1	BWR	PA									
PEACH BOTTOM 2 & 3	BWR	PA				1	0	13	209	71	39
SUSQUEHANNA 1 & 2	BWR	PA									
THREE MILE IS. 1, 2 & EPI	PWR	PA					1	4	3	17	16
MIDDLE ATLANTIC			**120**	**769**	**1383**	**1684**	**844**	**1545**	**616**	**311**	**1077**
HOPE CREEK 1	BWR	DE									
SALEM 1 & 2	PWR	DE							0	0	0
CALVERT CLIFFS 1 & 2	PWR	MD						8	9	22	28
NORTH ANNA 1 & 2	PWR	VA									15
SURRY 1 & 2	PWR	VA			0	1	7	8	19	19	4
BRUNSWICK 1 & 2	BWR	NC						0	19	246	91
HARRIS 1	PWR	NC									
MCGUIRE 1 & 2	PWR	NC									
CATAWBA 1 & 2	PWR	SC									
H.B. ROBINSON	PWR	SC		0	0	3	2	1	1	0	1
OCONEE 1, 2 & 3	PWR	SC				9	19	15	44	36	43
SUMMER 1	PWR	SC									
EDWIN I. HATCH 1 & 2	BWR	GA						0	3	2	2
VOGTLE 1	PWR	GA									
CRYSTAL RIVER 3	PWR	FL								3	7
ST. LUCIE 1 & 2	PWR	FL							2	25	29
TURKEY POINT 3 & 4	PWR	FL				1	5	13	16	23	24
SOUTH ATLANTIC				**0**	**0**	**14**	**33**	**46**	**112**	**377**	**244**
DAVIS-BESSE 1	PWR	OH								1	2
PERRY 1	BWR	OH									
BRAIDWOOD 1	PWR	IL									
BYRON 1 & 2	PWR	IL									
CLINTON 1	BWR	IL									

TABLE C-2 CONTINUED
AIRBORNE EFFLUENTS: TOTAL FISSION AND ACTIVATION GASES BY STATE AND REGION 1970-87
Figures represented in 1,000 curie units

Reactor Name	1979	1980	1981	1982	1983	1984	1985	1986	1987	TOTAL
MAINE YANKEE	2	4	0	0	0	0	0	1	1	22
VERMONT YANKEE	8	2	3	3	3	3	3	2		342
PILGRIM	14	26	5	19	20	0	3	0		1557
YANKEE ROWE	0	0	0	0	1	2	1	1	0	6
HADDAM NECK	6	3	2	1	3	8	3	2	4	36
MILLSTONE 1, 2 & 3	21	13	17	17	15	7	2	3	6	6762
NEW ENGLAND	**51**	**48**	**27**	**41**	**42**	**20**	**13**	**9**	**11**	**8726**
INDIAN POINT 1, 2 & 3	9	10	16	10	10	6	3	4	7	131
JAMES A. FITZPATRICK	3	77	200	211	86	34	15	3	5	710
NINE MILE POINT 1 & 2	1	1	1	0	0	1	1	0	0	3698
R.E. GINNA	1	1	1	2	1	0	0	0	0	27
SHOREHAM 1										
OYSTER CREEK 1	1010	31	53	23	2	4	42	77	3	5374
BEAVER VALLEY 1 & 2	2	0	1	0	0	1	0	0	0	5
LIMERICK 1								0	0	0
PEACH BOTTOM 2 & 3	190	15	16	13	35	81	129	28	12	851
SUSQUEHANNA 1 & 2				1	0	0	1	0	0	2
THREE MILE IS. 1, 2 & EPI	9972	47	0	1	0	0	0	4	1	10066
MIDDLE ATLANTIC	**11188**	**183**	**287**	**260**	**134**	**127**	**191**	**116**	**28**	**20863**
HOPE CREEK 1								0	1	1
SALEM 1 & 2	0	0	2	1	1	2	3	2	5	16
CALVERT CLIFFS 1 & 2	10	3	2	8	10	4	4	8	5	120
NORTH ANNA 1 & 2	6	4	5	4	22	18	8	6	1	89
SURRY 1 & 2	2	6	14	21	5	7	2	2	0	118
BRUNSWICK 1 & 2	116	69	522	465	487	167	18	45	26	2272
HARRIS 1									2	2
MCGUIRE 1 & 2			0	0	3	5	4	2	4	18
CATAWBA 1 & 2							0	3	5	8
H.B. ROBINSON	2	1	1	0	0	0	2	1	1	15
OCONEE 1, 2 & 3	48	19	16	24	24	23	24	24	11	379
SUMMER 1				0	0	0	0	0	1	1
EDWIN I. HATCH 1 & 2	2	38	28	5	32	13	13	20	21	179
VOGTLE 1									0	0
CRYSTAL RIVER 3	73	37	40	7	3	2	1	3	1	176
ST. LUCIE 1 & 2	15	9	23	23	23	43	60	43	15	311
TURKEY POINT 3 & 4	11	4	4	20	16	12	3	5	2	157
SOUTH ATLANTIC	**284**	**190**	**657**	**580**	**628**	**294**	**141**	**163**	**100**	**3863**
DAVIS-BESSE 1	2	3	1	1	1	1	0	0	0	12
PERRY 1								0	0	0
BRAIDWOOD 1									0	0
BYRON 1 & 2							0	1	1	2
CLINTON 1									0	0

TABLE C-2 CONTINUED
AIRBORNE EFFLUENTS: TOTAL FISSION AND ACTIVATION GASES BY STATE AND REGION 1970-87
Figures represented in 1,000 curie units
BWR = Boiling Water Reactor; PWR = Pressurized Water Reactor

Reactor Name	Type	ST	1970	1971	1972	1973	1974	1975	1976	1977	1978
DRESDEN 1, 2 & 3	BWR	IL	900	1333	1306	1720	725	889	484	833	891
LASALLE 1 & 2	BWR	IL									
QUAD CITIES 1 & 2	BWR	IL			132	900	950	110	34	26	32
ZION 1 & 2	PWR	IL				0	3	49	114	32	68
BIG ROCK POINT 1	BWR	MI	280	284	258	230	188	51	15	13	19
DONALD C. COOK 1 & 2	PWR	MI						0	1	4	49
FERMI 2	BWR	MI									
PALISADES	PWR	MI			0	0	0	3	0	0	0
KEWAUNEE	PWR	WI					3	2	1	2	0
LA CROSSE	BWR	WI	1	1	31	91	49	57	124	43	8
POINT BEACH	PWR	WI		0	0	6	10	45	2	1	1
EAST NORTH CENTRAL			**1181**	**1618**	**1727**	**2947**	**1928**	**1205**	**775**	**955**	**1070**
SEQUOYAH 1 & 2	PWR	TN									
BROWNS FERRY 1,2 & 3	BWR	AL					64	92	81	166	157
JOSEPH M. FARLEY 1 & 2	PWR	AL									4
GRAND GULF 1	BWR	MS									
EAST SOUTH CENTRAL							**64**	**92**	**81**	**166**	**161**
MONTICELLO	BWR	MN		76	751	870	1570	155	11	7	6
PRAIRIE ISLAND 1 & 2	PWR	MN				0	0	2	2	1	1
DUANE ARNOLD	BWR	IA						2	5	4	2
CALLAWAY 1	PWR	MO									
COOPER	BWR	NE					2	20	38	1	4
FORT CALHOUN 1	PWR	NE				0	0	0	2	4	1
WOLF CREEK 1	PWR	KS									
WEST NORTH CENTRAL				**76**	**751**	**870**	**1573**	**179**	**58**	**16**	**15**
ARKANSAS ONE 1 & 2	PWR	AR					0	1	6	14	8
RIVER BEND 1	BWR	LA									
WATERFORD 3	PWR	LA									
WEST SOUTH CENTRAL							**0**	**1**	**6**	**14**	**8**
FORT ST. VRAIN	GAS	CO									
PALO VERDE 1, 2 & 3	PWR	AZ									
MOUNTAIN											
WNP-2	BWR	WA									
TROJAN	PWR	OR								1	3	0
DIABLO CANYON 1 & 2	PWR	CA									
HUMBOLDT BAY 3	BWR	CA	540	514	430	350	572	297	93	0	0
RANCHO SECO	PWR	CA						0	0	2	7
SAN ONOFRE 1, 2 & 3	PWR	CA	0	0	0	11	2	1	0	0	2
PACIFIC			**540**	**514**	**430**	**361**	**574**	**298**	**94**	**5**	**9**

TABLE C-2 CONTINUED
AIRBORNE EFFLUENTS: TOTAL FISSION AND ACTIVATION GASES BY STATE AND REGION 1970-87
Figures represented in 1,000 curie units

Reactor Name	1979	1980	1981	1982	1983	1984	1985	1986	1987	TOTAL
DRESDEN 1, 2 & 3	69	43	37	10	8	2	3	0	0	9255
LASALLE 1 & 2				0	0	1	0	3	7	10
QUAD CITIES 1 & 2	35	22	32	12	12	6	3	1	0	2306
ZION 1 & 2	34	6	7	16	6	4	4	3	0	346
BIG ROCK POINT 1	7	22	20	13	11	141	63	68	8	1690
DONALD C. COOK 1 & 2	11	4	5	4	0	4	5	0	1	87
FERMI 2										
PALISADES	0	0	3	7	3	0	4	0	2	23
KEWAUNEE	0	0	0	0	0	0	0	0	0	11
LA CROSSE	10	5	5	4	7	11	9	4	2	462
POINT BEACH	1	0	1	1	1	0	0	0	0	67
EAST NORTH CENTRAL	**169**	**104**	**111**	**68**	**50**	**168**	**90**	**81**	**22**	**14271**
SEQUOYAH 1 & 2		3	9	6	4	7	5	0		33
BROWNS FERRY 1, 2 & 3	271	166	45	276	479	664	26	2	0	2490
JOSEPH M. FARLEY 1 & 2	3	19	0	42	23	8	2	3	2	106
GRAND GULF 1					0	0	0	0	0	1
EAST SOUTH CENTRAL	**274**	**188**	**54**	**323**	**506**	**679**	**33**	**6**	**2**	**2629**
MONTICELLO	4	4	4	7	3	1	3	3	4	3478
PRAIRIE ISLAND 1 & 2	1	0	0	1	0	0	0	0	0	8
DUANE ARNOLD	9	3	0	0	0	0	0	0	0	26
CALLAWAY 1						0	2	5	3	10
COOPER	30	5	2	14	2	1	1	2	1	125
FORT CALHOUN 1	1	0	1	0	1	2	1	1	0	15
WOLF CREEK 1							0	0	0	0
WEST NORTH CENTRAL	**45**	**12**	**8**	**22**	**6**	**4**	**8**	**10**	**9**	**3663**
ARKANSAS ONE 1 & 2	13	47	8	12	2	6	17	5	1	140
RIVER BEND 1								2	0	2
WATERFORD 3							8	11	6	25
WEST SOUTH CENTRAL	**13**	**47**	**8**	**12**	**2**	**6**	**25**	**18**	**6**	**167**
FORT ST. VRAIN	0	0	0	0	0	0	0	0	0	1
PALO VERDE 1, 2 & 3							0	5	7	12
MOUNTAIN	**0**	**0**	**0**	**0**	**0**	**0**	**0**	**5**	**7**	**13**
WNP-2						0	0	0	1	1
TROJAN	1	0	1	1	0	1	1	1	0	11
DIABLO CANYON 1 & 2						0	1	2	1	4
HUMBOLDT BAY 3	0	0	0							2796
RANCHO SECO	9	2	1	1	1	4	5	0	0	32
SAN ONOFRE 1, 2 & 3	1	1	0	0	7	40	29	9	23	127
PACIFIC	**10**	**3**	**3**	**2**	**8**	**45**	**36**	**12**	**24**	**2970**

TABLE C-2 CONTINUED
**AIRBORNE EFFLUENTS: TOTAL FISSION AND ACTIVATION GASES
BY STATE AND REGION 1970-87**
Figures represented in 1,000 curie units
BWR = Boiling Water Reactor; PWR = Pressurized Water Reactor

Reactors	Type	1970	1971	1972	1973	1974	1975	1976	1977	1978
TOTAL PRESSURIZED	PWR	0	0	0	32	66	175	242	236	330
TOTAL BOILING	BWR	1841	3253	5090	6333	6479	6216	2196	2652	2861
GRAND TOTAL	BOTH	1841	3253	5090	6365	6545	6392	2439	2887	3192
CUMULATED TOTAL	BOTH	1841	5094	10184	16549	23094	29485	31924	34811	38003

Reactors	1979	1980	1981	1982	1983	1984	1985	1986	1987	TOTAL
TOTAL PRESSURIZED	10234	235	168	224	183	210	205	157	110	12807
TOTAL BOILING	1800	540	988	1085	1195	1133	333	263	98	44356
GRAND TOTAL	12035	775	1156	1310	1378	1343	538	420	209	57165
CUMULATED TOTAL	50038	50813	51968	53278	54655	55998	56536	56956	57165	

TABLE C-3 LIQUID EFFLUENTS: MIXED FISSION AND ACTIVATION PRODUCTS (CURIES)
BY STATE AND REGION 1970-87

Reactor	St	Type	1970	1971	1972	1973	1974	1975	1976	1977	1978
MAINE YANKEE	ME	PWR			0.10	0.10	4.00	3.21	2.84	0.44	0.10
VERMONT YANKEE 1	VT	BWR				0.10		0.01	0.01	0.16	
PILGRIM 1	MA	BWR			1.50	0.90	4.20	8.01	2.33	3.41	1.77
YANKEE ROWE 1	MA	PWR	0.10	0.10	0.10	0.10	0.10	0.02	0.01	0.02	0.08
HADDAM NECK	CT	PWR	6.70	5.90	4.80	3.00	2.20	1.20	0.13	1.71	0.95
MILLSTONE 1	CT	BWR		19.70	51.50	33.40	198.00	199.00	9.65	0.53	0.18
MILLSTONE 2	CT	PWR						0.02	0.26	1.56	2.79
MILLSTONE 3	CT	PWR									
NEW ENGLAND			**6.80**	**25.70**	**58.00**	**37.60**	**208.50**	**211.47**	**15.23**	**7.82**	**5.87**
INDIAN POINT 1 & 2	NY	PWR				2.20	4.20	4.93	4.98	3.02	1.99
INDIAN POINT 3	NY	PWR									1.03
JAMES A. FITZPATRICK	NY	BWR						5.32	6.01	0.89	1.58
NINE MILE POINT 1	NY	BWR	28.00	32.20	34.60	40.80	25.60	21.00	2.14	0.30	
NINE MILE POINT 2	NY	BWR									
R. E. GINNA	NY	PWR	10.00	0.90	0.30	0.10	0.10	0.42	0.69	0.06	0.06
SHOREHAM 1	NY	BWR									
OYSTER CREEK 1	NJ	BWR	18.50	12.00	10.00	4.20	0.70	0.41	0.22	0.10	0.02
BEAVER VALLEY 1 & 2	PA	PWR							0.17	0.65	0.26
LIMERICK 1	PA	BWR									
PEACH BOTTOM 2 & 3	PA	BWR				0.10	0.90	0.93	3.38	2.23	5.11
SUSQUEHANNA 1 & 2	PA	BWR									
TMI 2/EPICOR	PA	PWR									
THREE MILE ISLAND 1	PA	PWR					1.30	0.07	0.10	0.19	0.61
THREE MILE ISLAND 2	PA	PWR									0.39
MIDDLE ATLANTIC			**56.50**	**45.10**	**44.90**	**47.40**	**32.80**	**33.08**	**17.69**	**7.45**	**11.06**
HOPE CREEK 1	DE	BWR									
SALEM 1	DE	PWR							0.01	2.88	4.02
SALEM 2	DE	PWR									
CALVERT CLIFFS 1 & 2	MD	PWR						1.44	1.18	3.48	6.13
NORTH ANNA 1 & 2	VA	PWR									0.27
SURRY 1 & 2	VA	PWR			0.20	0.10	3.80	9.27	33.70	65.50	2.41
BRUNSWICK 1 & 2	NC	BWR						1.89	3.29	6.22	3.48
HARRIS 1	NC	PWR									
MCGUIRE 1	NC	PWR									
MCGUIRE 2	NC	PWR									
CATAWBA 1	SC	PWR									
CATAWBA 2	SC	PWR									
H. B. ROBINSON 2	SC	PWR		0.70	0.80	0.60	2.50	0.45	0.38	0.33	0.18
OCONEE 1, 2 & 3	SC	PWR				2.80	1.90	5.05	7.93	36.20	6.51
SUMMER 1	SC	PWR									
EDWIN I. HATCH 1	GA	BWR						0.06	0.04	25.00	0.04
EDWIN I. HATCH 2	GA	BWR									

TABLE C-3 CONTINUED
LIQUID EFFLUENTS: MIXED FISSION AND ACTIVATION PRODUCTS (CURIES) BY STATE AND REGION 1970-87

Reactor	1979	1980	1981	1982	1983	1984	1985	1986	1987	Total
MAINE YANKEE	0.46	0.30	0.44	0.70	0.20	0.09	0.03	0.30	0.88	14.19
VERMONT YANKEE 1	0.00		0.01							0.29
PILGRIM 1	0.51	2.73	1.94	0.87	0.94	4.75	1.06	0.21	1.47	36.60
YANKEE ROWE 1	0.01	0.02	0.01	0.01	0.01	0.03	0.02	0.01	0.02	0.77
HADDAM NECK	0.87	0.28	0.71	0.07	0.48	0.26	0.08	0.31	0.43	30.08
MILLSTONE 1	0.21	0.72	0.39	1.15	0.81	0.04	0.47	0.77	1.14	517.65
MILLSTONE 2	4.87	2.81	4.18	13.90	7.81	3.55	4.60	4.49	4.49	54.91
MILLSTONE 3								3.01	5.40	8.41
NEW ENGLAND	**6.93**	**6.85**	**7.69**	**16.70**	**10.25**	**8.72**	**6.26**	**9.11**	**13.40**	**662.90**
INDIAN POINT 1 & 2	1.94	1.26	5.67	2.41	4.02	2.67	1.85	3.61	6.02	50.77
INDIAN POINT 3	0.40	2.90	2.62	0.55	0.54	1.26	0.42	0.20	0.35	10.26
JAMES A. FITZPATRICK	0.65	1.51	2.51	0.65	0.77	0.10	0.18	0.02	0.08	20.26
NINE MILE POINT 1	1.89		5.35	0.00	0.01			0.00		191.90
NINE MILE POINT 2									1.30	1.30
R. E. GINNA	0.09	0.02	0.04	0.62	0.19	0.17	0.52	0.06	0.06	14.40
SHOREHAM 1								0.01	0.00	0.01
OYSTER CREEK 1	0.01	0.51	0.25	0.08	0.00	0.01			0.01	47.00
BEAVER VALLEY 1 & 2	0.12	0.10	0.14	0.15	0.06	0.20	0.11	0.12	0.67	2.77
LIMERICK 1						0.00	0.02	0.01	0.07	0.10
PEACH BOTTOM 2 & 3	19.50	1.90	1.97	9.33	2.24	6.15	2.16	0.46	0.33	56.69
SUSQUEHANNA 1 & 2				0.20	2.49	0.15	0.64	0.79	0.31	4.57
TMI 2/EPICOR										0.00
THREE MILE ISLAND 1	0.49	0.18	0.09	0.05	0.08	0.03	0.01	0.01	0.04	3.27
THREE MILE ISLAND 2	0.33	0.00	0.00	0.00	0.00	0.00	0.00	0.00	0.00	0.72
MIDDLE ATLANTIC	**25.41**	**8.38**	**18.64**	**14.04**	**10.41**	**10.74**	**5.91**	**5.29**	**9.24**	**404.03**
HOPE CREEK 1								0.76	1.62	2.38
SALEM 1	3.98	2.65	2.80	3.22	2.97	3.31	2.88	4.35	3.33	36.40
SALEM 2		0.39	1.51	3.21	2.85	2.75	2.80	6.11	4.07	23.69
CALVERT CLIFFS 1 & 2	7.80	4.53	2.68	5.26	2.24	1.64	2.38	1.79	5.19	45.74
NORTH ANNA 1 & 2	0.59	1.05	0.68	1.32	5.88	4.51	5.07	0.94	1.33	21.63
SURRY 1 & 2	2.53	3.85	6.11	6.68	14.50	9.73	8.55	8.77	5.17	180.87
BRUNSWICK 1 & 2	5.10	1.26	2.20	2.32	1.08	0.57	0.12	0.13	0.72	28.36
HARRIS 1									0.91	0.91
MCGUIRE 1			0.39	1.75	1.87	1.51	0.62	0.77	1.57	8.49
MCGUIRE 2					1.87	1.51	0.62	0.77	1.57	6.34
CATAWBA 1							1.26	0.38	0.65	2.30
CATAWBA 2								0.38	0.65	1.04
H. B. ROBINSON 2	0.30	0.36	1.84	1.20	0.82	0.39	0.09	0.26	0.74	11.94
OCONEE 1, 2 & 3	0.92	1.54	1.75	1.04	1.43	1.58	4.16	3.02	2.90	78.73
SUMMER 1				0.00	1.47	4.54	0.71	0.33	0.49	7.53
EDWIN I. HATCH 1	0.05	0.07	0.37	0.70	0.91	1.05	0.48	0.49	0.69	29.94
EDWIN I. HATCH 2		0.05	0.16	0.18	0.33	0.27	0.26	0.30	0.13	1.68

TABLE C-3 CONTINUED

LIQUID EFFLUENTS: MIXED FISSION AND ACTIVATION PRODUCTS (CURIES) BY STATE AND REGION 1970-87

Reactor	St	Type	1970	1971	1972	1973	1974	1975	1976	1977	1978
VOGTLE 1	GA	PWR									
CRYSTAL RIVER 3	FL	PWR								0.02	0.03
ST. LUCIE 1	FL	PWR							0.08	5.80	2.80
ST. LUCIE 2	FL	PWR									
TURKEY POINT 3	FL	PWR									
TURKEY POINT 3 & 4	FL	PWR				0.10	1.60	3.07	8.65	8.90	3.32
TURKEY POINT 4	FL	PWR									
SOUTH ATLANTIC			**0.00**	**0.70**	**1.00**	**3.60**	**9.80**	**21.23**	**55.26**	**154.32**	**29.19**
DAVIS-BESSE 1	OH	PWR								0.03	0.09
PERRY 1	OH	BWR									
BRAIDWOOD 1	IL	PWR									
BYRON 1 & 2	IL	PWR									
CLINTON 1	IL	BWR									
DRESDEN 1	IL	BWR	8.20	6.20	6.80	9.20	6.90	0.84	0.36	0.60	0.33
DRESDEN 2 & 3	IL	BWR		23.00	22.00	25.90	33.10	0.81	1.21	0.44	0.40
LASALLE 1 & 2	IL	BWR									
QUAD CITIES 1 & 2	IL	BWR			2.40	21.40	38.80	17.10	6.99	1.34	2.24
ZION 1	IL	PWR				0.10	0.10	0.01	0.16	0.95	0.95
ZION 2	IL	PWR									
BIG ROCK POINT 1	MI	BWR	4.70	3.50	1.10	2.70	1.10	2.02	0.77	0.39	0.27
DONALD C. COOK 1 & 2	MI	PWR							0.26	1.87	1.52	1.48
FERMI 2	MI	BWR									
PALISADES	MI	PWR			6.80	27.80	5.90	3.45	0.44	0.09	0.10
KEWAUNEE	WI	PWR					0.40	0.72	2.83	1.26	0.70
LA CROSSE	WI	BWR	6.40	17.10	48.50	35.90	13.10	14.20	5.78	21.30	8.86
POINT BEACH 1 & 2	WI	PWR		0.10	1.50	0.80	0.20	2.34	3.24	1.50	0.69
EAST NORTH CENTRAL			**19.30**	**49.90**	**89.10**	**123.80**	**99.60**	**41.75**	**23.65**	**29.42**	**16.10**
SEQUOYAH 1 & 2	TN	PWR									
BROWNS FERRY 1, 2 & 3	AL	BWR					0.80	2.70	3.95	1.19	13.20
JOSEPH M. FARLEY 1	AL	PWR									0.10
JOSEPH M. FARLEY 2	AL	PWR									
GRAND GULF 1	MS	BWR									
EAST SOUTH CENTRAL			**0.00**	**0.00**	**0.00**	**0.00**	**0.80**	**2.70**	**3.95**	**1.19**	**13.30**
MONTICELLO	MN	BWR		0.10	0.10						
PRAIRIE ISLAND 1 & 2	MN	PWR				0.10	0.10	0.45	0.10	0.01	0.00
DUANE ARNOLD	IA	BWR						0.01	0.01	0.00	0.27
CALLAWAY 1	MO	PWR									
COOPER	NE	BWR					1.40	1.74	0.07	0.75	3.05
FORT CALHOUN 1	NE	PWR				0.10	2.30	0.36	0.55	0.36	0.60
WOLF CREEK 1	KS	PWR									
WEST NORTH CENTRAL			**0.00**	**0.10**	**0.10**	**0.20**	**3.80**	**2.56**	**0.73**	**1.13**	**3.92**

TABLE C-3 CONTINUED
LIQUID EFFLUENTS: MIXED FISSION AND ACTIVATION PRODUCTS (CURIES) BY STATE AND REGION 1970-87

Reactor	1979	1980	1981	1982	1983	1984	1985	1986	1987	Total
VOGTLE 1									0.58	0.58
CRYSTAL RIVER 3	0.42	0.15	0.13	0.11	0.15	0.23	1.51	0.81	0.96	4.50
ST. LUCIE 1	2.67	2.36	2.46	3.07	2.99	1.93	2.72	2.53	0.60	30.01
ST. LUCIE 2					0.44	1.93	2.75	2.43	0.54	8.09
TURKEY POINT 3							0.45	0.25	0.37	1.08
TURKEY POINT 3 & 4	0.41	0.68	0.30	1.68	1.13	0.23				30.07
TURKEY POINT 4							0.45	0.25	0.37	1.08
SOUTH ATLANTIC	**24.77**	**18.93**	**23.39**	**31.74**	**42.93**	**37.67**	**37.88**	**35.83**	**35.14**	**563.36**
DAVIS-BESSE 1	0.04	0.21	0.79	0.22	0.54	0.19	0.19	0.06	0.07	2.42
PERRY 1								0.00	0.01	0.02
BRAIDWOOD 1									0.05	0.05
BYRON 1 & 2							16.30	4.05	2.48	22.83
CLINTON 1									0.02	0.02
DRESDEN 1	0.03									39.45
DRESDEN 2 & 3	0.27	0.72	0.06	0.02	0.01	0.12	2.03	0.21	0.38	110.67
LASALLE 1 & 2				0.98	8.60	0.08	3.84	0.02	0.89	14.41
QUAD CITIES 1 & 2	1.31	13.10	3.27	0.40	0.14	0.07	1.46	0.24	0.07	110.33
ZION 1	0.70	0.47	1.61	0.72	1.50	6.82	0.32	0.56	0.75	15.73
ZION 2			1.05	1.65	1.15	7.06	2.05	1.04	0.82	14.82
BIG ROCK POINT 1	0.90	0.78	0.39	0.26	0.08	0.15	0.15	0.07	0.27	19.62
DONALD C. COOK 1 & 2	2.58	1.37	1.86	1.90	0.68	1.19	2.26	0.33	2.00	19.31
FERMI 2								0.00	0.02	0.02
PALISADES	0.13	0.01	0.03	0.13	0.07	0.04	0.06	0.14	0.09	45.28
KEWAUNEE	0.89	0.62	0.82	1.52	0.54	1.01	1.35	0.53	1.29	14.48
LA CROSSE	1.67	2.13	0.23	5.83	3.75	3.26	1.83	5.00	1.16	196.00
POINT BEACH 1 & 2	0.73	0.63	1.01	2.95	1.27	12.20	1.90	16.00	0.76	47.81
EAST NORTH CENTRAL	**9.24**	**20.03**	**11.12**	**16.58**	**18.34**	**32.19**	**33.74**	**28.26**	**11.13**	**673.25**
SEQUOYAH 1 & 2			2.76	9.82	4.61	3.23	1.45	0.17	0.47	22.50
BROWNS FERRY 1, 2 & 3	10.20	9.38	2.24	53.60	12.80	6.30	1.34	0.54	0.33	118.56
JOSEPH M. FARLEY 1	0.06	0.06	0.13	0.06	575.00	0.06	0.07	0.10	0.05	575.70
JOSEPH M. FARLEY 2			0.03	0.03	0.02	0.09	0.04	0.08	0.05	0.33
GRAND GULF 1					0.00	0.03	0.21	0.30	0.36	0.91
EAST SOUTH CENTRAL	**10.26**	**9.44**	**5.16**	**63.51**	**592.43**	**9.71**	**3.11**	**1.19**	**1.25**	**718.01**
MONTICELLO			0.00	0.00						0.20
PRAIRIE ISLAND 1 & 2	0.01	0.01	0.01	0.00	0.03	0.02	0.03	0.60	0.07	1.55
DUANE ARNOLD	0.00			0.00		0.00	0.00			0.30
CALLAWAY 1						0.00	0.00	0.04	0.49	0.54
COOPER	2.48	11.00	3.61	5.44	12.30	6.30	13.00	7.40	2.25	70.79
FORT CALHOUN 1	0.25	0.53	0.18	0.20	0.14	2.91	0.29	0.08	0.20	9.05
WOLF CREEK 1							0.64	2.26	0.29	3.19
WEST NORTH CENTRAL	**2.73**	**11.55**	**3.79**	**5.65**	**12.48**	**9.23**	**13.96**	**10.38**	**3.31**	**85.61**

TABLE C-3 CONTINUED
LIQUID EFFLUENTS: MIXED FISSION AND ACTIVATION PRODUCTS (CURIES) BY STATE AND REGION 1970-87

Reactor	St	Type	1970	1971	1972	1973	1974	1975	1976	1977	1978
ARKANSAS ONE 1	AR	PWR					6.50	3.11	13.10	4.50	6.05
ARKANSAS ONE 2	AR	PWR									
RIVER BEND 1	LA	BWR									
WATERFORD 3	LA	PWR									
WEST SOUTH CENTRAL			**0.00**	**0.00**	**0.00**	**0.00**	**6.50**	**3.11**	**13.10**	**4.50**	**6.05**
FORT ST. VRAIN	CO	GAS									
PALO VERDE 1	AZ	PWR									
PALO VERDE 2	AZ	PWR									
MOUNTAIN			**0.00**	**0.00**	**0.00**	**0.00**	**0.00**	**0.00**	**0.00**	**0.00**	**0.00**
WNP-2	WA	BWR									
TROJAN	OR	PWR							2.77	4.19	0.71
DIABLO CANYON 1 & 2	CA	PWR									
HUMBOLDT BAY 3	CA	BWR	2.40	1.80	1.40	2.40	4.40	3.79	0.99	0.92	0.20
RANCHO SECO 1	CA	PWR						0.01			
SAN ONOFRE 1	CA	PWR	7.60	1.50	30.30	16.00	5.00	1.22	7.43	9.84	11.80
SAN ONOFRE 2 & 3	CA	PWR									
PACIFIC			**10.00**	**3.30**	**31.70**	**18.40**	**9.40**	**5.02**	**11.19**	**14.95**	**12.70**
U.S. TOTAL			**92.6**	**124.8**	**224.8**	**231.0**	**371.2**	**320.9**	**140.8**	**220.8**	**98.2**
CUMULATIVE			**92.6**	**217.4**	**442.2**	**673.2**	**1044.4**	**1365.3**	**1506.1**	**1726.9**	**1825.1**

Reactor	1979	1980	1981	1982	1983	1984	1985	1986	1987	Total
ARKANSAS ONE 1	3.09	3.42	7.50	5.80	4.30	4.10	3.53	5.09	2.45	72.54
ARKANSAS ONE 2	1.30	4.13	2.95	5.90	3.70	2.48	4.36	3.43	1.85	30.10
RIVER BEND 1							0.11	0.08	0.19
WATERFORD 3						0.29	4.02	1.28	5.59
WEST SOUTH CENTRAL	**4.39**	**7.55**	**10.45**	**11.70**	**8.00**	**6.58**	**8.18**	**12.65**	**5.66**	**108.41**
FORT ST. VRAIN	0.00	0.00	0.00	0.00	0.02	0.00	0.00	0.00	0.00	0.02
PALO VERDE 1										0.00
PALO VERDE 2										0.00
PALO VERDE 3										0.00
MOUNTAIN	**0.00**	**0.00**	**0.00**	**0.00**	**0.02**	**0.00**	**0.00**	**0.00**	**0.00**	**0.02**
WNP-2						0.03	0.01	0.02	0.01	0.07
TROJAN	0.56	0.79	0.99	0.86	0.31	0.35	0.47	0.26	0.21	12.46
DIABLO CANYON 1 & 2						0.01	3.20	11.10	2.86	17.17
HUMBOLDT BAY 3	0.10	0.14	0.16	0.35	0.10	0.16	0.13	0.05	0.01	19.47
RANCHO SECO 1		0.00	0.59	0.22	0.28	0.63	0.01	0.00	0.00	1.75
SAN ONOFRE 1	11.00	11.20	3.64	2.15	1.22	2.74	7.79	0.85	0.84	132.12
SAN ONOFRE 2 & 3				0.63	2.79	13.00	11.20	0.82	0.54	28.98
PACIFIC	**11.65**	**12.13**	**5.38**	**4.20**	**4.70**	**16.93**	**22.80**	**13.11**		**4.47**	**212.02**
U.S. TOTAL	**95.4**	**94.9**	**85.6**	**164.1**	**699.6**	**131.8**	**131.8**	**115.8**	**83.6**	**3427.6**
CUMULATIVE	**1920.5**	**2015.4**	**2101.0**	**2265.1**	**2964.6**	**3096.4**	**3228.2**	**3344.0**	**3427.6**	

HOW THE NATIONAL CANCER INSTITUTE CONFIRMED THAT PROXIMITY TO REACTORS INCREASES BREAST CANCER RISK

A concerned Minnesota citizens group first used our breast cancer mortality database from the National Cancer Institute in legislative hearings on dry-cask storage at the Prairie Island reactor in May of 1994, as discussed in chapter 8. We offered them preliminary data showing a significant increase in the 12 rural counties near the 2 Minnesota reactors and an early version of table 7–2, in which we used data for 268 rural counties near reactors to show that most rural counties near reactor sites around the nation displayed such significant mortality increases.

Our use of the NCI database evidently caused some official concern. We are in possession of a confidential NCI memorandum dated January 5, 1995, by Dr. Charles E. Land, a health statistician in the Radiation Epidemiology branch. The memo was written to debunk our findings but unwittingly confirms them.

Land does this by providing two tables showing the age-adjusted white female breast cancer change for counties within 50 miles of each of 51 reactor sites. Happily, they replicated our methodology by using 1950 as the standard year for age-adjustment. So thorough was his analysis that he even noted that we had "incorrectly counted some counties twice. Although this error would have had a minor effect on the significance tests, it does suggest a lack of attention to detail."

His replication of our table yields precisely the same results we obtained, thus confirming the accuracy of our methodology. Here is a comparison of the trend over the three time periods: the NCI version of the combined rate for all 268 selected counties versus our original version. This and our current version, which extends the selection of nearby rural counties to 346, both show the same significant 10 percent increase since 1950–54 as compared with a 1 percent increase for the United States.

TABLE D-1 268 COUNTIES DOWNWIND OF 51 REACTOR SITES
Deaths per 100,000 Women

Tabulation	Age-Adjusted Mortality Rates			Percent Change 80-84/ 50-54	85-89/ 50-54	Number of Deaths		
	1950-54	80-84	85-89			50-54	80-84	85-89
NCI Tabulation	24.0	26.1	26.4	1.09	1.10	12518	30776	34244
U.S. Total	24.4	24.9	24.6	1.02	1.01	91392	167803	178868
Balance of U.S.	24.4	24.6	24.2	1.01	0.99	78882	137027	144624
RPHP Tabulation	24.0	26.1	26.4	1.09	1.10	13304	31744	35175
U.S. Total	24.4	24.9	24.6	1.02	1.01	91392	167803	178868
Balance of U.S.	24.4	24.6	24.2	1.01	0.99	78358	136059	143693

The reader should understand that hundreds of thousands of calculations are required to develop a database with the ability to secure age-adjusted mortality rates for any combination of counties. Not having access to the giant mainframe NCI computers, we performed our tedious computations over a period of many months with a personal computer. To have the NCI confirm the accuracy of our methodology in securing age-adjusted breast cancer rates, even for the United States as a whole—considering that such figures had never before been published—is, of course, extremely gratifying to us. The slight difference, due to some duplicated counties in the total number of deaths in the 268 counties, is seen not to affect the rates or the percent change over time.

But Land differs with our interpretation of the above results. In our selection of the 268 contiguous nearby counties we had obviously omitted the large urban counties within a 50-mile radius. Land suggests the "counties included in the Gould-Sternglass study may have been selected to produce a desired result."

If Land had the opportunity to read this book, he would know that this table was designed to show how the NCI definition of an exposed county was hopelessly limited. The NCI assumed that emissions from a reactor would affect only the rural counties in which the reactors were located. It is precisely because there was some early appreciation of the dangers of locating reactors close to population centers that most reactors (with the painful exception of the Indian Point and Brookhaven reactors in Westchester and Suffolk Counties) were located in low-population rural counties. This first table was designed to show that extending the NCI definition of "nuclear" counties to include additional neighboring rural counties could achieve the statistical significance that had previously eluded the NCI.

We were perfectly aware that this extension of the definition of proximity was itself limited and that it would be necessary to extend the definition to include nearby large urban counties, too.

This is precisely what Land does in his table 2, in which he applies our methodology ". . . to include all counties whose geographical centers were within 50 miles of the specified sites." We reproduce this table D-2, rounding off some decimal points to make it somewhat more readable.

This permits him to state that "the results in 'all sites' and 'balance of the U.S.,' especially for the 1980–84 vs. 1950–54 and 1985–89 vs. 1950–54 ratios, are opposite in direction to those in table 1, and in no way support the conclusions of Gould and Sternglass."

Consider what these results say about the importance of table D–2. Land has divided the nation into 2 sectors—a "nuclear" sector for counties within 50 miles of a reactor with an overall breast cancer mortality rate of about 27 deaths per 100,000—and a nonnuclear sector for all other counties with a rate of about 23 deaths per 100,000.

One need not be a statistician to realize that he has demonstrated that the risk of dying of breast cancer is significantly greater for women living within 50 miles of a reactor than for those living elsewhere. In statistical terms the difference is equivalent to 200 standard deviations, and the probability that it could be due to chance is too small to be even calculable! The fact that the difference was somewhat greater in 1950–54 does not mean that breast cancer mortality in the "nuclear"

TABLE D-2 NCI TABULATION OF WHITE FEMALE AGE-ADJUSTED BREAST CANCER MORTALITY RATES,1950-89
COUNTIES WITHIN 50 MILES OF EACH OF 51 REACTORS
Deaths per 100,000 Women

	Name of Facility	Age-Adjusted Mortality Rates			Percent Change		Deaths
		1950-54	80-84	85-89	80-84/ 50-54	85-89/ 50-54	Number per 85-89 Sq. Mi.
1	ARKANSAS ONE	16.2	18.3	17.4	1.13	1.07	197 0.079
2	BIG ROCK POINT	21.3	23.0	18.2	1.08	0.85	134 0.054
3	BROOKHAVEN	29.7	30.4	30.7	1.02	1.03	5571 2.228
4	BROWNS FERRY	17.0	23.3	21.4	1.37	1.26	539 0.216
5	BRUNSWICK	19.8	20.1	20.1	1.02	1.02	137 0.055
6	CALVERT CLIFFS	27.7	28.5	26.0	1.03	0.94	1058 0.423
7	COOPER STATION	22.3	22.8	17.7	1.02	0.79	139 0.056
8	DAVIS BESSE	27.2	27.0	27.0	0.99	0.99	2325 0.930
9	DRESDEN	28.7	28.2	28.3	0.98	0.99	5284 2.114
10	DUANE ARNOLD	21.2	23.8	23.9	1.12	1.13	435 0.174
11	FARLEY	19.3	15.1	16.8	0.78	0.87	129 0.052
12	FERMI	27.3	27.4	27.4	1.00	1.00	3152 1.261
13	FORT CALHOUN	26.2	36.7	23.8	1.40	0.91	557 0.223
14	FORT ST. VRAIN	27.0	23.3	23.1	0.86	0.86	930 0.372
15	GINNA	28.8	27.8	29.7	0.97	1.03	1149 0.460
16	HADDAM NECK	27.5	28.5	28.0	1.04	1.02	4897 1.959
17	HANFORD	14.6	19.7	23.6	1.35	1.62	138 0.055
18	HATCH	10.4	16.7	18.5	1.61	1.78	104 0.042
19	HUMBOLDT BAY	25.7	24.2	27.3	0.94	1.06	96 0.038
20	INDIAN POINT	31.2	29.9	29.4	0.96	0.94	13703 5.481
21	INEL	12.6	23.5	21.1	1.87	1.67	123 0.049
22	LA CROSSE	22.0	22.8	20.1	1.04	0.91	271 0.108
23	MAINE YANKEE	25.5	25.0	24.5	0.98	0.96	520 0.208
24	MCGUIRE	17.5	21.6	25.5	1.23	1.46	1202 0.481
25	MONTICELLO	29.4	24.2	23.4	0.82	0.80	1745 0.698
26	WEST VALLEY	29.6	28.8	30.5	0.97	1.03	1510 0.604
27	OAK RIDGE	18.1	20.2	19.7	1.12	1.09	655 0.262
28	OCONEE	16.8	22.5	23.7	1.34	1.41	631 0.252
29	OYSTER CREEK	28.7	29.2	29.7	1.02	1.03	4510 1.804
30	PALISADES	23.6	25.2	25.1	1.07	1.06	696 0.278
31	PATHFINDER	24.2	21.4	24.0	0.88	0.99	196 0.078
32	PEACH BOTTOM	25.9	25.5	26.8	0.98	1.03	3228 1.291
33	PILGRIM	28.0	29.3	29.4	1.05	1.05	3480 1.392
34	POINT BEACH	25.9	27.1	25.7	1.05	0.99	479 0.192
35	PRAIRIE ISLAND	28.9	24.9	26.3	0.86	0.91	1962 0.785
36	QUAD CITIES	25.4	24.6	22.0	0.97	0.87	536 0.214
37	RANCHO SECO	21.6	25.5	25.8	1.18	1.19	1213 0.485
38	ROBINSON	17.0	19.9	21.3	1.17	1.25	280 0.112
39	SALEM	27.5	28.2	28.2	1.03	1.03	4890 1.956
40	SAN ONOFRE	20.3	25.7	25.9	1.27	1.28	1556 0.622

TABLE D-2 CONTINUED
NCI TABULATION OF WHITE FEMALE AGE-ADJUSTED BREAST CANCER MORTALITY RATES,1950-89 COUNTIES WITHIN 50 MILES OF EACH OF 51 REACTORS
Deaths per 100,000 Women

Name of Facility	Age-Adjusted Mortality Rates			Percent Change 80-84/ 50-54	85-89/ 50-54	Deaths Number 85-89	per Sq. Mi.
	1950-54	80-84	85-89				
41 SAVANNAH RIVER	16.2	20.3	17.7	1.25	1.09	191	0.076
42 SEQUOYAH	18.4	21.1	20.7	1.15	1.13	525	0.210
43 BEAVER VALLEY	23.6	27.2	26.5	1.15	1.12	2850	1.140
44 ST. LUCIE	15.5	23.5	23.4	1.52	1.51	1226	0.490
45 SURRY	20.3	25.3	26.1	1.25	1.29	1200	0.480
46 THREE MILE ISLAND	25.2	25.8	26.1	1.02	1.04	2070	0.828
47 TROJAN	24.0	23.8	24.7	0.99	1.03	544	0.218
48 TURKEY POINT	19.9	23.9	23.2	1.20	1.17	1526	0.610
49 VERMONT YANKEE	26.6	27.8	26.3	1.05	0.99	1922	0.769
50 YANKEE ROWE	28.1	28.5	25.8	1.01	0.92	1123	0.449
51 ZION	29.9	28.2	28.1	0.94	0.94	6618	2.647
ALL 51 SITES	**27.4**	**27.0**	**26.9**	**0.99**	0.98	69554	
TOTAL U.S.	24.4	24.9	24.6	1.02	1.01	178868	
BALANCE OF U.S.	22.3	23.4	23.3	1.05	1.04	109319	

sector has improved over time but merely that even in the nonnuclear sector breast cancer mortality, while still relatively low, is also slowly increasing. The concept of proximity is seen to be purely relative. No one living in the United States can escape the possibility of ingesting some nuclear fission products.

Land is apparently not aware of the principal finding that emerges from our analysis of geographic differences in county cancer rates— namely the logarithmic shape of the dose response curve to radiation—which causes rural counties with low initial mortality rates to rise more rapidly than large urban counties. This makes for a gradual convergence of rural and urban mortality rates, as shown below by figures D-1 and D-2 based on Land's data.

First, for each of the reactor areas identified by number, we have correlated the ratio of change in mortality rates from 1950–54 to 1985–89 with the rate established in the initial period. We see in figure

D–1 the now familiar highly significant negative correlation, which shows that reactors located in rural areas with initial rates well below average have registered the greatest gains since 1950–54.

Specifically, we see that this is true for Hatch (#18), INEL (#21), Hanford (#17), and St. Lucie (#44), whereas Indian Point (#20), located in the large urban county of Westchester has registered no gain, but remains, along with Zion (#51), Monticello (#25), and Prairie Island (#35) with rates far above average.

Another way that Land's data show that women living in densely populated urban areas have the highest mortality rates is the significant positive correlation between current mortality rates and the current number of deaths per square mile in the 50-mile radius around each reactor, shown in figure D–2. Here the reactor areas with the highest mortality rates are those such as Brookhaven (#3) and Indian Point (#20) located in areas of greatest density and highest ratios of death per square mile.

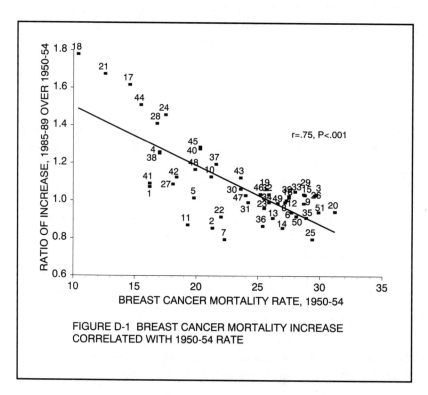

FIGURE D-1 BREAST CANCER MORTALITY INCREASE CORRELATED WITH 1950-54 RATE

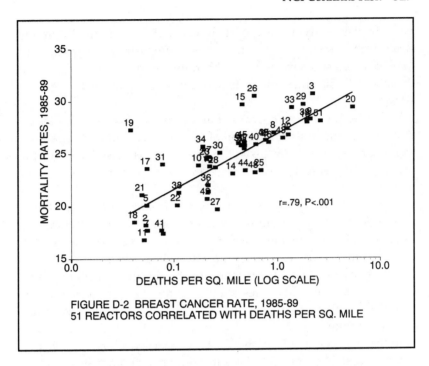

FIGURE D-2 BREAST CANCER RATE, 1985-89
51 REACTORS CORRELATED WITH DEATHS PER SQ. MILE

As we have shown in our final chapter and in appendix A, an even more extended definition of proximity to reactor emissions is to consider as "nuclear" those counties within 100 miles of each reactor site, which in effect divides the nation into a larger "nuclear" sector of 1,319 counties with an overall breast cancer rate close to 26 deaths per 100,000 as contrasted with the rate less than 23 deaths per 100,000 for the remaining rural counties lying mainly between the Rockies and the Mississippi River.

Using Land's 50-mile criterion of proximity to reactors, the effect of long chronic exposure to reactor emissions in rural areas can best be seen in the extraordinary long-term percent increases in breast cancer mortality shown in table D-2, for counties near the DOE reactor sites of Hanford (62 percent) and INEL (67 percent). No hint of such significant increases in breast cancer mortality appeared in the 1990 NCI study, *Cancer Mortality in Populations Near Nuclear Facilities*. We, of course, are delighted to acknowledge the support given in this confidential memo to the theme of our own study—that women living near reactors are at greater than average risk of dying of breast cancer. Land has helped demonstrate that this statement is true whether proximity to reactors is limited to those counties in which the reactors are located, or to those within 50 miles, or to those within 100 miles of the reactor sites.

The political sensitivity of Land's memo, which completely undermines the basic conclusion of the 1990 NCI study, can be seen from Land's failure to answer two questions raised by several investigative reporters to whom we have passed on copies of his memo.

First, how would he explain why nonurban counties, e.g., those within 50 miles of the oldest DOE reactor sites such as Hanford, INEL, Oak Ridge, Savannah River, and Brookhaven registered such large increases in breast cancer mortality since 1950?

Second, what were the reasons for the significant differences in breast cancer mortality rates shown in this table by large urban counties, particularly those within 50 miles of reactor sites, when compared with the significantly lower rates elsewhere? Surely, the National Cancer Institute should be concerned about the clearly environmental reasons for the wide regional differences in breast cancer mortality revealed by their own data.

Another question that should be put to Land is how he would explain the sharp changes in breast cancer mortality shown by his table 2 from 1980–84 to 1985–89, which could not possibly reflect sudden changes in genetic factors or exposure to toxic chemicals, but can be easily explained by the extreme changes in exposure to airborne I–131 and particulates shown in appendix C. For example, counties within 50 miles of the Point Beach–Kewaunee reactors recorded a peak in breast cancer mortality in 1980–84, but then by 1985–89 declined sharply to the 1950–54 level. This is in accordance with the far sharper decline of I–131 emissions shown in appendix C from these two reactors, from over 1.5 curies in the early 1970s to far lower levels in the early 1980s.

These questions will remain unanswered until the major media and Congress are ready to begin a long-delayed public debate on the health effects of all environmental carcinogens, including ionizing radiation.

For those unwilling to wait, useful videotapes on the health effects of both chemical pollutants and ionizing radiation, with particular attention to breast cancer, can be obtained from the Foundation for a Compassionate Society (512–441–2816) and EnviroVideos (800–ECO–TV46).

REFERENCES

1. Mitchell, W.C., *Types of Economic Theory: From Mercantilism to Institutionalism*, edited with an introduction by Dorfman, Joseph, New York: Augustus M. Kelley, 1967.

2. Gould, J.M., *Output and Productivity in the Electric and Gas Utilities*, New York: National Bureau of Economic Research, 1946.

3. Gould, J.M., *The Technical Elite*, New York: Augustus M. Kelley, 1968.

4. Veblen, T., *The Engineers and the Price System*, reprints of economic classics, New York: Augustus M. Kelley, 1965.

5. Sternglass, E.J., *Secret Fallout: Low-Level Radiation from Hiroshima to Three Mile Island*, New York: McGraw-Hill, 1981.

6. Gould, J.M., *Quality of Life in American Neighborhoods: Levels of Affluence, Toxic Waste, and Cancer Mortality in Residential ZIP Code Areas*, Boulder: Westview Press, 1986.

7. Carson, R., *Silent Spring*, Boston: Houghton Mifflin, 1962.

8. Gould, J.M., "Nuclear Emissions Take Their Toll," *Council On Economic Priorities Newsletter*, New York: December 1986.

9. Jablon, S., Hrubec, Z., Boice, J.D., and Stone, B.J., *Cancer in Populations Living Near Nuclear Facilities,* Washington: National Cancer Institute, National Institute of Health publication #90–874, July 1990.

10. Gould, J.M. and Sternglass, E.J., "Low-level Radiation and Mortality," *Chemtech,* American Chemical Society, January 1989.

11. Gould, J.M. and Goldman, B.A., *Deadly Deceit: Low-Level Radiation High Level Cover-Up,* New York: Four Walls Eight Windows, 1991.

12. Sternglass, E.J. and Gould, J.M., "Breast Cancer: Evidence for a Relation to Fission Products in the Diet," *International Journal of Health Service* 23, #4, 783–804, 1993.

13. Gould, J.M. and Sternglass, E.J., "Nuclear Fallout, Low Birthweight, and Immune Deficiency," *International Journal of Health Service* 24, #2, 311–335.

14. Mangano, J.J., "Cancer Mortality Near Oak Ridge, Tennessee," *International Journal of Health Service* 24, #3, 521–533, 1994.

15. Mangano, J.J., "A Response to Comments on 'Cancer Mortality Near Oak Ridge,'" *International Journal of Health Service* 25, #3, 1995

16. Sternglass, E.J. and Gould, J.M., "A Response to Comments on 'Breast Cancer: Evidence for a Relation to Fission Products in the Diet,'" *International Journal of Health Service* 25, #3, 1995.

17. Gould, J.M. and Sternglass, E.J., "Breast Cancer Mortality Near Nuclear Reactors," submitted to the Berlin Radiological Protection Society, April 30, 1995.

18. Mangano, J.J. and Reid, W., "Thyroid Cancer in America since Chernobyl," *British Medical Journal* 303, #7003, p. 511, August 1995.

19. Mangano, J.J., "A Post-Chernobyl Rise in Connecticut Thyroid Cancer," *European Journal of Cancer Prevention,* volume 5, #1, January 1996.

20. Sakharov, A., "Radioactive Carbon from Nuclear Explosions and Nonthreshold Biological Effects," *Soviet Journal of Atomic Energy*, volume 4, #6, July 1958. See also Sakharov, A., *Memoirs*, New York: Alfred Knopf, 1991.

21. Pauling, L., *No More War*, New York: Dodd Mead, 1958.

22. Sternglass, E.J. and Gould, J.M., "The Long Island Breast Cancer Epidemic: Evidence for a Relation to the Release of Hazardous Nuclear Waste," *CMA Occasional Paper*, Long Island University, School of Public Service, July 1994.

23. National Institute of Health, *Forty-five Years of Cancer Incidence in Connecticut*, NIH–86–2652, updated to 1990 via correspondence with Connecticut Department of Health.

24. *Washington Spectator*, volume 20, #13, July 1994.

25. "The Release of Radioactive Materials from Hanford, 1944–1972," *Hanford Health Information Network*, Seattle: 1994.

26. New York State Department of Health, *Annual Reports*, 1945–1970s.

27. *Vital Statistics of the U.S.*, Natality volumes, Washington, D.C., National Center for Health Statistics, 1950, 1951.

28. Whyte, R.K., "First-Day Neonatal Mortality since 1935: A Reexam-ination of the Cross Hypothesis," *British Medical Journal* 304, 343–346, 1992.

29. Miller, R., *Under the Cloud*, New York: The Free Press, 1986.

30. Norris, R.S., Cochran, T., and Arkin, W., "Known U.S. Nuclear Tests," Washington D.C.: Natural Resources Defense Council, 1988. See also *Natural Resources Defense Council: Nuclear Weapons Handbook*, volume IV, New York: Harper & Row, 1989.

31. Monthly milk radiation reports are available for selected cities from 1957 to 1974 from *Radiation Data and Reports* published by HEW. Since 1974, such reports have been available from the EPA as *Environmental Radiation Data*, but all measurements have been made at the same laboratory in Montgomery, Alabama.

32. Clapp, R., et al., "Leukemia Near Massachusetts Nuclear Power Plant," letter in *The Lancet*, December 5, 1987, 1324–1325.

33. Dobrynin, A., *In Confidence*, New York: Random House, 1995.

34. Riccio. J., "Westinghouse: Leaks and Lawsuits," *Public Citizen*, Washington, D.C.: June 2, 1994.

35. Feshbach, M., "Rising Infant Mortality in the USSR," Washington D.C., U.S. Census Bureau, Series P–25, #74, 1980.

36. Feshbach, M., *Ecocide in the USSR*, New York: HarperCollins, 1992.

37. Feshbach, M., ed., *Environmental and Health Atlas of Russia*, Moscow, PAIMS, 1995.

38. Herrnstein, R.J. and Murray, C., *The Bell Curve: Intelligence and Class Structure in American Life*, New York: The Free Press, 1994.

39. Sternglass, E.J. and Bell, S., *Fallout and the Decline of Scholastic Aptitude Scores*, paper presented at annual meeting, American Psychological Association, New York, September 3, 1979.

40. Pellegrini, R.J., "Nuclear Fallout and Criminal Violence: Preliminary Inquiry into a New Biogenic Predisposition Hypothesis," *International Journal of Biosocial Research* 9, #21, 125–143, 1987.

41. *U.S. Bureau of Labor Statistics*, Annual Labor Force Reports.

42. Buehler, J.W., Devine, O.J., Berkelman, R., and Chenarley, F.M., "Impact of the Human Immunodeficiency Virus Epidemic on

Mortality Trends in Young Men, U.S.," *American Journal of Public Health*, volume 80, #9, September 1990.

43. *Vital Statistics of the U.S. 1988*, volume 2.

44. National Cancer Institute, *Cancer Statistics Review, 1973–1988*, Bethesda: National Institute of Health Publication #91–2789.

45. Nuclear Regulatory Commission, *Radioactive Materials Released from Nuclear Power Plants*, 1987 Annual Report, Brookhaven National Laboratory, NUREG/CR–2907.

46. *New York Times*, March 10, 1994.

47. Gould, J.M., "Chernobyl—The Hidden Tragedy," *The Nation*, March 15, 1993.

48. Kliewer, E.V., Smith, K.R., "Breast Cancer Mortality Among Immigrants in Australia and Canada," *Journal of the National Cancer Institute* 87, 1154–1161, 1995.

49. Simonich, S.L. and Hites, R.A., "Global Distribution of Persistent Pesticides," *Science*, 269, 1851–1854, 1995

50. Greenberg, M.R., *Urbanization and Cancer Mortality*, New York: Oxford University Press, 1983.

51. Petkau, A., "Effect of 22Na on a Phosphilid Membrane," *Health Physics*, 22, 239244. See also, Petkau, A., "Radiation Carcinogenesis from a Membrane Perspective," *Acta Physiologica Scandinavia*, supplement, 492, 81–90, 1980.

52. Graeub, R., *The Petkau Effect*, New York: Four Walls Eight Windows, 1993.

53. Archer, V. E., "Association of Nuclear Fallout with Leukemia in the United States," *Arch. Env. Health*, 42, 263–271, 1987.

54. Sternglass, E.J., "Environmental Radiation and Human Health," *Effects of Pollution on Health*, proceedings of the sixth Berkeley Symposium on Mathematical Statistics and Probability, editor Lecam, L.M., Neyman, J., and Scott, E.L., Berkeley: University of California Press, 145–216, 1972.

55. Gofman, J.W., *Preventing Breast Cancer*, San Francisco: Committee for Nuclear Responsibility, 1995.

56. Resnikoff, M., *Deadly Legacy*, New York: Radioactive Waste Management Associates, 1990.

57. Lamont, L., *Day of Trinity*, New York: Atheneum, 1965.

58. Gordon, D.K, and Kennedy, R., *The Legend of City Water*, Garrison: The Hudson Riverkeeper Fund, 1991.

59. Henly, R., "Reservoirs At Risk," *Village Voice*, September 1, 1993.

60. *Environmental Radiation in New York State*, 1992 Annual Report, Albany: New York State Department of Health, Bureau of Environmental Protection, 1995.

61. Strand, J.A., et al., "Suppression of the Primary Immune Response in Rainbow Trout, Salmo Gardineri, Sub Lethaly Exposed to Tritiated Water during Embryogenesis," *Journal of Fish Research*, Board Canada 34, #1293, 1977 and *Radiation Research* 91, #533, 1982.

62. Saleska, S., "Nuclear Legacy," *Public Citizen Group*, Washington: September 1989.

63. Burrows, B.A. and Chalmers, T.C., "Cesium–137/Potassium–40 Ratios in Firewood Ashes as a Reflection of Worldwide Radioactive Contamination of the Environment," *Trends in Cancer Mortality in Industrial Countries*, editor Davis, D.L. and Hoel, D., New York Academy of Sciences, volume 609, 1990.

64. Leakey, R. and Lewin, R., *The Sixth Extinction: Patterns of Life and the Future of Mankind*, New York: Doubleday, 1995.

65. Udall, S.L., *The Myths of August: A Personal Exploration of Our Tragic Cold War Affair With the Atom*, New York: Pantheon, 1994.

66. Gould, J.M., "The Future of Nuclear Power," *Monthly Review*, 35, #9, 7–14, 1984.

67. Ford, D., *Cult of the Atom: The Secret Papers of the Atomic Energy Commission*, New York: Simon and Schuster, 1982.

INDEX

Illustrations are indicated in **bold type**.